The Dole Nutrition
HANDBOOK

WHAT TO EAT AND HOW TO LIVE FOR A LONGER, HEALTHIER LIFE

NUTRITION INSTITUTE

This book is intended as a reference volume only, not as a medical manual. The information given here is designed to help you make informed decisions about your health. It is not intended as a substitute for any treatment that may have been prescribed by your doctor. If you suspect that you have a medical problem, we urge you to seek competent medical help.

The information in this book is meant to supplement, not replace, proper exercise training. All forms of exercise pose some inherent risks. The editors and publisher advise readers to take full responsibility for their safety and know their limits. Before practicing the exercises in this book, be sure that your equipment is well-maintained, and do not take risks beyond your level of experience, aptitude, training, and fitness. The exercise and dietary programs in this book are not intended as a substitute for any exercise routine or dietary regimen that may have been prescribed by your doctor. As with all exercise and dietary programs, you should get your doctor's approval before beginning.

Mention of specific companies, organizations, or authorities in this book does not imply endorsement by the author or publisher, nor does mention of specific companies, organizations, or authorities imply that they endorse this book, its author, or the publisher.

Internet addresses and telephone numbers given in this book were accurate at the time it went to press.

© 2010 by Dole Nutrition Institute
All photographs courtesy Dole Nutrition Institute with the exception of the following:
age fotostock: pages 44, 113, 115, 130, 178, 210; Alamy; page 274; CMSP: page 245; Fotolia: pages 23, 50, 120, 172, 224; Getty Images: pages 10, 21, 22, 37, 46, 53, 58, 61, 65, 76, 84, 92, 112, 114, 115, 121, 122, 123, 124, 131, 135, 136, 141, 144, 149, 153, 157, 158, 165, 168, 176, 179, 181, 183, 191, 192, 193, 194, 203, 204, 207, 208, 213, 221, 222, 223, 227, 234, 235, 236, 237, 239, 250, 252, 260, 268, 273, 283; iStockfoto: pages 15, 17, 18, 19, 22, 23, 25, 26, 29, 30, 34, 39, 40, 41, 42, 43, 48, 49, 51, 54, 56, 60, 62, 63, 64, 70, 73, 74, 75, 76, 79, 80, 81, 90, 95, 96, 98, 100, 101, 102, 103, 104, 105, 106, 107, 108, 109, 110, 111, 112, 114, 115, 116, 117, 118, 119, 120, 121, 122, 123, 132, 133, 137, 138, 144, 147, 150, 151, 152, 154, 155, 156, 159, 162, 172, 175, 177, 186, 187, 189, 190, 197, 200, 212, 216, 219, 227, 230, 231, 232, 238, 248, 254, 255, 256, 264, 265, 266, 269, 271, 272, 282, 283, 286, 287, 290, 295; Penny Gentieu/Babystock: page 182; Illustrations by Bryon Thompson.

Printed in the United States of America

Book design by Rodale Inc.

The Library of Congress Catalog-in-Publication Data is on file with the publisher.

978-1-60529-295-3
1-60529-295-8

2 4 6 8 10 9 7 5 3 1

FOREWORD

BY ANDREW CONRAD, PHD

Aging may be inevitable—but science is revealing that we have far more control over the rate at which we age than previously believed. Many factors—environmental, behavioral and dietary—affect how quickly and how visibly we age. These same factors have bearing on our risk for disease. While symptoms of illness and signs of aging are the most outward aspects in the process of getting older, the true measure of health may be gauged by the body's ability to repair and protect its DNA.

As the Chief Scientific Officer of the North Carolina Research Campus, my role is to work with the leading scientific experts we have gathered to explore how nutrition and other factors impact both the preventable and genetic aspects of disease. For example, a study we're conducting with the University of North Carolina is looking at how childhood, or even prenatal, diets can program stem cells early on in life to reduce the risk for disease. You see, we all share a common genetic code. But every person has errors—like typos—in the code. What we eat has the power to either compensate for these errors, or make them worse. Eating more antioxidant-rich fruits and vegetables can protect our brain cells from dying too soon and our skin from wrinkling too fast.

A study we're doing with Duke University asks how we, through "personalized medicine," can develop earlier diagnostics and cures for obesity-related diabetes, heart disease, liver disease, cancer, Alzheimer's, arthritis and multiple sclerosis.

Another study we're doing at North Carolina State University looks at plant genetics. How can we grow a healthier blueberry? How can we help farmers grow hardier crops or have longer growing seasons?

And a study we're doing at Appalachian State University is examining variations between individual metabolisms and how exercise affects weight loss and our immunity to certain diseases. Our scientists are currently studying how certain nutrients—quercetin, in particular—can protect combat soldiers from infection.

My own research has focused on the idea of measuring the rate of DNA breakdown. Clearly, certain factors can accelerate this damage (UV radiation, cigarette smoke, chronic stress and a poor diet). But more important, certain factors may have protective effects, which increase antioxidant levels and perhaps the rate of repair through other means of intervention. What you *don't* want is to accumulate DNA damage faster than you're able to repair it.

Here's an analogy: Think of your body as a bathtub. The rate of DNA damage is the faucet filling up the tub. The drain is the rate of DNA repair. In order to keep the tub from overflowing, you've got to either reduce the flow from the spigot, or ensure that the drain is fully open. In order to help people preserve this balance, we created a test that actually measures the rate at which DNA damage is accumulating. Not only is this a powerful diagnostic tool—but it's also a means of prevention. It's one thing to tell people that smoking or using tanning beds is bad for their health. It's another thing entirely to show them how they're actually accelerating their own aging process with such behaviors.

Knowing what you're doing wrong is only part of the equation. The chapters ahead will tell you which nutrients, from which foods, and which behaviors will help you live better—and longer.

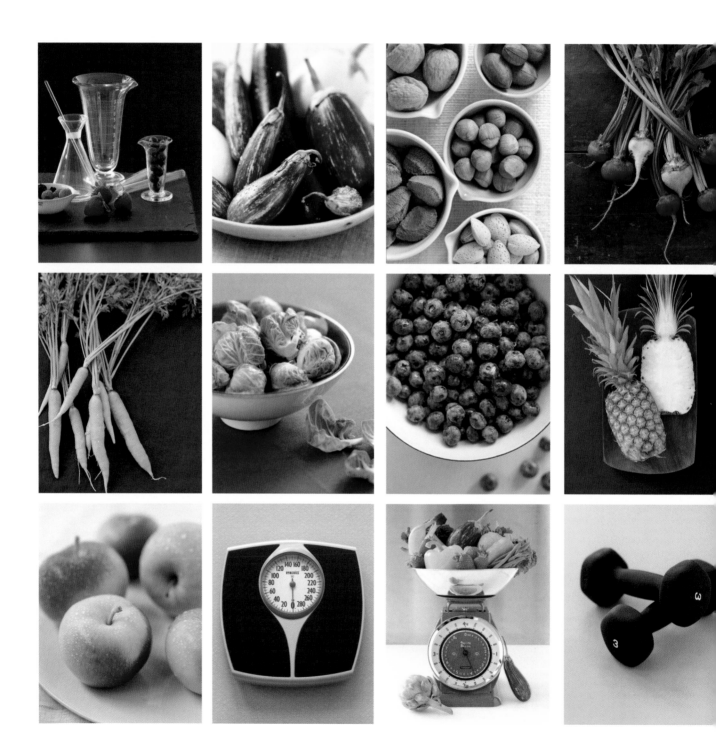

INTRODUCTION
Knowledge Is Power *by David H. Murdock* **6**

PART I
WHAT YOU NEED TO EAT EVERY DAY

CHAPTER 1
The Nutrients You Need **12**

CHAPTER 2
Next Nutrition Frontier **66**

CHAPTER 3
Superfoods **86**

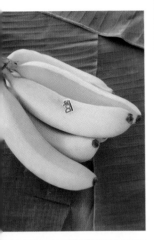

PART II
TOTAL HEALTH FROM HEAD TO TOE

CHAPTER 4
You Are What You Eat **126**

CHAPTER 5
Heart Health **142**

CHAPTER 6
Eye Health **160**

CHAPTER 7
Pregnancy Health **170**

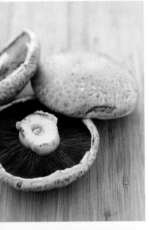

CHAPTER 8
Brain Health **184**

CHAPTER 9
Joint Health **198**

CHAPTER 10
Bone Health **214**

CHAPTER 11
Immunity **228**

PART III
SLIM DOWN, SHAPE UP WITH THE DOLE DIET AND FITNESS PLAN

CHAPTER 12
Health Risks of Excess Weight **242**

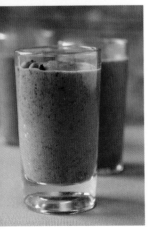

CHAPTER 13
Diet Myths and Weight-Loss Facts **262**

CHAPTER 14
Exercise Your Health **276**

CHAPTER 15
The Dole Diet **296**

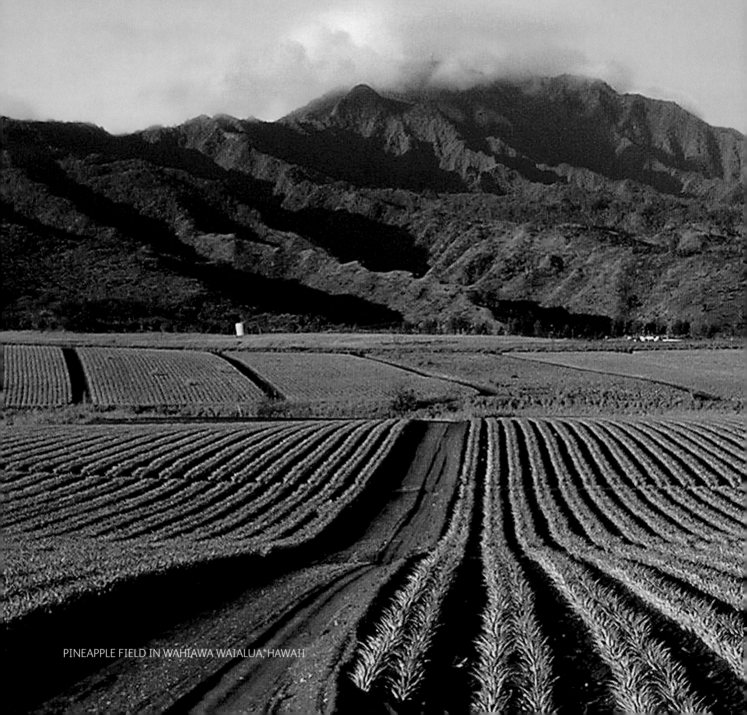

Knowledge Is Power

by David H. Murdock

PINEAPPLE FIELD IN WAHIAWA WAIALUA, HAWAII

Is it possible to live to the age of 125 or maybe even 150? It certainly is, as I recently discussed with Oprah Winfrey on her show on longevity. Oprah visited me at my farm to learn how, at 86, I'm enjoying the robust health, energy and mental creativity of someone many decades younger. My secret: large quantities of fruit and vegetables, plus an hour of daily exercise.

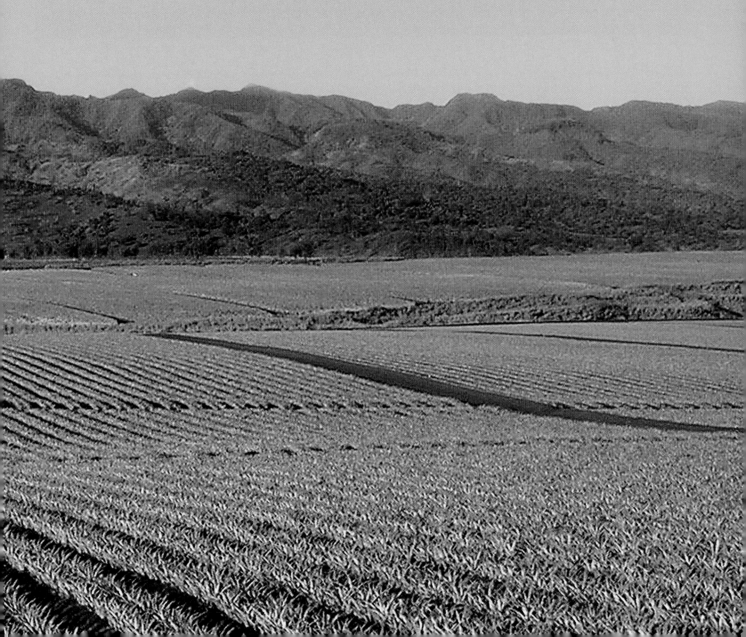

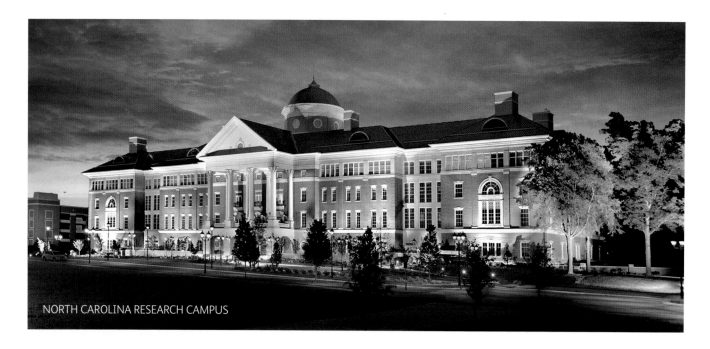

NORTH CAROLINA RESEARCH CAMPUS

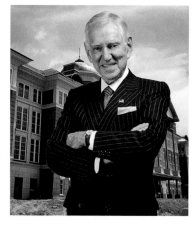

DAVID H. MURDOCK
AT THE
NORTH CAROLINA
RESEARCH CAMPUS

No pills, not even aspirin, and certainly no supplements ever enter my mouth—everything I need comes from my pescatarian diet, which incorporates 30 to 40 different kinds of fruit and vegetables every week. Even though I am Chairman of Dole Food Company, I do most of my own grocery shopping, and I even took Oprah on an impromptu trip to Costco, in a day that also included bike riding, exercising in the gym and juicing vegetables in the kitchen.

Oprah marveled at how I can eat so much, yet never gain a pound. In fact, I expend a lot of energy in my 50 to 60 minutes of cardio and strength training every day. Plus, there's the fact that fruits and vegetables tend to be lower in calories—but higher in filling fiber and other nutrients that help you feel satisfied—than other foods.

By eating many fruits and vegetables in place of fast food and junk food, people can avoid obesity. We're doing research on both the causes and effects of obesity—and the benefits of all different kinds of fruits and vegetables—at our North Carolina Research Campus in Kannapolis.

We've gathered a comprehensive array of famous scientists and scientific equipment under one roof, including a two-story, 950 megahertz, 8-ton superconducting magnet. It's the largest and most powerful magnet in the world, and it will help us look at both plant and human cells at the most minute level.

Together with Dole, the North Carolina Research Campus has given a $35 million grant to Duke University for the creation of the MURDOCK study, which actually stands for Measurement, Understanding and Reclassification of Disease of Cabarrus and Kannapolis counties. Researchers plan to study a group of 50,000 people from the area where the campus is located to determine why some people get sick and others don't. They're going to investigate which part of disease is controlled by DNA, and which part we must achieve through healthy living, regardless of our genetics.

At Dole's North Carolina Research Campus, we're also doing research that can help people who want to lose weight and have tried different diets but can't keep off the pounds. Professor Mary Ann Lila, who holds the David H. Murdock Chair for Nutrition at North Carolina State University and contributes her insights in the pages ahead, says, "People tend to eat the same volume of food every day." If you eat mostly fruits, vegetables, nuts, fish, whole grains and beans, you will never be hungry. If you eat high calorie snacks, junk food and fast food, that same volume of food will add up to thousands more calories than you need, and it will leave you hungry at the end of the day.

Another scientist at Dole's North Carolina Research Campus, professor David Nieman of Appalachian State University, has performed a series of studies which show that the key to long-term weight loss is calorie awareness and portion control. Professor Nieman—and many other top scientists from the North Carolina Research Campus—reveals his wisdom in the chapters that follow.

One of my commitments in life is to share this knowledge with others so that they too can live more vital, active and satisfying lives. Since acquiring major interests in Dole 26 years ago, my mission has been to educate the public on proper diet—and that has constituted the agenda of the Dole Nutrition Institute since its founding in 2003. We publish *Dole Nutrition News,* which is enjoyed by 2.5 million subscribers (sign up at www.dole.com). We create cooking and nutrition videos, cookbooks, brochures and other educational materials. We also provide educational support to teachers, parents and kids through www.dolesuperkids.com.

The culmination of all these activities is this book: a layman's guide that sifts through and simplifies some highly technical information so that you can become the master of your own health.

Like any educational endeavor, learning what you need to eat progresses from the simple to the complex. Consequently, so do the chapters that make up Part I of this book. We begin with answers to some basic questions: What do I need for health? What are nutrients? Why are they important? What foods supply the nutrients I need? Beyond basic nutrition, this section also includes a chapter on phytochemicals, natural compounds found in fruit, vegetables and other plants.

In Part II, we present simple "super chapters" on different parts of the body and aspects of health. Each chapter includes an interview with a leading scientific and nutrition expert from our North Carolina Research Campus.

Part III includes a two-week weight-loss plan based on total nutrition. Here, we pull together all of the information we've laid out in the first two sections of the book, translating it into an actual diet, meal plans and recipes. The Dole Diet is based on the philosophy that total nutrition supports weight loss by curbing deficiency-fueled overeating.

I've always believed that in order to achieve any goal, you need to define the problem, come up with the solution and then execute it. It's my hope that this book will help readers do just that—and realize their goals of living long, healthy and happy lives.

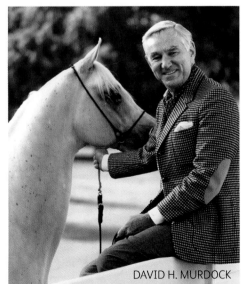

DAVID H. MURDOCK

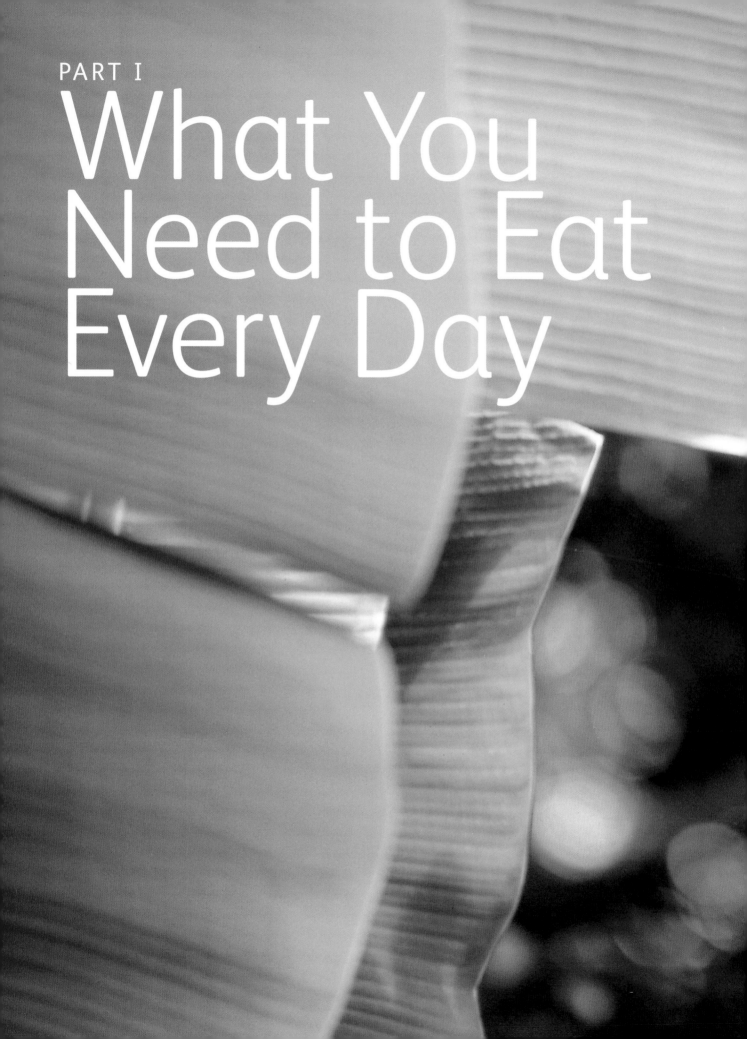

PART I

What You Need to Eat Every Day

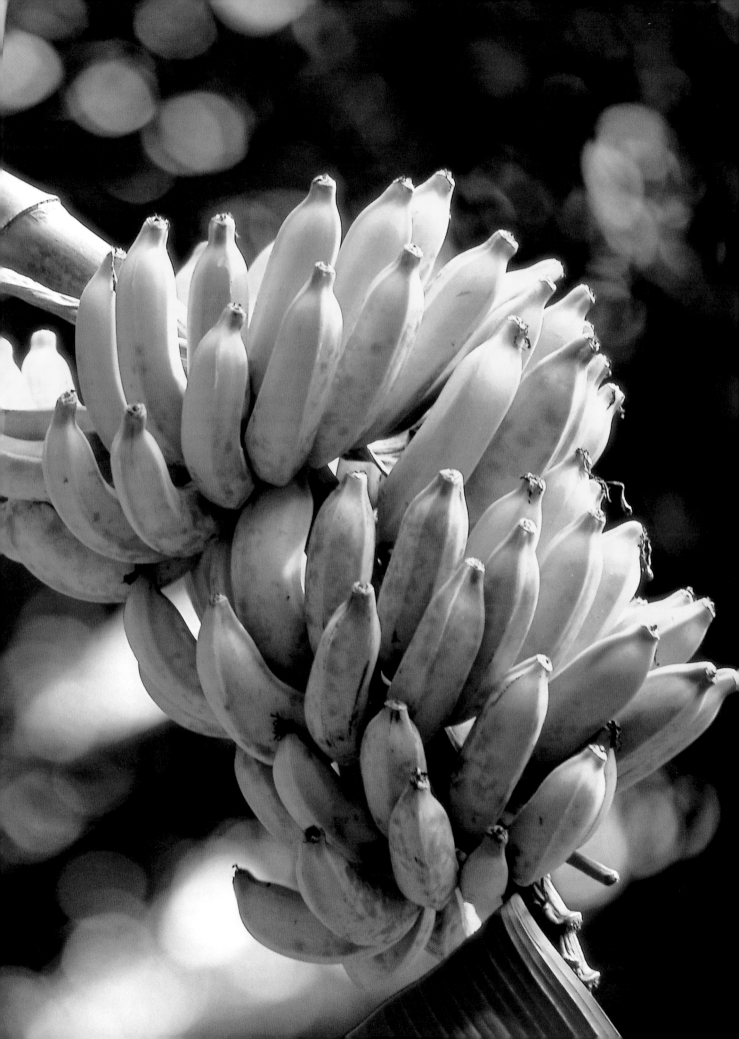

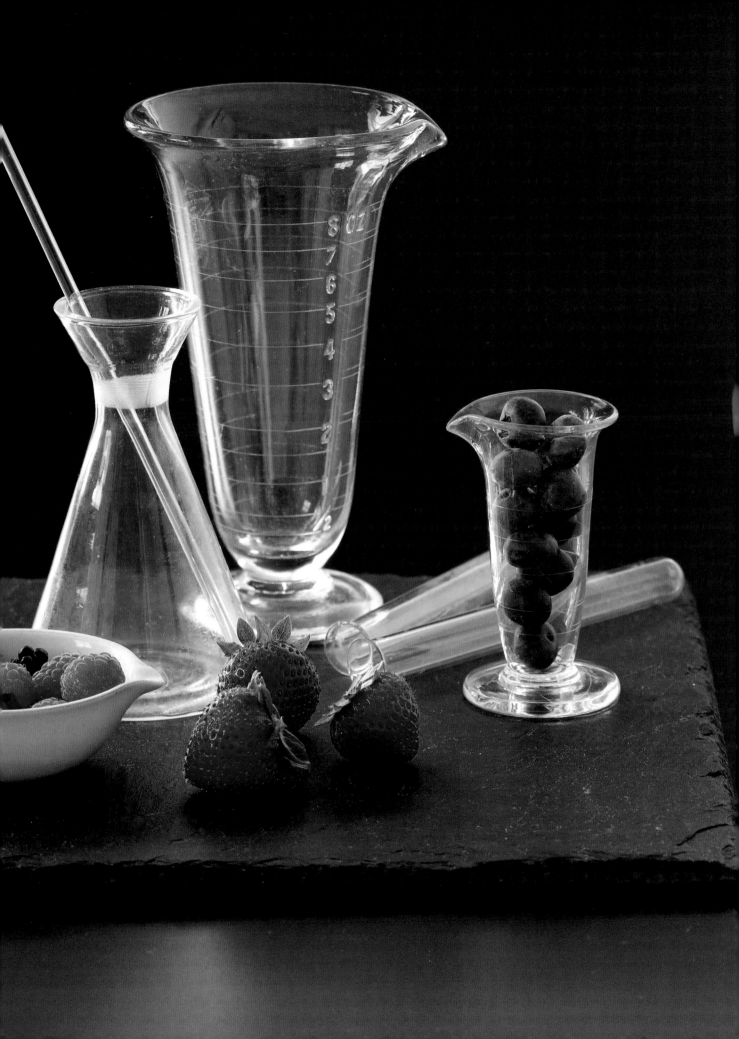

CHAPTER 1

The Nutrients You Need

Americans are overweight and undernourished. This seeming paradox results from the fact that while we gorge on unhealthy foods—sweetened beverages, pastries, junk food and fast food—we skimp on nutrient-dense, low-calorie fruits and vegetables. Less than a quarter of us consume five servings of fruits and vegetables a day—far fewer than the U.S. Department of Health and Human Services' recommended five to 13 servings a day (depending on your targeted caloric level). In fact, the average American eats just 1.4 servings of fruit per day. And only 7 percent of us receive the recommended three or more daily servings of whole-grain products.

We also take in far too many calories. Our average daily consumption has increased nearly 25 percent—530 calories, or almost the equivalent of a single Big Mac (540 calories)—since 1970. These days, adult men and women receive between 36 and 42 percent of their calories from sugar, fats and alcohol. Our average intake of added fats and oils has soared 67 percent, and while we tend to think of the 1950s as the "meat and potatoes" era, our meat consumption has increased a whopping 30 percent since then! In 2000, the average American consumed 152 pounds of sugar (and other caloric sweeteners). We're overdosing on fat, added sugar and sodium, and falling short on more than three-quarters of the 40 or so vitamins and minerals required for good health. In the pages that follow, you'll get a snapshot of each of those basic nutrients. You'll find out why you need them, where you can get them and what can happen if you don't get an adequate supply of them.

Our objective isn't to shock or frighten you, but rather to warn you of easily preventable problems so you can take action now. Heart disease—the ailment most firmly linked by established research to dietary problems—is America's number one killer, playing a role in one out of every three deaths. A close runner-up is cancer, which accounts for one in four deaths and is poised to overtake heart disease as the number one killer in the near future. Dietary changes could prevent about a third of those fatalities, according to the American Institute for Cancer Research.

A Quick Fix?

The desire to believe that proper nutrition can be achieved by popping vitamin, mineral and antioxidant pills has turned the dietary supplement business into a multibillion-dollar industry in recent years. Experts estimate that half of the American population takes multivitamins, and yet, as J. Michael McGinnis, MD, a senior scholar with the Institute of Medicine observes: "The bottom line is that we don't know for sure if they are benefiting from them." A spate of studies indicates that supplements are no substitute for nutrition derived from food. An editorial in the March 2009 issue of the *Journal of the National Cancer Institute* begins by stating, "The prospects for cancer prevention through micronutrient supplementation have never looked worse," and goes on to cite several large, randomized trials that reported no reduced cancer risk from micronutrient supplementation—as well as growing evidence that supplementation may actually be harmful. The previous month, in an *Archives of Internal Medicine* report, Women's Health Initiative researchers analyzed data from nearly 162,000 women and concluded that the multivitamins taken by 40 percent of them over nearly a decade had little or no effect on the risk of common cancers, cardiovascular disease or death among postmenopausal women.

One possible explanation is that the nutrients—vitamins, minerals and phytochemical antioxidants—within whole foods work synergistically. For instance, some antioxidants act as "big brother" to other nutrients, shielding them from oxidative damage so they can do their job. When supplements isolate these essential vitamins and minerals from their natural plant matrix, it can change the way they're processed in the body and interfere with their ability to work effectively. Supplementation and hyperfortification also make it easy to exceed daily nutrient requirements, which in some cases can lead to toxicity and liver damage. That's why, on the pages that follow, along with information on each essential nutrient, we've included a list of top whole food sources that contain it. The next chapter focuses on nutrients and highlights the power foods you need for total health.

But first, professor Bruce Ames shares his expert insights regarding the importance of meeting nutrient needs.

Dietary changes could prevent about a third of the most common fatalities, according to the American Institute for Cancer Research.

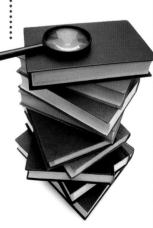

▶ Bruce Ames

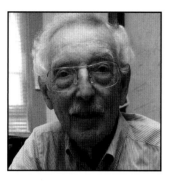

Bruce Ames is the director of the Nutrition and Metabolism Center at Children's Hospital Oakland Research Institute, Oakland, California. Having authored more than 500 scientific publications, he is among the most-cited scientists in any field. Recently he published his triage theory of DNA damage, in which he proposes that nutritional deficiencies cause our bodies to sacrifice long-term health in order to attend to the immediate needs of daily living. He also believes that such nutrient deficiencies may contribute to obesity by interfering with the satiety signals that the body needs to stop eating.

Bad diets are bad for a number of reasons—they include too much sugar, sodium, unhealthy fat and carbohydrates, and not enough protein and fiber. An additional characteristic of a bad diet is insufficient intake of essential micronutrients.

There are about 40 micronutrients in all, which include the essential vitamins and minerals. Proteins, fats and carbohydrates are considered macronutrients. Micronutrients have many important functions in the body, but one of the most vital is to help enzymes—proteins that keep all of our organs functioning—do their jobs. The body and brain can't function without enzymes.

Countless problems can arise from not getting enough of these micronutrients in the diet. Here are just a few:

Iron deficiency is the most widespread nutrition problem in the world. Iron is not only required by hemoglobin in red blood cells to carry oxygen throughout the body, it's also an essential constituent of many enzymes, including those involved in energy production and brain function. Iron deficiency results in anemia (a shortage of red blood cells), which is estimated to cost the world economy billions of dollars each year in lost productivity. Iron deficiency is also thought to have long-term adverse consequences; for example, causing poor cognitive function in children who are deprived of sufficient iron during critical periods of brain growth.

Magnesium deficiency is common in the United States, especially among the poor, obese, elderly and African-Americans. It has been associated with colorectal and other cancers, hypertension, osteoporosis, diabetes and metabolic syndrome (a prediabetic condition frequently accompanying obesity). In one large study more than 4,000 men were followed for 18 years to see if differences in blood concentrations of magnesium observed at the beginning of the study influenced future disease outcomes. The findings: Men with higher magnesium levels at the beginning of the study lived longer and had a lower incidence of heart disease and cancer than those with the lowest concentrations.

Vitamin D deficiency is associated with various cancers and ailments. Vitamin D is an unusual micronutrient for a couple of reasons. First, it doesn't just come from the diet (though a few foods, such as fresh or canned salmon, sardines and cod-liver oil contain a form of vitamin D); it's produced in the skin from exposure to sunlight. Second, the chemical form of vitamin D present in some foods and the form produced in the skin are not the active form of vitamin D, called calcitriol, which must be synthesized in the body from these precursor molecules. Because many of us spend most of our time indoors and don't

> One of the vital roles of micro-nutrients is to help enzymes do their job to keep our organs functioning properly.

get enough vitamin D from dietary sources, this deficiency is widespread. It's even more prevalent and severe in the United States among people with dark skin, such as African-Americans—although dark skin protects against excessive sun exposure in the tropics, it can be too protective in more northern latitudes where sun exposure is limited.

Vitamin D is associated with colon, breast, pancreatic and prostate cancer, as well as a variety of other ailments, including heart disease. Some scientists have suggested that vitamin D may inhibit cancer-cell growth and activate the immune system so it can fight infections.

Magnesium and vitamin D deficiencies are only two of the many micronutrient deficiencies associated with increased cancer risk. But it's very important to remember that when two things are associated (such as micronutrient deficiency and cancer, for example), it just means that they are often found together; it does not necessarily mean that one thing *causes* the other. Even when micronutrient deficiency is found to precede the onset of disease, it still does not prove that the deficiency *caused* the disease.

How might micronutrient deficiencies be linked to chronic diseases such as cancer? A clue comes from lab experiments in which researchers have observed that cells with an insufficient supply of some micronutrients continue to make energy and carry out normal "housekeeping" functions, but they can't protect their genetic material (DNA), which leaves them vulnerable to damage—thus accelerating the type of damage that accumulates over time, causing these cells to age faster than cells that receive a normal supply of micronutrients.

Cancers develop over many years, and the damage that builds up in DNA (which makes up chromosomes) is believed to play a causal role. Chromosome breakdown also appears to accompany aging. It's as though, when the availability of a micronutrient is limited, cells may have to forego some nonessential functions (such as keeping damage from slowly building up in DNA) in order to carry out more crucial duties (such as using oxygen to make energy). This theoretical analysis remains to be proven, but mounting evidence points in this direction.

The bottom line: Micronutrient deficiencies are prevalent across all ages and racial groups, and immediate action is called for. Here are two steps that can be taken right away.

(1) Changing from a "bad diet" to a "good diet": A diet containing fewer refined foods and more fruits, vegetables, fish and whole grains will help restore micronutrients and fiber to recommended levels—and is very likely to lead to weight loss. (The American Heart Association guidelines for physicians who treat obesity emphasize that the key to successful weight loss is decreasing energy intake. While we do not disagree that decreasing energy intake will lead to weight loss, we think the major focus should be on changing dietary habits; weight loss will then very likely be a pleasant side effect.)

(2) Increasing activity: A healthy diet needs to be supplemented with regular exercise. If you don't have a regimen already, choose an activity you enjoy (e.g., walking, running, playing tennis, working out in the gym, etc.) and start arranging your schedule to do it at least three times a week.

Cells with an insufficient supply of micronutrients are unable to protect their genetic material from damage.

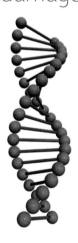

DNA STRAND

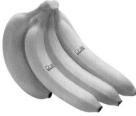

BANANAS

Carbohydrates

FUNCTION

Carbohydrates are the primary energy source for the brain, which is the only carbohydrate-dependent organ in the body. Carbohydrates also provide energy for normal activity and exercise. Since roughly 45 to 65 percent of total daily calories should come from carbohydrates, it's important to choose healthy sources.

CARBOHYDRATES

Recommended Dietary Allowance (RDA)
130g per day

Healthy Sources	Quantity	Grams of Carbs
Navy Beans	1 cup	47
Bananas	1 large banana	31
Whole Wheat Bread	2 slices	24
Raspberries	1 cup	15
Unhealthy Sources		
Pancakes, with syrup	1 pancake	45
Sodas	1 can	35
Doughnuts	1 doughnut	34
White Bread	1 slice	25

GOOD VERSUS BAD CARBS

Carbohydrates are classified as either simple or complex. Simple carbohydrates include sugars, such as glucose and fructose (found primarily in fruits), lactose (found in dairy products) and sucrose (found in table sugar). Complex carbohydrates include starch and fiber, which are digested more slowly, providing a sustained energy source without spiking insulin levels (or raising diabetes risk). While some carbohydrates are essential to health, others offer little more than empty calories. Good carbohydrates—like those found in fruits and vegetables—are rich in nutrients, low in calories, high in fiber and slowly digested, leaving you feeling fuller longer. Bad carbohydrates break down quickly, resulting in a blood sugar spike that makes you hungry in a shorter amount of time.

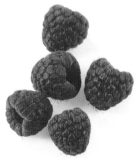

VS.

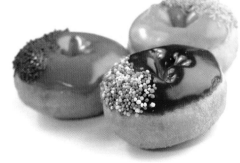

RASPBERRIES   DOUGHNUTS

Low-Carb Diet Dangers

Fad diets that severely restrict carbohydrates while promoting meat pose many health risks. Reasons to steer clear of these include the following:

Diet Rebound: Dieters often regain lost weight.

Free-Radical Damage: Metabolic imbalances from insulin shifts leave DNA more vulnerable to harm.

Cancer Risk: Studies indicate that low-fiber and high-meat consumption may increase the risk of colon cancer.

Calcium Depletion: Excessive protein intake can increase calcium excretion in the urine.

Gout and Kidney Stones: Too much protein can prompt the overproduction of uric acid that may lead to gout and kidney stones.

Reduced Antioxidants: A lack of fruits and vegetables cheats the body of disease-fighting phytochemicals.

Constipation: A low intake of dietary fiber interferes with the regularity of bowel function.

Diverticulitis: Fruits, vegetables and whole grains protect against developing this often-painful intestinal disorder.

Diminished Athletic Performance: Depleted carbohydrate-glycogen stores in the liver and muscles can impair strength and endurance.

Breath Odor: Bad breath and body odors result from low-carb-induced ketosis, a condition that also includes weakness, nausea and dehydration.

Fiber
FUNCTION

There are two types of dietary fiber: soluble and insoluble. All fiber-containing foods contain a combination of both, and both are beneficial. Water-soluble fiber helps lower cholesterol by binding with it during digestion and flushing it from your system. Insoluble fiber absorbs water during the digestion process, and thus helps prevent constipation.

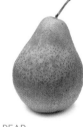
PEAR

FIBER

Adequate Intake (AI)
38g per day (men)
25g per day (women)

Tolerable Upper Intake Level (UL)
None established

Top Sources	Quantity	Daily Value (Men)	Daily Value (Women)
Lentils	1 cup	41%	62%
Artichokes	1 cup	38%	58%
Dates	1 cup	37%	57%
Beans	1 cup	33–50%	50–76%
Raspberries	1 cup	21%	32%
Blackberries	1 cup	20%	30%
Oat Bran	1 cup	15%	23%
Parsnips	1 cup	15%	23%
Collard Greens	1 cup	14%	21%
Pears	1 pear	13%	20%

Certain kinds of dietary fiber can defend against foodborne pathogens by selectively feeding "good" gut bacteria, which form a barrier to infection.

WEIGHT MANAGEMENT

Study after study reveals an inverse correlation between fiber intake and body weight. Fiber helps puts the brakes on overeating by delaying gastric emptying of the stomach into the small intestine, which increases the sensation of fullness. This delay can also help stabilize blood-glucose levels by moderating the amount of sugar released into the bloodstream.

PROSTATE HEALTH

There are also signs that fiber protects the prostate. A study published in the *International Journal of Cancer* monitored vegetable fiber intake and incidence of prostate cancer among 1,294 men over a period of 11 years, and found that those who consumed the most vegetables were 18 percent less likely to develop prostate cancer.

DIGESTIVE HEALTH

Japanese researchers have found an even stronger correlation between dietary fiber intake and rates of colon and colorectal cancers. Study participants with the highest fiber intake had a 27 percent reduced risk for colorectal cancer and a 42 percent reduced risk for colon cancer. Researchers speculate that these results are due to the tendency of insoluble fiber to promote regularity.

BREAST-CANCER PROTECTION

Fiber consumption may also help reduce breast-cancer risk, according to a Swedish study of 11,700 postmenopausal women in which researchers found that those with the highest fiber intake had a 40 percent lower risk of breast cancer.

GALLSTONE PREVENTION

Data analysis from the Nurses' Health Study indicates that insoluble fiber may reduce the risk of having to undergo gallstone surgery. In this landmark study, women with the highest insoluble fiber intake were 17 percent less likely to require gallstone surgery than those with the lowest fiber intake. Researchers suspect that by regulating cholesterol levels, fiber may prevent cholesterol from accumulating in the gallbladder and crystallizing into gallstones.

Fight Cardiovascular Disease with Fiber

Are you among the 96 percent of Americans who don't get enough fiber? And among the one in three who suffer from cardiovascular disease? Well, there may be a correlation. A Tulane University study of 10,000 women found that those with the highest fiber intake had a 15 percent lower risk of heart disease. In addition, after analyzing the dietary data of 6,000 men and women, French researchers found that those with the highest intake of insoluble fiber had lower blood pressure, cholesterol, triglycerides and homocysteine levels.

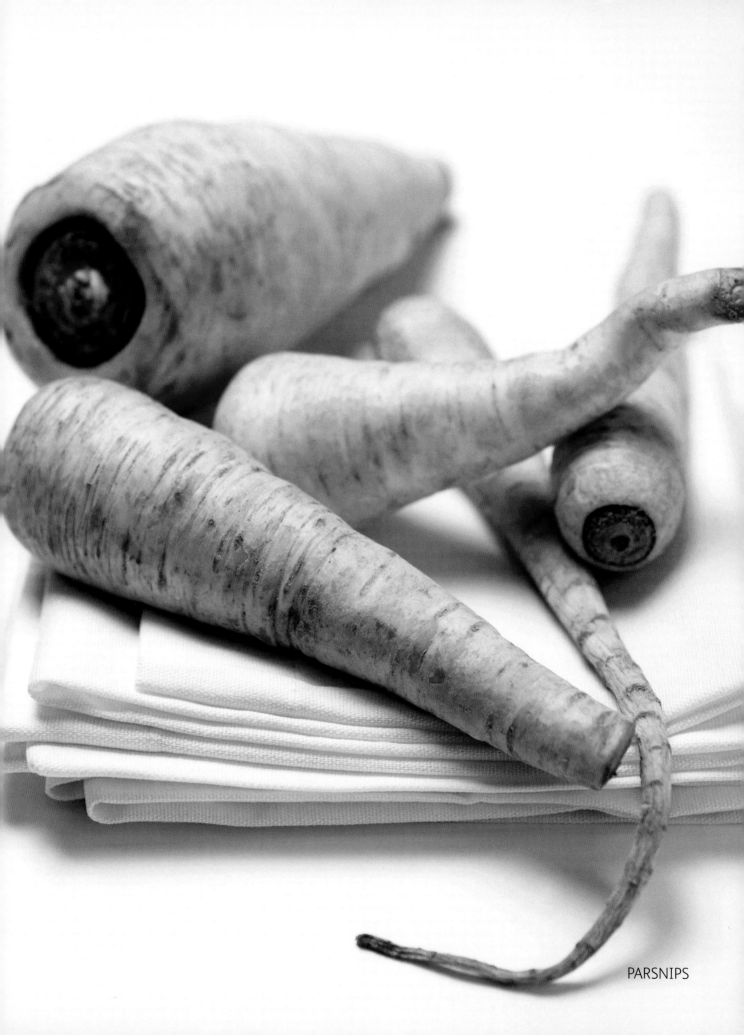

PARSNIPS

Fats

FUNCTION

Although almost every cell in the body contains some fat in the form of cell membranes, fat is not an essential nutrient. That's because the body is able to make the fat it needs—and then some! The fats we consume in food are used primarily as an energy source. Each gram of fat has 9 calories—nearly double that of carbohydrates and protein. The *Dietary Guidelines for Americans, 2005,* recommends that 20 to 35 percent of your daily calories come from fats, which equates to between 44 and 78 grams per day for a 2,000 calorie diet. There are "good" and "bad" fats, however: You need to be sure that the fat in your diet is the good kind.

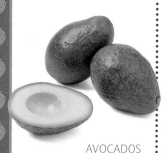

AVOCADOS

FATS

Fat Intake Limits:
44–78g total fat per day
16g saturated fat per day

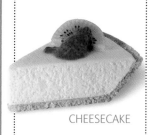

CHEESECAKE

Healthy Sources	Quantity	Fat, grams	Saturated/ Unsaturated*
Pecans	1 oz	20	9% / 87%
Sunflower Seeds	1 oz	15	9% / 81%
Avocado	½ fruit	15	15% / 79%
Wild Salmon	6 oz	14	15% / 73%
Less Healthy Sources			
Hamburger	7.5 oz	33	36% / 51%
Cheesecake	3 oz	18	44% / 45%
Butter	1 Tbsp	12	63% / 30%
Whole Milk	1 cup	8	57% / 31%

*The percentage of saturated and unsaturated fats doesn't add up to 100%, because other lipids (e.g., cholesterol, phytosterols, etc.) don't qualify as either, but they still count toward the total amount of fat.

GOOD AND BAD FATS

The amount and type of fat you ingest makes a significant difference to your health. Good fats of the polyunsaturated and monounsaturated variety may help lower cholesterol in the blood when consumed in place of bad fats. Bad fats include saturated fats, derived mainly from animal sources, such as meat, cheese and other whole-milk dairy products. Even less healthy are trans fats, which are primarily produced through hydrogenation—a process that turns liquid vegetable oils into solids such as the shortening and margarine often used in baked goods and snack foods. In general, fried food and fast food tend to be high in trans fats. Saturated-fat intake should not exceed 7 percent of daily calories (16 grams per day), and the latest research suggests trans fat consumption should be reduced to 1 percent of calories, if not avoided completely.

Fight Fat with Fish

Here's another reason to distinguish between "good" and "bad" fats: The former may actually help keep off pounds. So suggests a new animal study from the University of Georgia in which omega-3 fatty acids were found to intervene in fat formation by either stunting or killing off cells that would have otherwise matured into adipocytes (fat cells). While more research is needed to confirm the antiobesity potential of omega-3s in humans, conscientious dieters should opt for fish and other omega-3 sources.

Protein

FUNCTION

Although proteins themselves are the main structural component of all cells in the body, dietary proteins have a dual function. They can act as an energy source (dietary guidelines recommend that proteins make up 10 to 35 percent of daily calories), and they also provide the building blocks (amino acids) of muscles, membranes and some hormones.

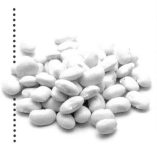

WHITE BEANS

PROTEIN

Acceptable Macronutrient Distribution Range (AMDR)
50–175g per day

Adequate Intake (AI)
0.8g per kg per day;
e.g., 180 lb human =
65g per day

Healthy Sources	Quantity	Protein	Fat
Turkey Breast	6 oz	52g	1g
Tuna/Halibut	6 oz	51g / 45g	2g/5g
White Beans	1 cup	17g	<1g
Less Healthy Sources			
Fried Chicken	1 piece	36g	31g
Duck	6 oz	32g	49g
Cheddar Cheese	1.5 oz	11g	14g
Hamburger	1 burger	32g	33g

HEART HEALTH

British researchers have found that people who get more protein from nonmeat sources (vegetables, grains, legumes, nuts, etc.) tend to have lower blood pressure than their more carnivorous peers. These results may help explain why a Mayo Clinic analysis found a 30 percent lower risk of death from heart disease among postmenopausal women who consumed high amounts of vegetarian protein sources.

Choose Healthy Proteins

"Not all proteins are equal in their health effects," notes Linda E. Kelemen, RD, ScD and assistant professor of epidemiology at the Mayo Clinic. "Vegetable proteins may deliver minerals and antioxidants that the body benefits from or contain substances that affect our hormones in healthier ways." By contrast, excessive intake of red meat is linked to increased risk of colorectal and lung cancer. Also, certain protein sources can make you feel fuller for longer. Fish is more filling than beef—with half the calories and a tenth of the saturated fat. A Swedish study published in the *European Journal of Clinical Nutrition* found that those who lunched on fish, instead of beef, consumed 10 percent fewer calories at dinner.

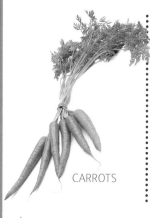

CARROTS

Vitamin A

FUNCTION

Vitamin A (or retinol) supports healthy vision, gene expression, reproduction, embryonic development, growth and immune function. Vitamin A comes in two forms: preformed vitamin A and provitamin A carotenoids. Preformed vitamin A is found only in animal products and is immediately available to the body upon ingestion. Provitamin A carotenoids are found in fruits and vegetables, and come from a type of antioxidant that can be converted into vitamin A by the body. The foods listed in the chart below are top sources of provitamin A carotenoids. About half of all Americans fail to get enough vitamin A.

VITAMIN A

Recommended Dietary Allowance (RDA)
900mcg per day (men)
700mcg per day (women)

Tolerable Upper Intake Level (UL)
3,000mcg per day

Top Sources	Quantity	Daily Value (Men)	Daily Value (Women)
Sweet Potato, baked with skin	1 medium	122%	157%
Carrots, raw	1 medium	72%	93%
Kale	⅔ cup	66%	85%
Butternut Squash	½ cup	64%	82%
Spinach, raw	3 cups	47%	60%
Collard Greens	½ cup	43%	55%
Green Leaf Lettuce	2½ cups	35%	45%
Cantaloupe	⅓ melon	25%	32%
Pumpkin	⅓ cup	23%	29%
Red Bell Peppers	1 small	13%	17%

EYE HEALTH

The retina, the part of the eye that transforms light into electrical signals to be sent to the brain, requires preformed vitamin A to enable vision in dim light. A deficiency can lead to poor vision or night blindness and contribute to age-related macular degeneration.

SKIN HEALTH

Vitamin A is involved in the formation, maintenance and repair of our skin. A deficiency can lead to impaired functioning of the outer layer of cells, resulting in a dry skin condition called xerosis.

IMMUNITY

Vitamin A plays a role in the development of immune and mucosal cells (cells that line the airways and the urinary and digestive tracts). These tissues are the body's first line of defense against colds and viruses. Vitamin A also helps support the formation of white blood cells, which the body marshals to fight infection.

PREGNANCY HEALTH

In a Polish study, researchers found that infants born to mothers who ranked in the lowest third of vitamin A intake during the year preceding pregnancy experienced significant adverse pollution-induced birth outcomes, as far as weight and length were concerned, while those with higher levels of vitamin A had completely normal babies.

FOOD TIP

Cooked carrots provide slightly more vitamin A than raw carrots. Why? Because heat breaks down the cell walls, making the nutrient contents more available.

GREEN PEAS

Thiamin

FUNCTION

Also known as vitamin B1, thiamin supports metabolism and regulates the flow of electrolytes in and out of muscle and nerve cells. We need increased thiamin during strenuous exertion, fever, pregnancy, breast-feeding and adolescent growth. While most Americans get more than enough thiamin, a deficiency of it sometimes occurs in third world countries, among alcoholics and gastric bypass patients. Severe thiamin deficiency causes the disease beriberi, a condition that eventually leads to nerve damage.

THIAMIN (VITAMIN B1) Recommended Dietary Allowance (RDA) 1.2mg per day Tolerable Upper Intake Level (UL) None established	Top Sources	Quantity	Daily Value (Men)	Daily Value (Women)
	Yellowfin Tuna	6 oz	71%	77%
	Wild Salmon	6 oz	39%	43%
	Navy Beans	1 cup	36%	39%
	Green Peas	1 cup	35%	38%
	Cereal	½ cup	30–130%	33–142%

Mental Health

Thiamin may help support emotional health and mental acuity. In a Welsh study researchers reported increased cognitive function among 127 young adults who took in 10 times the recommended dietary allowance (RDA). And, in a study at the University of California, Davis, 80 elderly women who ingested seven times the RDA of thiamin experienced improved sleep patterns, increased energy levels and feelings of general well-being.

Sports Recovery

Thiamin is needed to process lactic acid buildup after exercise. In a small Dutch study, athletes deprived of thiamin, among other B vitamins, experienced diminished exercise performance in a matter of weeks compared with those with normal levels of thiamin. They also experienced faster blood lactate buildup, meaning that their muscles could no longer deal with the lactic acid being produced. In another study, from Japan, researchers found that athletes supplemented with 100 times the thiamin RDA had fewer fatigue complaints immediately after exercise.

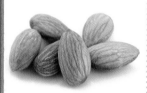

ALMONDS

Riboflavin

FUNCTION

Riboflavin is integral to the body's antioxidant defense systems. It activates the liver's Phase II enzymes, which neutralize and flush toxins from the body. Though rare, riboflavin deficiency can cause a sore throat, cracked lips, a magenta-colored tongue and anemia.

RIBOFLAVIN (VITAMIN B2)

Recommended Dietary Allowance (RDA)
1.3mg per day (men)
1.1mg per day (women)

Tolerable Upper Intake Level (UL)
None established

Top Sources	Quantity	Daily Value (Men)	Daily Value (Women)
Wild Salmon	6 oz	64%	75%
White Mushrooms, cooked	1 cup	36%	43%
Almonds	1 oz	22%	26 %
Cereal	¾ cup	20–160%	24–190%
Turkey Breast	6 oz	18%	21%
Spinach, raw	3 cups	13%	15%

NUTRITION TIP
A Belgian study found that sufferers of recurrent migraines experienced fewer headache days after significantly increasing riboflavin intake for a period of three months.

METABOLISM AND EXERCISE
Riboflavin supports metabolism of carbohydrates, fats and proteins. It can be depleted during exercise, so very active people need to make sure they get enough of this vitamin.

EYE HEALTH
Researchers have shown that those in the top fifth of riboflavin intake have a 30 to 50 percent lower risk of cataracts than those in the bottom fifth.

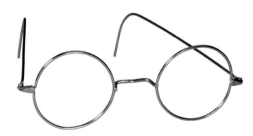

Niacin

FUNCTION

Niacin is a B vitamin that helps activate over 200 enzymes, the majority of which regulate the breakdown of carbohydrates, fats and proteins, which the body then uses for energy and for keeping the nervous system, digestive system, skin, hair and eyes healthy. Most people get about twice as much niacin as they need from their diet. Cereals are fortified with niacin and are probably part of the reason that there's no apparent niacin deficiency in the U.S. population. Deficiency still occurs in developing countries, however, causing pellagra—which is characterized by gastrointestinal problems, skin rashes and mental disorders.

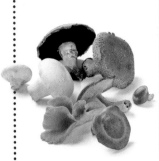

MUSHROOMS

NIACIN (VITAMIN B3)	Top Sources	Quantity	Daily Value (Men)	Daily Value (Women)
	Yellowfin Tuna	6 oz	127%	145%
Recommended Dietary Allowance (RDA) 16mg per day (men) 14mg per day (women)	Wild Salmon	6 oz	107%	122%
	Turkey	6 oz	81%	93%
	Halibut	6 oz	76%	86%
	Rainbow Trout	6 oz	61%	70%
Tolerable Upper Intake Level (UL) None established for food; 35mg per day for supplements	Portobello Mushrooms	1 cup	45%	51%
	Cereal	½ cup	25–125%	29–140%
	Button Mushrooms, raw	1 cup	22%	25%
	Peanuts	1 oz	21%	24%

BRAIN HEALTH

Niacin may help reduce the risk of Alzheimer's disease. A Rush Institute for Healthy Aging study found that people in the top fifth of niacin intake had an 80 percent lower risk of developing Alzheimer's, with the risk reduction stronger for food sources of niacin, as opposed to those who took it in its supplement form.

HEART HEALTH

Some doctors prescribe high dosages of niacin to lower LDL (bad) cholesterol and increase HDL (good) cholesterol. Unfortunately, the dose needed to have an effect is 30 to 100 times the amount of niacin you get from foods, and is high enough to cause side effects and even liver problems.

NUTRITION TIP

Although there is no known toxicity in humans from natural sources of niacin, supplements and fortification can push you over your limit. Side effects, such as flushed skin, can occur in those who have ingested as little as 30 milligrams per day.

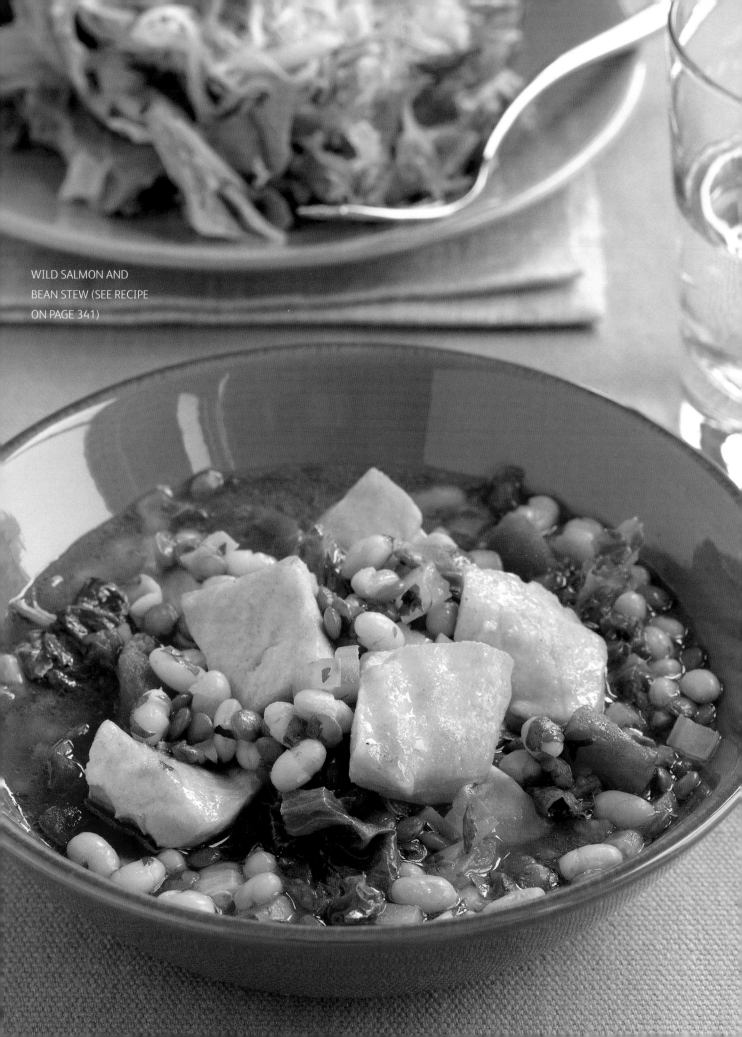

WILD SALMON AND
BEAN STEW (SEE RECIPE
ON PAGE 341)

Vitamin B5

FUNCTION

Pantothenic acid, also called vitamin B5, is required by dozens of enzymes that either produce energy from food or synthesize useful substances for the body (essential fats, cholesterol, steroids, neurotransmitters, red blood cells, etc.). Though rare, deficiency symptoms include headaches, fatigue and insomnia.

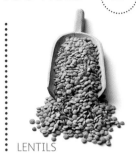

LENTILS

Hair Repair?

A study at the University of California, Los Angeles, found that mice exhibited skin irritation and loss of hair color in cases of severe B5 deficiency. Extrapolating from such results, some hair-care companies began to put pantothenic acid into their products, claiming it could help restore natural hair color, though clinical trials have failed to bolster such claims.

VITAMIN B5
(PANTOTHENIC ACID)

Adequate Intake (AI)
5mg per day

Tolerable Upper Intake Level (UL)
None established

Top Sources	Quantity	Daily Value
Liver	3 oz	112%
Wild Salmon	6 oz	65%
Mushrooms	1 cup	40–104%
Lentils	1 cup	25%
Turkey Breast	6 oz	25%
Cereal	½ cup	10–200%

Don't "B" Stressed

Pantothenic acid plays an essential role in the body's ability to regulate the stress hormone cortisol. When you're experiencing emotional conflict you overproduce stress hormones, which in turn depletes vitamin B5 stores. Adding more B5 sources, such as lentils, salmon and mushrooms, to your diet can help you restore balance.

Vitamin B6

FUNCTION

Vitamin B6 supports more than 100 enzymes that perform a variety of essential functions in the body, including the release of stored glucose (glycogen) from muscles, the synthesis of both the "feel-good" neurotransmitter serotonin and the oxygen transport protein hemoglobin, and the lowering of homocysteine levels in the blood (which, when elevated, increase the risk for bone fractures, heart disease and stroke). Most people get more than enough B6, though the elderly may not reach the higher recommended intake of 2 milligrams per day set for their population group. Though rare, a B6 deficiency can result in anemia, skin rash, seizures, depression and impaired immune function.

RED BELL PEPPER

VITAMIN B6
(PYROXIDINE)

Recommended Dietary Allowance (RDA)
1.3mg per day

Tolerable Upper Intake Level (UL)
100mg per day

Top Sources	Quantity	Daily Value
Yellowfin Tuna	6 oz	136%
Wild Salmon	6 oz	123%
Turkey Breast	6 oz	73%
Russet Potato, baked with skin	1 medium potato	47%
Banana	1 medium banana	33%
Cereal	½ cup	30–277%
Sweet Potato, baked with skin	1 medium potato	25%
Chickpeas	1 cup	18%
Red Bell Pepper	1 small pepper	17%
Spinach, raw	3 cups	14%

Tinkering with Immunity

Vitamin B6 may help maintain immune function as you age. Tufts University researchers found that seniors with depleted vitamin B6 levels had impaired immune response, including significant drops in the numbers of lymphocytes (white blood cells) and interleukin levels (immune response signaling cells). Doubling the RDA of B6 helped boost immune function back to baseline levels.

HEART HEALTH

Vitamin B6 helps lower levels of homocysteine, an amino acid linked to an increased risk of cardiovascular disease, by facilitating its conversion into a harmless and even useful amino acid that's used as a building block in most proteins.

CANCER PREVENTION

Scottish researchers discovered that patients diagnosed with colorectal cancer had lower vitamin B6 intakes than a control group. The effect was dose dependent: The higher the intake, the lower the risk. The greatest protection (a 30 percent risk reduction) came from dietary intakes of more than 3.26 milligrams per day, about two-and-a-half times the recommended daily amount.

DNA Repair

Vitamin B6 is emerging as a player on the DNA maintenance team. It helps convert folate—another B vitamin—into thymine, a component of DNA. When you're running low on B6, DNA can't be repaired, and the cumulative effect of breaks in DNA leads to the negative effects of aging and development of disease. In fact, in a Washington State University study, after just one month, participants on a low B6 diet exhibited 75 percent more DNA-strand breaks than when the study began. This could well be why B6 has been linked with lower risk of various cancers, including colon, prostate, lung, gastric and pancreatic.

Biotin

FUNCTION

Biotin is a water-soluble B vitamin that supports the metabolism of carbohydrates, fats and amino acids. Though rare, a biotin deficiency can result in hair loss and rashes around the eyes, nose and mouth, as well as an increased vulnerability to bacterial and fungal infections.

DIABETES PREVENTION

Type 2 diabetics often have low levels of biotin, which seems to interfere with the body's ability to properly utilize glucose. Researchers believe that biotin is involved in the synthesis and release of insulin, and preliminary studies suggest that it may help improve blood sugar control.

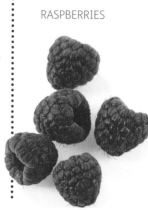

RASPBERRIES

BIOTIN
(VITAMIN B7,
ALSO KNOWN AS
VITAMIN H)

Adequate Intake (AI)
30mg per day

Tolerable Upper
Intake Level (UL)
None established

Top Sources	Quantity	Daily Value
Beef Liver	3 oz	90%
Egg, cooked	1 large	43–83%
Wild Salmon	3 oz	13–17%
Avocado	1 whole	7–20%
Whole Wheat Bread	1 slice	1–20%
Cauliflower	1 cup	1–13%
Raspberries	1 cup	1–7%

Hoof and Hand?

Animal husbandry researchers found that fortifying feed with biotin helped treat hoof abnormalities in horses and hogs. Could biotin also strengthen brittle nails among humans? Researchers found that increased biotin intake did indeed thicken nails by 25 percent. Aim to get your biotin from your diet since no safe upper limit has been established.

Folate

FUNCTION

Folate (or folic acid, as it's referred to in fortified foods and supplements) is a B vitamin that supports the proper formation of red blood cells. Folate is particularly important for pregnant women, as a deficiency of it may cause birth defects (such as spina bifida). This is what led the U.S. Food and Drug Administration (FDA), beginning in January 1998, to require all enriched cereal-grain products in the United States be fortified with folic acid.

Like vitamins B6 and B12, folate also lowers homocysteine levels in the blood, helping to reduce the risk of heart attack, stroke, cancer and bone fractures.

BONE HEALTH

Researchers in the United States and Holland reported the results of two separate studies in the *New England Journal of Medicine* linking the risk of bone fractures in elderly subjects to elevated homocysteine levels. Both reports suggested that folic acid and other homocysteine-lowering B vitamins may play a key role in helping to prevent bone fractures.

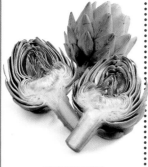

ARTICHOKES

FOLATE
(VITAMIN B9)

Recommended Dietary
Allowance (RDA)
400mcg per day

Tolerable Upper Intake
Level (UL)
1,000mcg per day

Top Sources	Quantity	Daily Value
Lentils	1 cup	90%
Spinach, cooked	1 cup	66%
Black, Navy and Pinto Beans	1 cup	64–74%
Beef Liver	3 oz	55%
Collard Greens	1 cup	44%
Cereal, fortified	¾ cup	40–200%
Artichokes	1 cup	38%
Beets	1 cup	34%
Brussels Sprouts	1 cup	24%

Fortification Fears

In the decade since the FDA mandated the folate fortification of breads, cereal and pasta, neural tube defects have plummeted 30 percent, sparing a thousand babies from spina bifida and anencephaly. But immediately following fortification, colon cancer rates reversed their steady decline, climbing by 12 percent (resulting in an additional 15,000 cases a year), according to a Tufts University study, which speculates that excessive supplementation may accelerate the growth of already existing precancerous cells.

HEART HEALTH

The Nurses' Health Study reported that women ages 27 to 44 who consumed at least 1,000 micrograms a day of total folate (two-and-a-half times the RDA) had a 46 percent lower risk of developing hypertension than those who consumed less than 200 micrograms a day.

CANCER PREVENTION

Folate levels that are too high—or too low—could raise your cancer risk. An Italian study linked a 50 percent reduction in precancerous lesions on the larynx of subjects with higher folate intake. And, according to Canadian animal researchers, low folate may actually *initiate* the development of colorectal cancer tumors. However, researchers caution that while folate may play an important role in preventing the development of colorectal cancer tumors, excessive supplementation may actually increase the replication of precancerous cells. The best way to ensure that your folate level is neither too high—nor too low—is to favor whole food sources over supplements and fortified products.

HEARING

Dutch scientists have linked low folate levels to age-related hearing loss, finding that an increase in folic acid slowed down low-frequency hearing loss in a cohort of people ages 50 to 70.

NUTRITION TIP
Nutrition knowledge can whet your appetite for healthy foods. Researchers at Monell Chemical Senses Center found that gaining a better understanding of why certain foods are good for you can make you more receptive to foods that once turned you off. So broaden your nutrition horizons by signing up for *Dole Nutrition News* at www.dole.com.

Melancholic? Check Your Folic

Folate plays an important role in regulating neurochemical reactions that affect mood. Tufts University researchers analyzed folate levels in nearly 3,000 study subjects and found deficiencies in a large proportion of those who suffered from depression.

Cereal Overload

In the mid-20th century, public health officials fortified cereals in response to widespread niacin deficiency caused by the modernized grain-milling process. The government mobilized bread and cereal manufacturers to start adding niacin, other B vitamins and some minerals to their products. Today, scientists are grappling with the possibility that cereal fortification has gone too far. The FDA has found that fortified cereal labels often underestimate nutrient content. Moreover, men tend to serve themselves over 250 percent more cereal than the recommended 30 gram serving size—and women over 180 percent more—upping some vitamin intakes by as much as 400 percent of the daily value. Such excessive intake puts consumers at risk of far exceeding toxicity limits for a number of nutrients, including folate and iron.

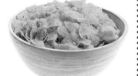

CEREAL

Vitamin B12

FUNCTION

The last of the B vitamins to be discovered, vitamin B12 has two main roles: protein synthesis and energy production from fats and proteins. Vitamin B12 is only available from animal sources, which is why vegetarians often rely on fortified cereals to meet their nutrient needs. The earliest sign of B12 deficiency is anemia. Over a longer duration, B12 deficiency leads to nerve damage that starts with tingling and numbness and can progress to difficulty walking and mental disorders. As we get older we make less stomach acid, which is needed to absorb B12. The elderly and those taking drugs that lower stomach acid should take extra precautions to get enough vitamin B12.

VITAMIN B12

Recommended Dietary Allowance (RDA)
2.4mcg per day

Tolerable Upper Intake Level (UL)
None established

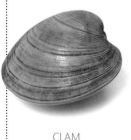

CLAM

Top Sources	Quantity	Daily Value
Clams	3 oz	3,503 %
Oysters	3 oz	1,020 %
Alaskan King Crab	6 oz	815 %
Cereal	¾ cup	250 %
Wild Salmon	6 oz	216 %
Soy Milk	1 cup	125 %
Halibut	6 oz	97 %
Nonfat Yogurt	1 cup	48 %
Yellowfin Tuna	6 oz	43 %
Turkey Breast	6 oz	28 %

HEART HEALTH

One of vitamin B12's metabolic functions is to help convert homocysteine, an amino acid that in excess ups the risk for cardiovascular disease, to a useful amino acid needed for protein synthesis. Although vitamin B12 (as well as vitamin B6 and folate) supplementation can effectively reduce homocysteine levels, so far taking it in supplement form has not been found to curb cardiovascular disease.

BRAIN HEALTH

A French review of studies on diet and dementia highlights the fact that Alzheimer's sufferers almost *always* have low vitamin B12 levels. In a Swedish study, 370 subjects with low serum levels of B12 actually doubled their risk of developing Alzheimer's. And a study at the University of Oxford in England demonstrated that people with below-average B12 levels were six times more likely to experience "brain shrinkage." While the precise mechanism of this effect is not thoroughly understood, researchers believe that low levels of B12 may inhibit proper DNA repair, which over time can lead to memory loss.

HEALTH TIP
Gain a rosy outlook by listening to the blues. Researchers found that by regularly listening to music, pain sufferers reduced discomfort by 20 percent, while also alleviating depression. Soothe your mood and manage chronic pain by listening to your favorite tunes.

Mood Boost

University of North Carolina researchers showed that 30 percent of patients who were hospitalized for depression had low levels of vitamin B12. Researchers speculate that this vitamin may help synthesize serotonin, one of the feel-good neurotransmitters in the brain. Antidepressant medicines (selective serotonin reuptake inhibitors or SSRIs) attempt to elevate these same feel-good compounds by inhibiting the breakdown of serotonin.

BONE HEALTH

Vitamin B12 deficiency has also been shown to increase the risk for bone fractures. Tufts University researchers found that men and women with low-plasma vitamin B12 levels had lower bone-mineral density at the hip and spine, respectively. The link was still significant even after adjusting for homocysteine (a risk factor for bone fracture), which suggests that modifying vitamin B12 levels could help prevent osteoporosis.

PINEAPPLES

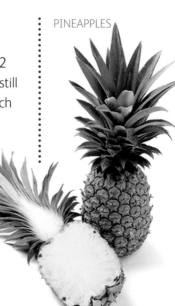

Vitamin C

FUNCTION

Although severe vitamin C deficiency, which causes scurvy, is rare, 40 percent of Americans are moderately deficient in this powerful antioxidant. Vitamin C enhances iron absorption, supports collagen formation and strengthens immune function.

VITAMIN C
(ASCORBIC ACID)

Recommended Dietary
Allowance (RDA)
90mg per day (men)
75mg per day (women)

Tolerable Upper Intake
Level (UL)
2,000mg

Top Sources	Quantity	Daily Value (Men)	Daily Value (Women)
Acerola Cherries	1 cup	1,827%	2,192%
Red Bell Pepper	1 medium	169%	203%
Kiwifruits	2 medium	157%	188%
Broccoli, cooked	1 cup	112%	135%
Brussels Sprouts	1 cup	107%	129%
Papaya	1 cup	96%	115%
Strawberries	1 cup	94%	113%
Pineapple	2 slices	70%	84%

HEART HEALTH

USDA researchers have linked low vitamin C with elevated C-reactive protein, an inflammatory marker for heart disease. Vitamin C also combats the oxidation of LDL (bad) cholesterol, preventing deposits and facilitating blood flow.

BONE AND JOINT HEALTH

Research shows vitamin C may support bone health by promoting collagen formation. According to a Boston University study, people who got less than 150 milligrams daily of vitamin C had faster cartilage breakdown. Studies have linked higher levels of vitamin C with greater forearm bone-mineral content in postmenopausal women.

Fight Fat with Vitamin C

Research from Arizona State University shows that raising vitamin C intake boosts your body's ability to burn fat. The study followed 20 obese subjects on a low-fat diet, which provided about two-thirds of daily vitamin C needs. The intervention group increased its vitamin C intake by 500 milligrams per day, and four weeks later they were able to oxidize 30 percent more fat during moderate exercise than the control group was. Scientists point to vitamin C's role in the manufacture of the amino acid carnitine, which helps flush fatty acids from the body.

LUNG HEALTH

Vitamin C could help alleviate symptoms of respiratory ailments like cystic fibrosis and asthma by loosening viscous secretions in the air passage, which lowers the risk of infection and makes breathing easier. Because smokers and people exposed to secondhand smoke tend to have deficient vitamin C levels in the blood, the Food and Nutrition Board recommends that they consume an additional 35 milligrams of vitamin C per day. Some studies have suggested that even higher amounts may be required to achieve the same levels as in nonsmokers.

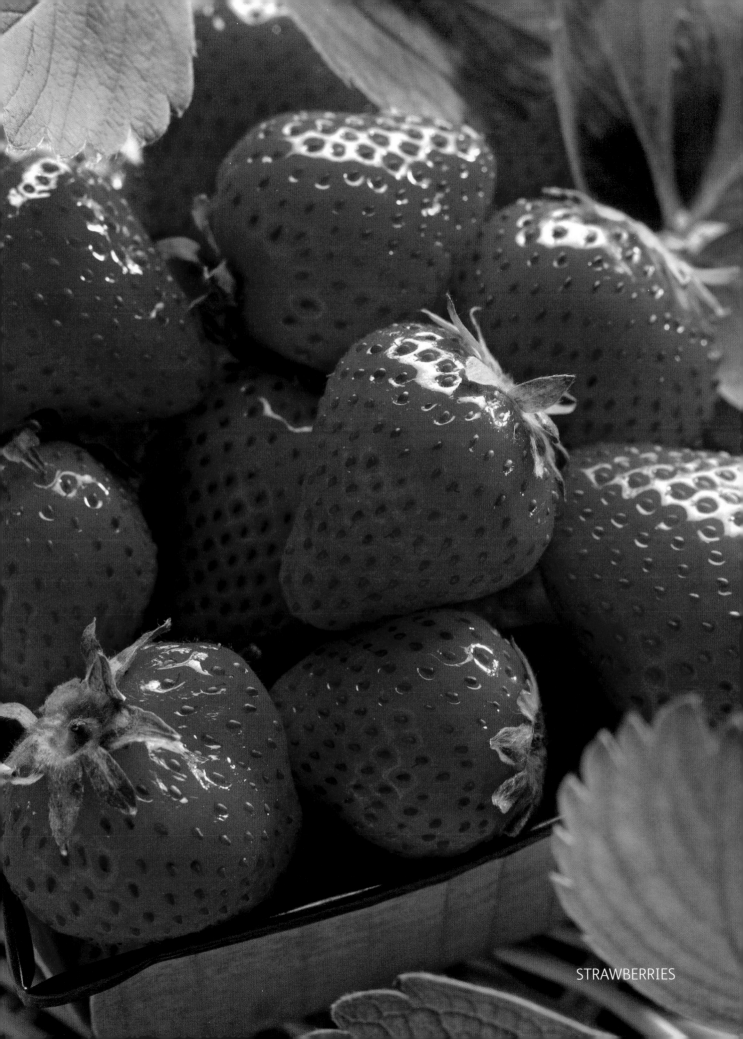

STRAWBERRIES

NUTRITION TIP
Exceeding the upper limit for vitamin C—2,000 milligrams per day—can cause diarrhea and gastrointestinal distress. This is worth watching out for, since many popular supplements contain 1,000 milligrams—more than 10 times the RDA.

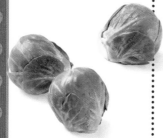

BRUSSELS SPROUTS

STOMACH HEALTH

In a 2004 trial, a team of Finnish and American researchers found that fruit and vitamin C consumption was associated with an approximately 45 percent reduction of risk in noncardia cancer, the most common form of stomach cancer in most parts of the world.

SKIN HEALTH

New British research looked into the dietary habits of more than 4,000 American women and found that those who got the most vitamin C from their diets had smoother, moister and more youthful-looking skin. Not only did the study find more signs of aging—wrinkles, dryness, thinning skin—among those with lower vitamin C intakes, it concluded that a high-fat diet also tended to make women look old for their age.

Choline

FUNCTION

Choline is needed for the formation of neurotransmitters and for strengthening cell walls. Intakes of choline in the U.S. population are not well documented, so it's hard to assess the prevalence of a deficiency. Inadequate choline intake can result in a condition called fatty liver, which arises when the phospholipids required to transport fat away from the liver are in short supply. As the organ becomes congested with excess fat, severe liver damage occurs. At the same time, exceeding the upper level intake (UL) of 3.5 grams per day is likely to lead to a dramatic drop in blood pressure, profuse sweating and diarrhea.

CHOLINE

Adequate Intake (AI)
550mg per day (men)
425mg per day (women)

Tolerable Upper Intake Level (UL)
3,500mg per day

Top Sources	Quantity	Daily Value (Men)	Daily Value (Women)
Beef Liver	3 oz	65%	84%
Wheat Germ	1 cup	31%	40%
Cod	6 oz	26%	33%
Egg, boiled	1 large	21%	27%
Wild Salmon	6 oz	20%	26%
Soybeans	1 cup	15%	19%
Navy Beans	1 cup	15%	19%
Brussels Sprouts	1 cup	12%	15%
Broccoli, cooked	1 cup	11%	15%

HEART HEALTH

Along with vitamins B6, B12 and folate, choline helps regulate levels of the amino acid homocysteine, helping to ward off cardiovascular disease.

Choline Cuts Breast Cancer Risk

Women with the highest choline intake have a 24 percent reduced risk of developing breast cancer, according to a National Institutes of Health–funded study. Researchers looked at 3,000 women and found a protective effect among those with an average choline intake of 455 milligrams per day (a little higher than the established adequate intake of 425 milligrams per day) compared with those with the lowest intake (average of 196 milligrams per day).

Earlier research had found that egg-eating adolescent girls reported less incidence of breast cancer later on in life. A single, large poached egg contains about 100 milligrams of choline.

BRAIN HEALTH

Choline is needed to make acetylcholine, a neurotransmitter that helps brain cells communicate. Research has shown that Alzheimer's patients are often deficient in acetylcholine, suggesting that adequate levels of its precursor, choline, may help maintain mental acuity.

Feed Your Brain

Researchers at the University of North Carolina at Chapel Hill fed pregnant rats either a high-choline or low-choline diet to see how it would impact their offspring. During a critical period of about five days (the equivalent development time of the human memory center at 25 weeks) in the 21-day rat gestation period, a little extra choline in the mother's diet resulted in a 30 percent improvement in memory that lasted for the offspring's entire lifetime. Two additional studies suggest that women with diets low in choline have a greater risk for having a baby with several kinds of birth defects.

Vitamin D

FUNCTION

Vitamin D is a fat-soluble vitamin that aids in the absorption and use of calcium and phosphorus, and thus plays an important role in maintaining healthy bones and teeth. The nutrient is unique in that, although you can ingest it from food, it can also be synthesized in the body upon exposure of your skin to the sun. Thus, extreme northern or southern latitudes, prolonged winter months, smog and dark skin can inhibit vitamin D production. Vitamin D deficiency is widespread in the United States, particularly among people with dark skin, such as African-Americans. Deficiency can cause rickets, which is characterized by the stunting and warping of the long bones.

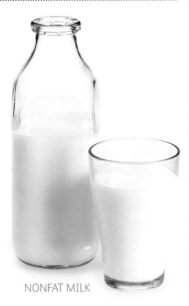

NONFAT MILK

VITAMIN D

Adequate Intake (AI)
5mcg per day

Tolerable Upper
Intake Level (UL)
50mcg per day

DOLE PORTOBELLO
MUSHROOMS

Top Sources	Quantity	Daily Value
Salmon, canned	3 oz	266%
Sardines, canned	3 oz	116%
DOLE Portobello Mushrooms	1 cup	100%
Sunshine	15 minutes per day	100%
Nonfat Milk, fortified	1 cup	50%
Cereal, fortified	1 cup	20–26%
Egg Yolk	1 egg	11%
Button Mushrooms	1 cup	9%

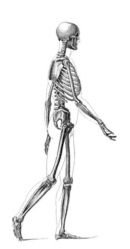

HEALTHY BONES

DIET TIP

A vegetarian diet
could add years to
your life! A review
of six studies in the
*American Journal
of Clinical Nutrition*
found that a nearly
meatless diet may
extend your life by
as many as three-
and-a-half years.

BONE AND DENTAL HEALTH

A Harvard University study of more than 72,000 postmenopausal women found that those
who consumed double the RDA of vitamin D had a 37 percent lower chance of hip fracture.
Additionally, investigators from the Humboldt University of Berlin in Germany, Harvard
University and Tufts University reviewed periodontal records of more than 11,000 men and
women and found that those over the age of 50 with the lowest levels of vitamin D suffered
about 25 percent more tooth loss than those with the highest levels. Researchers attributed
this in part to vitamin D's role in achieving optimal bone-mineral density (weaker bones are
less able to hold teeth in place), but they also speculate that it may have an anti-inflammatory
effect that counters the inflammation characteristic of gum disease.

JOINT HEALTH

Further indication of vitamin D's possible anti-inflammatory benefits comes from
studies showing that people who meet their daily requirement for vitamin D are less
likely to experience arthritis pain. For example, a study at the University of Iowa found
that the risk of rheumatoid arthritis was 33 percent lower among women ages 55 to 69
with the highest vitamin D intake.

HEART HEALTH

Low vitamin D levels raise the risk of peripheral artery disease (a narrowing of the arteries
in the legs, arms and areas other than the heart and brain), as well as of heart attack and
stroke. One study showed double the risk of heart failure among those with low vitamin D
levels. Vitamin D also affects hypertension (high blood pressure), which may be why Dutch
researchers found that exposure to sunlight just three times a week reduced both diastolic
and systolic blood pressure by about 5 to 8 percent.

Megavitamin Mushroom

In a dazzling dietary breakthrough, Dole food researchers have figured out how to naturally boost vitamin D levels in mushrooms to 100 percent of daily requirements. It turns out that humans aren't the only light-triggered generators of vitamin D: Mushrooms also produce the nutrient upon exposure to light. Starting with portobellos, Dole pioneered a process of using an ordinary flashbulb (similar to the sort used in cameras) to boost the mushrooms' vitamin D content without compromising freshness or food safety.

CANCER PREVENTION

Researchers began to look more deeply into vitamin D's possible chemo-protective benefits after observing higher cancer rates in northern latitudes, where sunlight—and therefore sun exposure—is limited. A study of women from over 100 countries found breast-cancer rates were nine times higher for those who lived in areas with the least light. Researchers at the University of California, San Diego, demonstrated that an additional 25 micrograms of vitamin D per day (five times the RDA) could reduce the risk of colon cancer by 50 percent, and breast and ovarian cancers by 30 percent. Another study at Northwestern University showed that just 10 micrograms of vitamin D per day (double the RDA) reduced the risk of pancreatic cancer by 43 percent.

MENTAL HEALTH

A newly discovered link between low levels of vitamin D and depression may shed light on why winter's wan sun leaves some feeling glum. A Dutch study of more than 1,200 seniors found 14 percent lower levels of vitamin D among those reporting more feelings of loneliness and listlessness. Other research has found that chronic pain problems are more prevalent among those lacking vitamin D. For instance, in a University of Delaware study, vitamin D deficiency doubled women's risk of serious lower back pain.

DIABETES

Low-serum vitamin D levels are also associated with an increased risk of diabetes. In a Finnish study, women with the lowest vitamin D levels were 14 percent more likely to develop type 2 diabetes, while men's increased risk was double that amount.

MULTIPLE SCLEROSIS

Numerous studies have linked low vitamin D levels to multiple sclerosis (MS). In fact, MS is virtually unknown in equatorial regions, where sun exposure is high; and its prevalence increases with latitude, as sun exposure diminishes. Norway, where the diet is high in vitamin D–rich fatty fish and cod-liver oil, is an exception, particularly in coastal towns where fish consumption is the highest. In a Harvard School of Public Health study, those with highest vitamin D levels demonstrated a 62 percent lower risk of MS.

DIET TIP

Drive-through dining adds up to empty calories, leaving you overfed, undernourished and more apt to overeat. Researchers have found an inverse relationship between the number of fast-food visits and dietary intake of vitamins C and A, beta-carotene, calcium, magnesium and phosphorus. They also report that frequent fast-food consumers drink twice the amount of carbonated soft drinks as fast-food abstainers.

NUTRITION TIP
Extensive data
shows that people
with the lowest
vitamin D levels are
26 percent more
likely to die from any
cause than those
with highest levels.

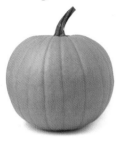

PUMPKIN

PMS SYMPTOMS

Scientists at the University of Massachusetts kept tabs on more than 3,000 participants over a period of 10 years in the long-running Nurses Health Study and found that women in the top fifth of vitamin D intake experienced a 41 percent reduction in premenstrual tension.

IMMUNITY

Scientists at Harvard Medical School and Children's Hospital Boston have linked low vitamin D levels with a higher risk of cold and flu infections. The link was even stronger in individuals with asthma.

Vitamin E

FUNCTION

Vitamin E is a potent antioxidant that may help slow the aging process. In addition to protecting cells from oxidation, vitamin E also shields other nutrients—such as vitamins A and C—from free-radical damage.

VITAMIN E

Recommended Dietary
Allowance (RDA)
15mg per day

Tolerable Upper Intake
Level (UL)
1,000mg per day

Top Sources	Quantity	Daily Value
Sunflower Seeds	1 oz	63%
Almonds	1 oz	50%
Hazelnuts	1 oz	28%
Beet, Dandelion and Turnip Greens	1 cup	17–18%
Broccoli, cooked	1 cup	15%
Pumpkin	1 cup	13%
Red Bell Pepper	1 medium pepper	13%
Spinach, raw	3 cups	12%

Reduce Bladder Cancer Risk

Dietary vitamin E could protect against bladder cancer, according to researchers from the University of Texas M.D. Anderson Cancer Center in Houston. Their 2004 study found that subjects who consumed the most vitamin E from food alone (9 milligrams—not even topping the daily recommended intake) reduced their risk for bladder cancer by 42 percent.

Food, Not Supplements

The jury is still out on the efficacy—indeed, the safety—of vitamin E supplementation, particularly at high levels. A disturbing report published in the *Journal of Clinical Investigation* found that vitamin E pills actually increased LDL (bad) cholesterol in animal studies. In an accompanying editorial, Dr. Ronald Krauss, director of atherosclerosis research at the Children's Hospital Oakland Research Institute, said: "One should rely on eating foods that are rich in antioxidants and not rely on taking supplements to prevent heart disease."

IMMUNE HEALTH

In a study published in the *Journal of the American Medical Association*, seniors who were given synthetic vitamin E (90 milligrams, which is six times the RDA) were nearly 20 percent less likely to catch a cold in a 12-month period than those given a placebo.

BRAIN HEALTH

Researchers in Chicago showed that seniors in the top fifth of vitamin E intake from food (less than 4.7 milligrams per day) had a 70 percent lower risk of developing Alzheimer's. The authors noted that there was no protective effect from supplemental vitamin E.

In addition, a Canadian study found that increased vitamin E intake reduced the frequency of seizures in epileptic children.

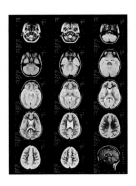

BRAIN SCAN

Vitamin K
FUNCTION

The name *vitamin K* comes from the German word *koagulation,* in reference to the vitamin's first-known biological role in blood clotting. While blood has the remarkable ability to remain liquid even though it's loaded with all sorts of solid material—red and white blood cells, protein, vitamins, minerals and fat —it can also become solid within seconds when a blood vessel breaks. This particular ability can spell the difference between life and death if you're seriously injured—and it requires vitamin K, which your body needs to make several blood proteins involved in clotting. If your body is short of vitamin K, your blood will clot very slowly, and you might develop symptoms, such as easy bruising, frequent nosebleeds or cuts that won't stop bleeding.

This fat-soluble vitamin also helps strengthen bones, fight cancer and prevent heart disease. Vitamin K comes in a number of forms, including K1, which is found in plants, and K2, which is found in meats and eggs. Although K1 is the main dietary source for humans, K2 is the form found in the human body. Scientists suspect that the body converts K1 into K2. Unfortunately, 80 percent of men and 59 percent of women fail to get enough of this vital nutrient. Vitamin K deficiency is associated with bruising, extremely heavy menstrual periods and nosebleeds.

NUTRITION TIP
Like other fat-soluble nutrients, (e.g., vitamins A, D and E), vitamin K isn't absorbed well in the absence of dietary fat. Make sure you choose the healthy kind, as in olive oil, avocados and nuts.

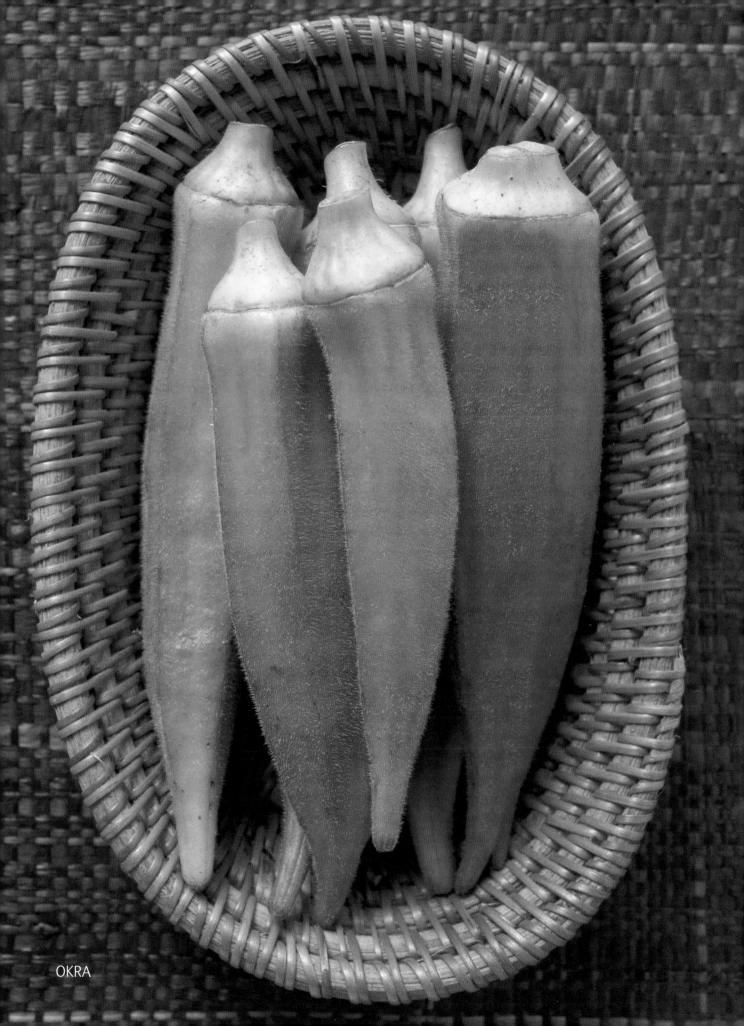

OKRA

VITAMIN K

Adequate Intake (AI)
120mg per day (men)
90mg per day (women)

Tolerable Upper Intake
Level (UL)
Not established

DANDELION GREENS

Top Sources	Quantity	Daily Value (Men)	Daily Value (Women)
Kale	½ cup	443%	590%
Spinach, raw	3 cups	362%	483%
Collard Greens	½ cup	348%	464%
Beet, Dandelion and Turnip Greens	½ cup	220–290%	294–387%
Cabbage	1 cup	136%	181%
Broccoli, raw	1½ cups	125%	167%
Green Leaf Lettuce	1½ cups	122%	162%
Brussels Sprouts	½ cup	91%	122%
Scallions	½ cup	86%	115%
Romaine Lettuce	1¾ cups	73%	97%
Okra	½ cup	27%	36%
Celery	½ cup	12%	16%

BONE HEALTH

Vitamin K is needed to create two proteins found in bone and plays a significant role in activating osteoblasts (bone-forming cells). Without it, bones produce an abnormal form of these proteins that can't bind to the minerals that normally form them.

One Japanese study suggests that low vitamin K levels play a role in the breakdown of bone after menopause. Some researchers contend that postmenopausal women are at risk for a low-level vitamin K deficiency that the traditional blood-clotting test would not detect. In addition, the Framingham Heart Study found that seniors with a high dietary intake of vitamin K had a 65 percent lower risk of hip fractures.

CANCER PREVENTION

Encouraging research suggests that vitamin K2 may play a role in inhibiting the growth of tumors and cancer cells. Several studies have linked higher levels of supplemental vitamin K2 intake with stabilization of liver cancer. For example, a Japanese study showed that women who consumed 45 milligrams of vitamin K2 per day were 80 percent less likely to develop liver cancer than those in the control group. This amount is several hundred times higher than the RDA for vitamin K, but single servings of some foods (particularly leafy greens) provide equivalent amounts. For example, a cup of cooked spinach provides nearly 1,000 percent of the recommended daily intake of Vitamin K.

HEALTH TIP

Could the way to a man's heart actually be through his mind? According to the National Cancer Institute, men are significantly less likely than women to recognize the health benefits of fruits and vegetables, such as their role in reducing the risk of many cancers, diabetes, high blood pressure and heart disease. So, it follows that the way to lower their risk for heart disease is by raising their health awareness.

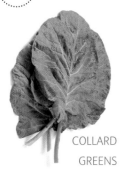

COLLARD
GREENS

Calcium

FUNCTION

Calcium is essential for strong bones and teeth, which is where 99 percent of this mineral is stored in the body. Calcium also plays a role in nerve-impulse transmission and in the constriction and relaxation of blood vessels and muscles. Approximately 88 percent of adult females and 63 percent of adult males don't get enough calcium.

CALCIUM

Adequate Intake (AI)
1g per day

Tolerable Upper Intake Level (UL)
2.5g per day

Top Sources	Quantity	Daily Value
Nonfat Milk	1 cup	31%
Collard Greens	1 cup	27%
Turnip Greens	1 cup	20%
Canned Salmon	3 oz	18%
Beet Greens	1 cup	16%
Dandelion Greens	1 cup	15%
Navy Beans	1 cup	13%
Kale	1 cup	9%

NUTRITION TIP

Better together: calcium and inulin. In addition to helping your body resist foodborne pathogens, the dietary fiber inulin aids calcium absorption. So try mixing and matching calcium sources (nonfat milk, kale, canned salmon and black-eyed peas) with inulin sources (bananas, leeks, onions, garlic, asparagus and artichokes).

BONE HEALTH

One of the most serious consequences of a calcium deficiency is that the body will actually leach needed calcium from the bones, which can lead to osteoporosis. A British study showed that risk of fracture was 75 percent higher in women whose dietary calcium intakes were less than 525 milligrams per day than for those whose intakes were over 1,200 milligrams per day.

CANCER PREVENTION

A study of nearly half a million people by the National Institutes of Health found that diets rich in calcium from food sources may help protect against over 10 different types of cancer, the most common being prostate, breast, lung and colorectal.

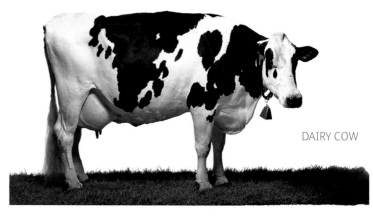

DAIRY COW

CALCIUM FROM FOOD, NOT SUPPLEMENTS

One of the biggest investigations into the efficacy of calcium supplementation among postmenopausal women (the population most vulnerable to osteoporosis) concluded that supplements had little impact on bone density and, in fact, were associated with the increased incidence of kidney stones. Furthermore, researchers at the Washington University in St. Louis School of Medicine found that women who get calcium from food, rather than from supplements, actually have higher bone-mineral densities, even when their total intakes are less.

Calcium and Weight Management?

When you're calcium deficient, your body is more disposed to create fat cells than when you're getting an adequate amount of calcium. Researchers at the University of Tennessee found that high calcium, and especially high-dairy diets, seemed to enhance weight loss among obese individuals who were already following a low-calorie regimen—but other investigators have had difficulty duplicating these results.

Molybdenum

FUNCTION

Molybdenum is an essential trace element required for the activity of several enzymes, including an enzyme that's involved in the body's production of genetic material and proteins; another that helps the body produce uric acid, which helps eliminate waste; and a third that helps the body detoxify sulfites, which are found in protein-rich foods and used as chemical preservatives in some foods and drugs. Certain people are extremely sensitive to the sulfites used as additives and have trouble breaking them down, which causes a toxic buildup in the body and can lead to asthma and other life-threatening breathing problems.

Currently, data on molybdenum content from foods is scarce (which is why the table gives such a broad indication of molybdenum sources). Cases of deficiency or toxicity have not been reported, but excessive intake, in rare cases, can increase uric acid levels and potentially trigger gout. Also, because molybdenum interferes with the absorption of copper, long-term supplementation could, in theory, result in a copper deficiency.

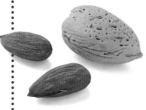

ALMONDS

MOLYBDENUM	Top Sources	Quantity
Recommended Dietary Allowance (RDA) 45mcg per day	Legumes	High
	Whole Grains	Good
	Nuts	Good
Tolerable Upper Intake Level (UL) 2,000mcg per day	Fruits	Low
	Dark Green, Leafy Vegetables	Low

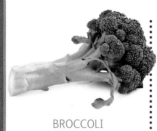

BROCCOLI

Chromium

FUNCTION

Chromium is a trace mineral required in minute quantities for glucose metabolism. Its role in regulating insulin helps normalize blood sugar levels, which may help keep appetite in check. In one study, men with higher chromium intakes were found to have lower blood sugar and improved insulin resistance than those with lower chromium intakes—which is consistent with the link various studies have found between low chromium intake and diabetes and cardiovascular disease.

CHROMIUM	Top Sources	Quantity	Daily Value (Men)	Daily Value (Women)
Adequate Intake (AI) 35mcg per day (men) 25mcg per day (women)	Broccoli	1 cup	63%	88%
	Grape Juice	1 cup	21%	30%
Tolerable Upper Intake Level (UL)	English Muffin	(1) 2.5 oz	10%	14%
None established	Potatoes	1 cup	8%	11%

SUPPLEMENTAL DANGER

Chromium supplements are often advertised as fat-burning and muscle-building, but several studies have found that they have no such effect, and supplement companies have lost lawsuits for failing to supply scientific evidence for such claims. In fact, one study showed that chromium picolinate, the supplemental source of chromium, actually damages animal DNA.

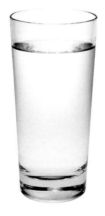

WATER

Fluoride

FUNCTION

Fluoride prevents dental cavities. It can be dangerous, even toxic, at levels above the tolerable upper limit. Levels of more than 5 milligrams per kilogram of body weight can trigger nausea, abdominal pain and vomiting.

FLUORIDE	Top Sources	Quantity	Daily Value (Men)	Daily Value (Women)
Adequate Intake (AI) 4mg per day (men) 3mg per day (women)	Sardines	3.5 oz	5–10%	7–13%
	Tap Water	1 cup	5%	6%
Tolerable Upper Intake Level (UL)	Chicken	3 oz	2–3%	2–3%
10mg per day	Fish (in general)	3 oz	1–4%	1–6%

It's in the Water

In the United States the local water districts maintain the fluoride content of water at between 0.7 and 1.2 milligrams per liter, which is enough to prevent dental decay. But not all water sources are equal. Water from wells may not be fluoridated, and some home water-treatment systems actually remove fluoride. (Brita-type filters that affix to the faucet do not.)

BONE AND TEETH HEALTH

Fluoride stabilizes bone mineral and hardens tooth enamel. In fact, 95 percent of the body's fluoride is stored in the bones and teeth. Fluoride has been used as a therapeutic agent in the treatment of osteoarthritis, and doses of it in the range of more than 10 times the RDA have been successful in increasing bone mass in the lumbar region of the human spine.

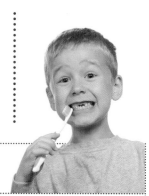

Don't Eat the Toothpaste, Children!

Children who swallow toothpaste can overdose on fluoride, putting them at risk of dental fluorosis, a white speckling of the teeth. Toothpastes in kid-pleasing flavors—from bubble gum to apple—increase this danger. Supervise your kids' brushing to make sure such tube treats remain a spur to better dental care, rather than an invitation for ingestion.

Copper

FUNCTION

Copper plays a role in energy production, connective tissue formation, iron metabolism and central nervous system function. It also helps activate antioxidant enzymes and regulate gene expression. Though deficiency is rare, symptoms include immunity dysfunction and anemia. Copper is toxic at very high levels.

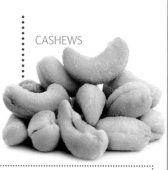

CASHEWS

Copper Caper?

Anemia (a shortage of red blood cells) can be a clinical clue to copper deficiency. When copper is low, iron accumulates in the liver instead of being transported to the bone marrow, where it is used to form new red blood cells.

COPPER

Recommended Dietary Allowance (RDA)
900mcg per day

Tolerable Upper Intake Level (UL)
10,000mcg per day

Top Sources	Quantity	Daily Value
Oysters	3 oz	411%
Lobster	3 oz	183%
Shiitake Mushrooms	1 cup	144%
Alaskan King Crab	3 oz	111%
Roasted Chestnuts	1 cup	81%
Soybeans	1 cup	78%
Dry-Roasted Cashews	1 oz	70%
Sunflower Seeds	¼ cup	66%
Clams	3 oz	66%
Baked Beans	1 cup	61%

NUTRITION TIP
High zinc intake can interfere with copper absorption. How? Excess zinc boosts the production of a protein in the intestinal wall that binds tightly with copper, thus limiting its bioavailability.

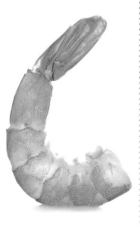

SHRIMP

SKIN HEALTH

Copper is involved in an enzyme reaction that cross-links collagen and elastin, giving skin its youthful elasticity and plumpness. It also supports melanin formation, essential for pigmentation of skin.

BONE HEALTH

Copper helps link the long strands of proteins that make up the connective tissue throughout the body. It's essential to bone formation, and studies show that it can help prevent loss of bone calcium when dieting. A small study found that dieting women with higher copper intakes (about 3 milligrams per day) kept more calcium in their bones than those with lower intakes (just over 1 milligram per day).

PREGNANCY HEALTH

In a 2006 China Medical University study, researchers found that mothers of premature babies were low on copper, suggesting that deficient copper could undermine collagen production and contribute to a more precarious pregnancy. Other animal research suggests copper deficiency during pregnancy could lead to lower levels of certain enzymes needed for infants' brain development.

Iodine
FUNCTION

Iodine is a trace element required for the synthesis of thyroid hormones, which regulate growth, development, metabolism and reproduction. Prevalent in underdeveloped countries, iodine deficiency is typified by a goiter (enlarged thyroid gland). Deficiency during pregnancy is the most common cause of mental retardation globally.

Iodine Overload?

The average American's intake of iodine is roughly 300 micrograms—double the RDA. In some regions of Japan, where seaweed is a dietary staple, intakes can range up to 80,000 micrograms per day. But even these levels are below the gram quantities that would induce acute iodine toxicity.

IODINE

Recommended Dietary Allowance (RDA)
150mcg per day

Tolerable Upper Intake Level (UL)
1,100mcg per day

Top Sources	Quantity	Daily Value
Seaweed	1 oz	High and variable
Cod	3 oz	66%
Salt, iodized	⅛ tsp	51%
Navy Beans	1 cup	43%
Potato, baked with skin	1 medium	40%
Shrimp	3 oz	23%
Turkey Breast	3 oz	23%

The "I" in Soil

The amount of iodine in fruits, vegetables and legumes largely depends on the iodine content of the soil in which they are grown, which makes consistent measurements difficult. The iodine content in seafood depends on its environment as well, because fish, crustaceans and seaweed absorb iodine from salt water.

Phosphorus

FUNCTION

Phosphorus, in the form of calcium phosphate, forms much of the structural component of bones and teeth, and, in the form of phospholipids, of cell membranes. Studies have linked low dietary intake of phosphorus with osteoporosis. But, while an estimated 40 percent of young women do not get enough phosphorus, deficiency symptoms—including anemia, muscle weakness and bone pain—are only observed in instances of near starvation.

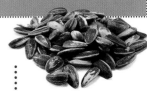

SUNFLOWER SEEDS

NUTRITION TIP

Excess phosphate usually gets excreted, but those with kidney problems may accumulate too much of this mineral, which can start to calcify body tissues.

PHOSPHORUS

Recommended Dietary
Allowance (RDA)
700mg per day

Tolerable Upper Intake
Level (UL)
4,000mg per day

Top Sources	Quantity	Daily Value
Oat Bran	1 cup	99%
Halibut	6 oz	65%
Wild Salmon	6 oz	61%
Soybeans	1 cup	60%
Sunflower Seeds	¼ cup	53%
Lentils	1 cup	51%
Crab	1 cup	50%
Cereal	½ cup	49%

NUTRITION TIP

Some antacids hinder
phosphorus intake by
forming aluminum
phosphate, which is
insoluble and cannot
be absorbed.

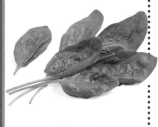

SPINACH

ENERGY AND METABOLISM

Phosphorus is essential for pH balance (i.e., the level of acidity in the body). Phosphorus regulates pH balance by soaking up or freeing particular molecules that can tip the scales toward acidity or alkalinity.

Iron
FUNCTION

Two-thirds of the body's iron is found in hemoglobin, a blood protein that transports oxygen from the lungs to the rest of the body. Any blood loss results in a loss of iron, which is why 15 percent of premenopausal women fall short on this mineral. Mothers-to-be and toddlers are also at high risk of deficiency. Iron deficiency is *the* most common nutrient deficiency worldwide. However, too much iron can also be damaging. This is why vitamin pills for premenopausal women contain iron, but those for others do not.

A University of Michigan study found that iron-deficient babies grew up with lower motor skills and mental measures. Symptoms of iron deficiency include low energy, difficulty maintaining body temperature and impaired immune response. Among pregnant women, iron deficiency may result in premature deliveries and low birth weights.

Overweight and Anemic

New research suggests that absent nutrients—not just excess calories—may be contributing to childhood obesity. In a national sample of nearly 10,000 subjects, between the ages of 2 and 16, University of Rochester researchers found a significantly higher prevalence of iron deficiency among obese children. In fact, the obesity-iron deficiency link was so strong that the authors of the study recommend that an elevated body mass index (BMI) be considered an independent risk factor in anemia screening. And a Yale University study demonstrated that iron deficiency is twice as common in overweight versus healthy-weight teens.

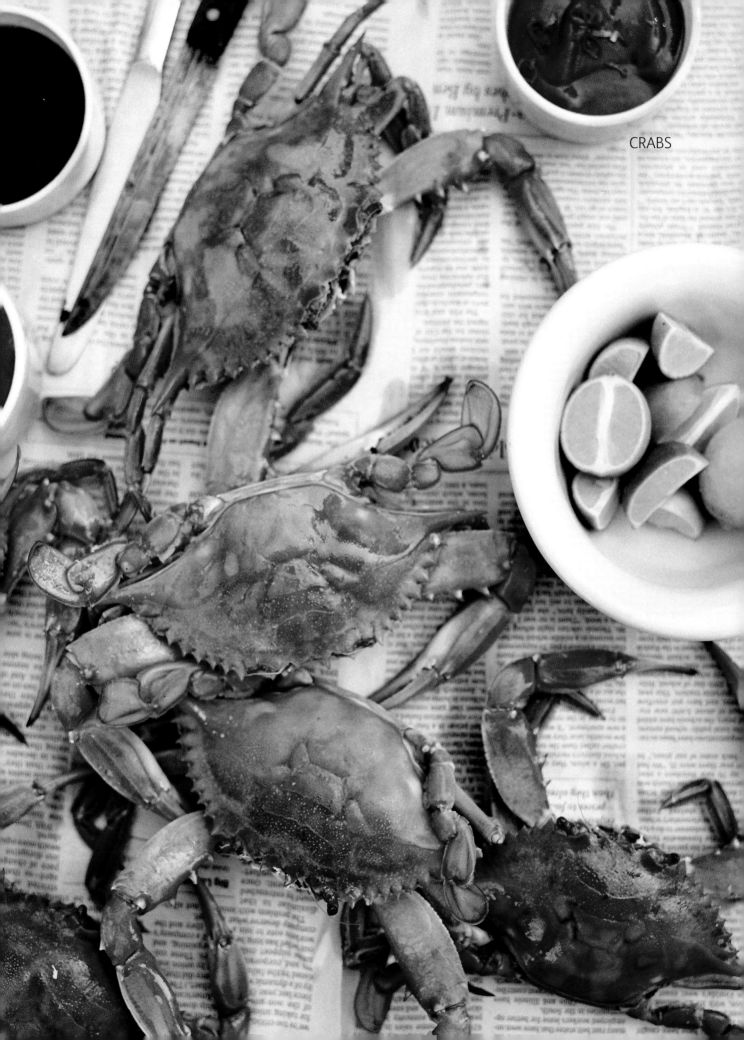

CRABS

IRON

Recommended
Dietary Allowance
(RDA)
8mg per day
(men)
18mg per day
(women)

Tolerable Upper
Intake Level (UL)
45 mg per day

Top Sources	Quantity	Daily Value (Men)	Daily Value (Women)
Clams	3 oz	297%	132%
Cereal	1 cup	279%	124%
Soybeans	1 cup	111%	49%
White Beans	1 cup	98%	44%
Lentils	1 cup	82%	37%
Spinach	1 cup	80%	36%
Oysters	3 oz	74%	33%
Liver	3 oz	70%	31%
Oat Bran	1 cup	64%	28%
Soy Milk	1 cup	34%	15%

NUTRITION TIP
Several studies
suggest that iron
deficiency may
raise the risk of lead
poisoning among
children, because
low iron levels
actually increase the
intestinal absorption
of lead.

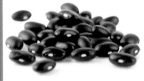

BLACK BEANS

FOR VEGETARIANS

Animal-derived iron is more easily absorbed than iron from plant sources. Vegetarians need to make a conscious effort to incorporate plenty of healthy iron sources into their diet. Foods rich in vitamin C can help enhance iron absorption, whereas the phytic acid found in soy inhibits it. In addition, foods containing prebiotic fiber help increase the bioavailability of iron and other minerals. A Cornell University animal study found that prebiotic fiber increased iron absorption by 28 percent.

FOR ATHLETES

Regular endurance exercise can increase your iron needs by as much as 30 percent. Workouts that push the body beyond its normal limit can lead to blood loss via microscopic tears in the gastrointestinal tract.

Magnesium

FUNCTION

Magnesium is responsible for hundreds of biochemical reactions, among them the contraction and relaxation of muscle and blood vessels, the synthesis of protein and DNA, and the production and transport of energy from carbohydrates, fats and proteins. About two-thirds of all adults fall short on magnesium.

SOYBEANS

Top Sources	Quantity	Daily Value (Men)	Daily Value (Women)
Halibut	6 oz	43%	57%
Spinach, cooked	1 cup	37%	49%
Soybeans	1 cup	35%	46%
Black Beans	1 cup	29%	38%
Brazil Nuts	1 oz	25%	35%
Beet Greens	1 cup	23%	31%
Navy Beans	1 cup	23%	30%
Oat Bran, cooked	1 cup	21%	28%
Artichokes	1 cup	17%	22%

MAGNESIUM

Recommended Dietary Allowance (RDA)
420mg per day (men)
320mg per day (women)

Tolerable Upper Intake Level (UL)
None established (from food)

HEART HEALTH

Researchers at the Medical University of South Carolina found that levels of C-reactive protein (a marker for heart disease) were three times higher among those with low magnesium intakes. Magnesium also helps maintain normal blood pressure levels by supporting the proper dilation of blood vessels.

CANCER PREVENTION

Given magnesium's role in regulating cell growth, some researchers believe the mineral may have a chemo-protective effect. In fact, in the Paris Prospective Study 2, French researchers tracked more than 4,000 men for nearly two decades and found a 50 percent reduced risk of death by cancer among those with the highest magnesium levels. And consumption of magnesium-rich foods cut the number of colon tumors by 34 percent in a Swedish study.

All-Cause Mortality

Reports from the Paris Prospective Study 2 indicate that high blood levels of magnesium are linked to a 40 percent lower risk of death from any cause. High serum levels of copper and zinc, however, seem to increase the risk of death from all causes.

Get Magnesium, Stop Gallstones

Simply meeting daily magnesium needs can slash men's gallstone risk by a third. The University of Kentucky Medical Center analyzed dietary data for over 42,000 men and found that those who consumed adequate magnesium from diet alone enjoyed a 32 percent lower risk of developing gallstones than those in the bottom fifth of magnesium intake. Researchers speculate that magnesium deficiency may cause problems with triglyceride and cholesterol levels, which in turn may raise gallstone risk.

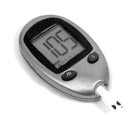

BLOOD-GLUCOSE
MONITOR

DIABETES PREVENTION

Harvard Medical School researchers used data from the Women's Health Study, which tracked more than 39,000 women—age 45 and older—over an average period of six years, and found that the risk of developing diabetes was 11 percent lower among those with the highest magnesium intake. (Other large studies have placed the protective benefit of magnesium at more than double that rate.) But administering megadoses isn't necessary to achieve healthy levels: The researchers also found that overweight women who had only adequate magnesium levels reduced their diabetes risk by more than 20 percent compared with overweight women with low magnesium levels.

BRAIN HEALTH

About half of all migraine sufferers have low magnesium levels. Research suggests that increased magnesium intake during an attack can yield dramatic and sustained relief.

Manganese

FUNCTION

Manganese is an essential trace mineral that helps activate powerful antioxidant enzymes, convert fats and proteins into energy, and support cartilage and bone formation. Manganese deficiency is rare, but symptoms can include loss of bone mass and stunted growth in children.

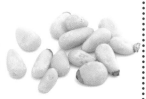

PINE NUTS

Damage Control

Manganese is crucial in protecting mitochondria—the power plants of the cells—from free-radical damage. Since mitochondria process 90 percent of the oxygen that enters the body, they need the best defense against oxidative damage. Manganese supplies this in the form of manganese superoxide dismutase—the fastest reacting antioxidant enzyme that exists.

MANGANESE

Adequate Intake (AI)
2.3mg per day (men)
1.8mg per day (women)

Tolerable Upper Intake Level (UL)
11mg per day

Top Sources	Quantity	Daily Value (Men)	Daily Value (Women)
Oats	1 cup	333%	426%
Pine Nuts	1 oz	108%	139%
Brown Rice	1 cup	77%	98%
Roasted Chestnuts	1 cup	73%	94%
Spinach, cooked	1 cup	73%	94%
Pineapple	1 cup	59%	75%
Lima Beans	1 cup	42%	54%
Raspberries	1 cup	36%	46%
Cereal	1 cup	35–97%	44–124%

WOUND HEALING

Healing wounds requires increased production of cartilage and collagen. Manganese helps support this demand, which makes adequate dietary manganese especially important during recovery from injury. A Polish study found that certain cancer-fighting drugs that impair collagen synthesis and delay wound healing work by immobilizing manganese, so that it can't activate the collagen-building enzyme.

BONE HEALTH

Manganese helps activate enzymes required for creating cartilage and collagen to support normal bone growth. In a study at the University of California, San Diego, researchers found that while calcium slowed spinal bone-mineral loss in postmenopausal women, a mineral combination of zinc, copper and manganese actually stopped it. Additional studies show that women with osteoporosis have decreased manganese levels.

BRAIN HEALTH

When Colombian scientists reviewed several human studies comparing manganese levels among epileptics and a control group, they found that seizure sufferers had particularly low levels. More research is needed to determine whether manganese deficiency is a cause—or effect—of epilepsy.

NUTRITION TIP
Although there is no known dietary manganese toxicity in healthy individuals, those with liver disease may need to take care. A Vanderbilt University study suggests that manganese can concentrate in the blood and brains of those with liver ailments or those on IV support (e.g., comatose patients). This may be dangerous because neurotoxicity results from the inhalation of this mineral.

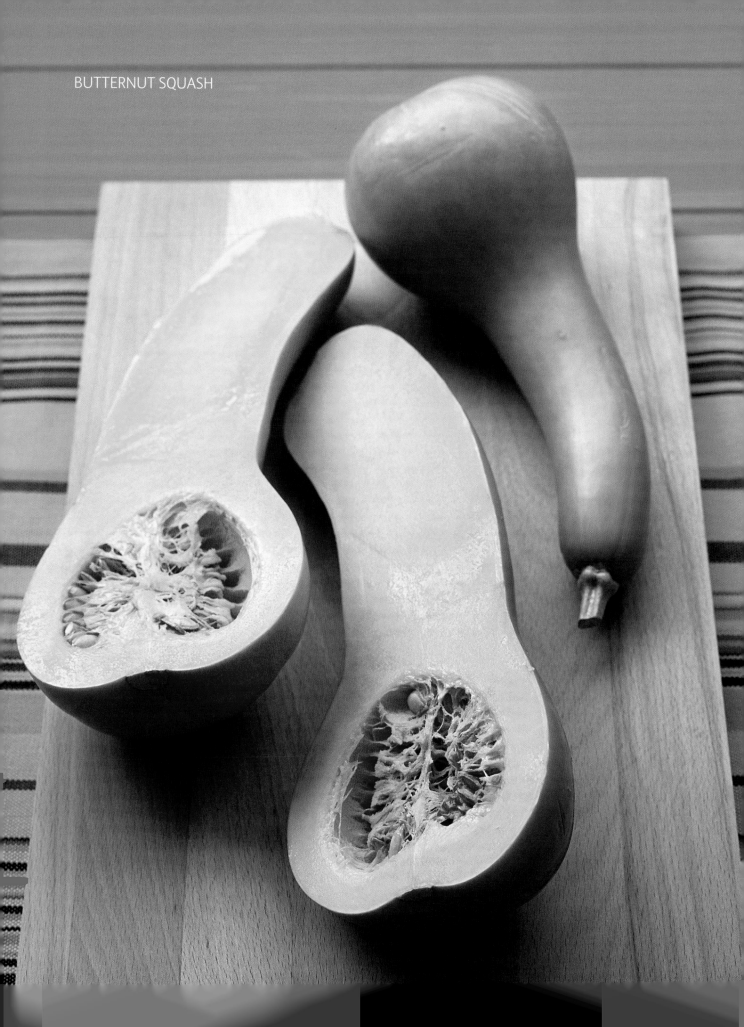

BUTTERNUT SQUASH

Potassium

FUNCTION

Potassium plays a key role in blood pressure, muscle contraction, nerve impulses, kidney function and maintenance of fluid balance in the body. Potassium, like sodium, is an electrolyte. Most of us get far too little potassium and far too much sodium. With too little potassium to blunt the effect of excess sodium, the body loses the electrolyte balance necessary to keep the blood pressure on an even keel. Potassium deficiency has also been linked to risk for kidney stones, osteoporosis and stroke. Almost 100 percent of Americans do not get enough potassium.

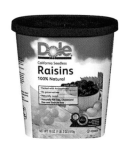

POTASSIUM

Recommended Dietary Allowance (RDA)
4,700mg per day

Tolerable Upper Intake Level (UL)
Not set, due to normal ability to excrete excess in urine

Top Sources	Quantity	Daily Value
Potato, baked with skin	1 large	35%
White Beans	1 cup	21%
Lima Beans	1 cup	20%
Soybeans	1 cup	19%
Beet Greens	½ cup	14%
Prunes	½ cup	14%
Butternut Squash	1 cup	12%
Raisins	½ cup	12%
Spinach, raw	1 cup	11%
Banana	1 large	10%

HEART HEALTH

Potassium can reverse rising blood pressure. Study participants who increased their fruit and vegetable consumption from 9 to 11 servings per day were able to lower their blood pressure levels within two weeks. Researchers believe the high potassium content of produce was among the primary causes of this turnaround. In addition, Harvard researchers demonstrated that those who consume diets rich in potassium (about 4,300 milligrams per day) were 48 percent less likely to have a stroke than those consuming 2,400 milligrams or less per day.

BABY BANANAS

NUTRITION TIP
Research shows that seniors with higher potassium intakes have more lean muscle mass than their potassium-poor peers. Potassium helps maintain the body's alkaline balance, thus preventing the muscle breakdown that occurs to counter excess acidity.

It's a Boy!

A higher potassium intake during pregnancy was linked to an 11 percent increased likelihood of having a son, bolstering the old wives' tale that links eating bananas with having boys. Mothers of boys consumed 300 milligrams more potassium on average per day compared with those who gave birth to girls. One banana contains 450 milligrams of potassium.

BONE HEALTH

Several studies have linked potassium intake with reduced osteoporosis risk in elderly men and women in all stages of life (pre-, peri- and post-menopausal). One Tufts University study also showed that higher potassium (and fruit and vegetable) intakes slowed age-related bone-mineral decline.

Selenium

FUNCTION

Selenium helps activate the body's own antioxidant enzymes. The average American gets nearly twice the daily requirement of selenium. Selenium intakes marginally above the upper limit (400 micrograms per day) can cause selenosis, characterized by brittleness and loss of hair and nails. Significantly higher intakes can be fatal.

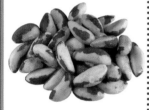

BRAZIL NUTS

SELENIUM

Recommended
Dietary Allowance
(RDA)
55mcg per day

Tolerable Upper
Intake Level (UL)
400mcg per day

Top Sources	Quantity	Daily Value
Brazil Nuts	1 oz	989%
Oysters, cooked	3 oz	238%
Halibut	6 oz	145%
Yellowfin Tuna	6 oz	145%
Lobster	3 oz	91%
Oat Bran	1 cup	77%
Shrimp	3 oz	61%
Shiitake Mushrooms, cooked	1 cup	65%
Sunflower Seeds	¼ cup	34%
Cereals	1 cup	20–30%

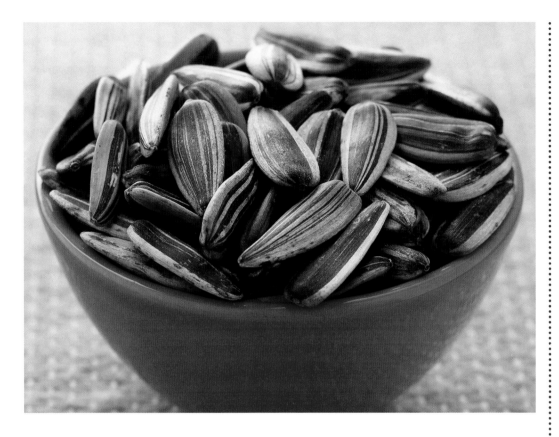

SPRINKLE SOME
SUNFLOWER SEEDS
ON A SALAD—OR
GRAB A HANDFUL
FOR AN ON-THE-GO
SNACK—AND FILL
HALF YOUR SELENIUM
NEEDS FOR THE DAY.

BONE AND JOINT HEALTH

Selenium counters the inflammation associated with the progression of osteoarthritis and rheumatoid arthritis. A University of North Carolina study found that men and women with high dietary selenium intakes were 40 percent less likely to develop osteoarthritis in their knees than those with lower intakes of selenium. And in a Belgian study, 15 women with rheumatoid arthritis who increased selenium intake for four months experienced significant improvement in joint movement and strength.

BRAIN HEALTH

Inadequate selenium can also take a toll on your brain. An Indiana University School of Medicine study looked at 2,000 men and women, age 65 and older, and found that those with the highest selenium intake had the cognitive ability of someone 10 years younger.

CANCER PREVENTION

A University of Arizona study of nearly 1,000 men found that those who took 200 micrograms of selenium developed 63 percent fewer cases of prostate cancer compared with a placebo-control group. Selenium has also shown potential to reduce the risk of lung, liver and colorectal cancers. One study, however, found an increased risk of a type of skin cancer (squamous cell carcinoma) in people taking selenium supplements. Also, in preliminary findings from a double-blind study of people who took 200 micrograms of selenium per day for several years to prevent recurrences of skin cancer, the incidence of diabetes was higher in those who received selenium than in those who received a placebo.

NUTRITION TIP
Plants obtain most of their selenium from the soil in which they are grown. For example, Brazil nuts that are grown in the selenium-rich soils of Brazil can contain double or even triple your daily value, with 140 micrograms in just a couple of nuts. So, eat them in moderation. At that rate, only five nuts would bring you close to the tolerable upper intake of 400 micrograms per day.

Salt at Fault

Reducing salt intake by a mere 15 percent could translate into nearly 9 million fewer deaths caused by the complications brought on by high blood pressure, or hypertension. A large-scale analysis of studies from 23 countries found that cardiovascular disease caused more than three-fourths of preventable deaths and identified salt as the culprit in 81 percent of those cases.

IMMUNE FUNCTION

Studies indicate that selenium deficiency may impair immune function. For example, a lack of dietary selenium can allow an otherwise harmless virus to undermine heart muscle, possibly explaining the prevalence of a cardiac ailment know as Keshan's disease in rural areas of China, where local soils lack selenium content.

Sodium

FUNCTION

Sodium helps regulate blood pressure, electrolyte balance and nerve impulses. Deficiency is not the problem with sodium. In fact, women consume more than double—and men more than triple—the recommended adequate intake of sodium. More than 75 percent of this comes from processed foods and restaurant meals—a fast-food hamburger can contain more than 1,000 milligrams of sodium, roughly the same amount found in a half teaspoon of table salt. Excessive sodium intake can cause elevated blood pressure, insomnia, pregnancy complications, kidney stones, respiratory problems and loss of bone mass.

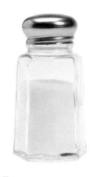

SALT

SODIUM

Adequate Intake (AI)
1.5g per day

Tolerable Upper Intake Level (UL)
2.3g per day

Top Sources	Quantity	Daily Value
Onion Soup, from mix	1 package	209 %
Table Salt	1 tsp	155 %
Dry Bread Crumbs, seasoned	1 cup	141 %
White Flour	1 cup	106 %
Sauerkraut, canned	1 cup	104 %
Tomato Sauce, canned	1 cup	86 %
Ham, cured	3 oz	75 %
Baked Beans	1 cup	74 %
Hamburger, fast-food	4 oz	73 %

BLOOD PRESSURE

Sodium helps maintain fluid balance in the body. It's the main electrolyte outside the cells, and when present in excess, water is pulled from inside the cells to dilute the outer sodium concentration—which increases blood volume and, in turn, raises blood pressure.

KIDNEY HEALTH

Too much salt in your diet could raise your risk of developing kidney stones. Harvard researchers, monitoring over 90,000 women, found that those who consumed more than three times the adequate intake of sodium daily were 30 percent more likely to suffer from kidney stones than those who consumed the adequate intake (1.5 grams per day). Why might this be? Excessive salt increases the urinary excretion of calcium—a main component of kidney stones—and the excess calcium may then build up as it passes through the kidneys.

NUTRITION TIP

Just when you've memorized the low-salt mantra, a U.S. study found that men eating less than 2.3 grams of sodium per day were 37 percent more likely to die from cardiovascular disease and 28 percent more likely to die from any cause compared with those eating more than this amount.

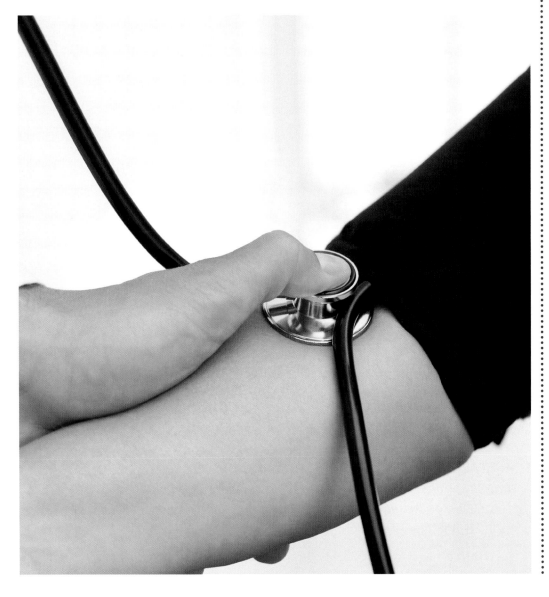

SODIUM HELPS REGULATE BLOOD PRESSURE, BUT EXCESSIVE AMOUNTS CAN SEND IT SOARING.

Zinc

FUNCTION

Zinc supports healthy skin, cell structure, immunity, neurological functions and reproduction. While most Americans get enough zinc, one-third of those over 70 years old are zinc deficient. Zinc intake of more than 40 milligrams per day begins to interfere with copper absorption, and intake of more than 200 milligrams per day can cause abdominal pain, diarrhea and vomiting.

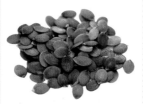

PUMPKIN SEEDS

ZINC

Recommended Dietary Allowance (RDA)
11mg per day (men)
8mg per day (women)

Tolerable Upper Intake Level (UL)
40mg per day

Top Sources	Quantity	Daily Value (Men)	Daily Value (Women)
Oysters	3 oz	257 %	353 %
Alaskan King Crab	3 oz	59 %	81 %
Lobster	3 oz	56 %	77 %
Baked Beans	1 cup	53 %	72 %
Lentils	1 cup	23 %	31 %
White Beans	1 cup	22 %	31 %
Clams	3 oz	21 %	29 %
Cereal	1 cup	20–40 %	25–190 %
Pumpkin Seeds	1 oz	19 %	26 %
Oat Bran, cooked	1 cup	11 %	15 %

HEART HEALTH

A Turkish study looked at 56 heart failure patients and 30 healthy volunteers and found that the serum zinc levels were 11 percent lower in the afflicted group.

IMMUNE FUNCTION

Various studies show zinc-deficient people experience more frequent infections due to impaired immune function, similar to that seen in age-related immune decline. Tufts University researchers showed that nursing home residents, ages 65 and older, with low-serum zinc levels were twice as likely to develop pneumonia.

SKIN HEALTH

A University of Washington study found that adequate dietary zinc intake was significantly associated with a 54 percent reduced risk of malignant melanoma, a rare but deadly type of skin cancer.

Zinc Rethink

The popularity of zinc supplements may encourage some consumers to exceed the upper limit. Excessive zinc intake interferes with copper absorption and can increase magnesium excretion. By taking zinc lozenges for colds, you can get almost four times the upper limit. Studies of the effectiveness of zinc lozenges on cold symptoms are inconclusive, with only half showing any positive effect.

BRAIN HEALTH

British scientists have found that dyslexic children often have lower levels of zinc in their sweat (which is thought to be a more useful measure than that in blood serum). In addition, animal studies have shown that zinc deficiency during pregnancy can result in learning impairment for the offspring.

NUTRITION TIP

If you take a lot of aspirin, you may be lowering your levels of folic acid, vitamin B12, zinc and vitamin C. There's little you can do to counteract aspirin's diuretic influence, but you can get more folate from spinach, more B12 from salmon, more C from pineapple and more zinc from oysters.

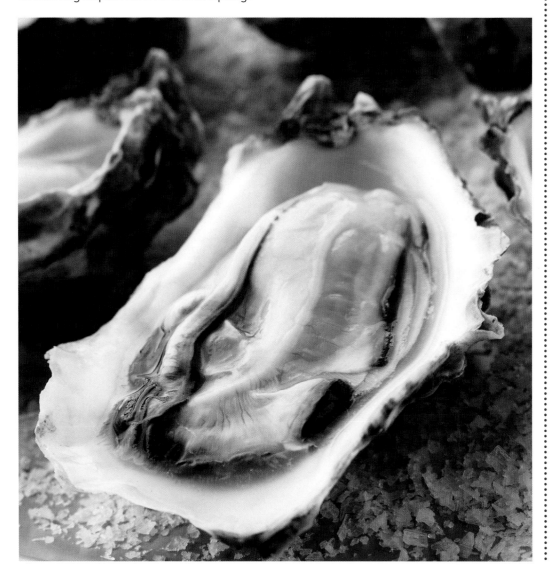

OYSTERS ARE A TOP WHOLE FOOD SOURCE FOR ZINC.

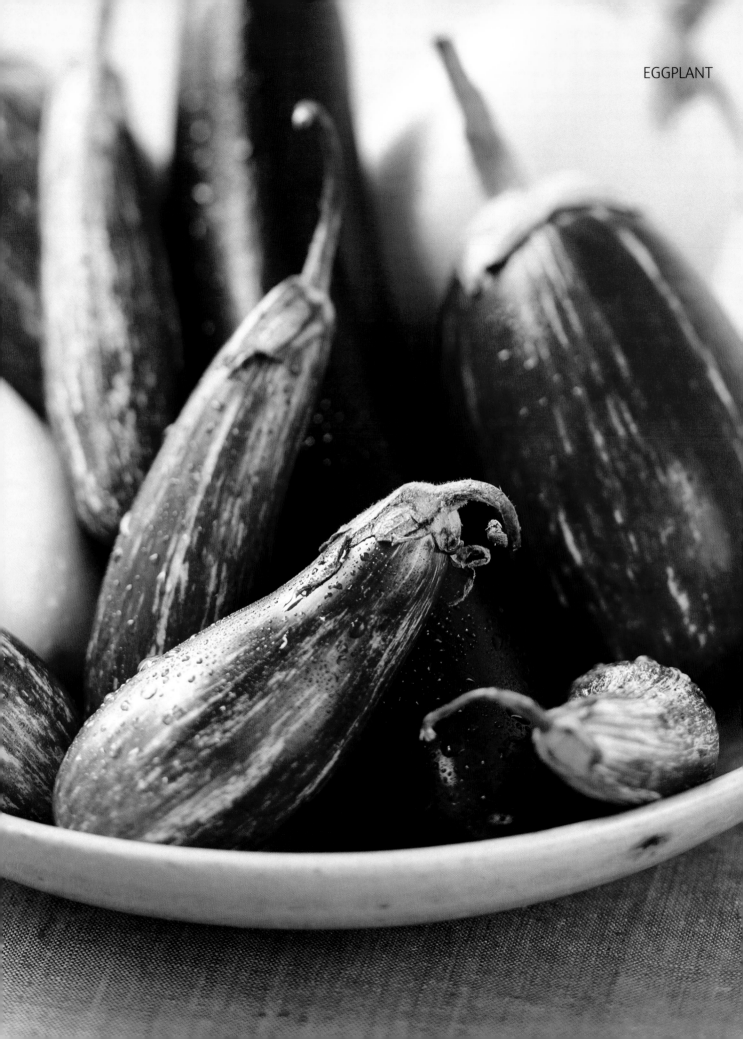

CHAPTER 2

Next Nutrition Frontier

The Phytochemicals You Need for Optimum Health

Beyond the many vitamins and minerals you've just read about exists a galaxy of compounds called phytochemicals that give healthful foods their protective properties. What are phytochemicals? In the simplest sense, they are any plant chemical (the prefix *phyto* derives from the Greek word for *plant*). To nutritionists, phytochemicals are plant compounds that are not already classified as vitamins or minerals. Several thousand have been identified, and certainly many more await discovery. What makes this area of nutrition research so exciting is that not only does the list keep growing, but researchers are also continually learning more about how important these compounds are to human health.

Known phytochemicals have a broad range of protective benefits, from reducing inflammation and speeding healing to preventing infection and fighting cancer. Phytochemicals are not essential to humans—i.e., not required by the body to sustain life—but they are essential to plants such as fruits and vegetables. They are plants' self-protection program, helping shield young buds and sprouts from predators, pollution, the elements and more. When we eat fruits and vegetables, they pass along many of these protective benefits to us.

Many phytochemicals are antioxidants. Lycopene, quercetin and beta-carotene are some of the better-known antioxidant phytochemicals. Other phytochemical subcategories include plant enzymes (such as pineapple's bromelain); phytoestrogens (in soy), which mimic human hormones; and glucosinolates (in broccoli, cabbage and cauliflower), which activate the body's detoxifying enzymes. As yet, there are no official dietary requirements for phytochemicals—no established upper limit for lycopene, no recommended intake for quercetin. Scientists are steadily addressing this void, and as they isolate, identify and study phytochemicals, they hope to gather sufficient data to make dietary recommendations. In the following pages, you can explore those phytochemicals that have thus far been identified as the most beneficial to human health.

Carotenoids

FUNCTION

Among the growing list of identified phytochemicals, carotenoids are the best studied. There are currently more than 700 known carotenoids, the most common being the compounds that produce the red, yellow and orange pigments found in colored fruits and vegetables. The best-known, carotene, was first isolated in carrots and gives them their bright orange color.

BETA-CAROTENE

Beyond its essential function as the raw material for vitamin A (often referred to as a provitamin A carotenoid), beta-carotene has many other health benefits. It's a powerful antioxidant capable of mopping up free radicals, and it's thought to reduce the risk of cardiovascular disease as well as several types of cancer. Research has linked higher blood levels of beta-carotene with lower levels of C-reactive protein, a marker of inflammation and a known risk factor for heart disease. Other research has found that beta-carotene inhibits collagen breakdown and defends epithelial cells against the kind of UV radiation that can lead to wrinkles and age spots, thus acting as a kind of internal sunscreen.

NUTRITION TIP
Additional carotenoids include phytoene, phytofluene, zeta-carotene, gamma-carotene and neurosporene. These exotic-sounding carotenoids have been identified in tomatoes and tomato products, and they may provide additional protection against oxidative cell damage, which left unchecked can contribute to the development of certain forms of prostate cancer.

CARROTS

Beta-Carotene

Top Dietary Sources	Quantity	mcg
Sweet Potato, with skin	1 medium	13,120
Carrots, cooked	1 cup	12,998
Spinach, cooked	1 cup	11,318
Kale, cooked	1 cup	10,625
Carrots, raw	1 cup	10,108
Butternut Squash, cooked	1 cup	9,368
Collard Greens, cooked	1 cup	9,147
Cantaloupe	1 cup	3,232
Green Leaf Lettuce	2 cups	3,199
Red Bell Pepper	1 medium	1,933

NUTRITION TIP

Keep in mind that cooking releases lutein from the cell walls of food, making it more available to the body. Also, adding a bit of healthy fat (the monounsaturated and polyunsaturated kind) helps enhance the body's ability to absorb lutein.

ALPHA-CAROTENE

A 2006 Japanese study published in the *Journal of Epidemiology* found that alpha-carotene reduces the risk of death by cardiovascular disease even more effectively than beta-carotene.

Top alpha-carotene sources include butternut squash, carrots, pumpkins and persimmons

BETA-CRYPTOXANTHIN

The last of the carotenoids that can be converted directly into vitamin A is beta-cryptoxanthin. In a British study, intake was associated with a 50 percent reduced risk of polyarthritis (arthritis affecting two or more joint groups). Harvard researchers have also linked this carotenoid to a reduced risk of lung cancer, and Australian scientists have shown beta-cryptoxanthin to be nearly as effective as lycopene (see below) in protecting against prostate cancer.

Top beta-cryptoxanthin sources include butternut squash, pumpkins, red bell peppers and tangerines

LYCOPENE

This carotenoid promotes heart health by preventing LDL (bad) cholesterol oxidation and reducing inflammation, which is a marker of heart disease. Harvard University researchers have found that eating seven or more servings per week of tomatoes (including tomato sauce) might reduce the risk of cardiovascular disease by 30 percent.

Studies also indicate that this colorful carotenoid may keep the prostate healthy and lower the risk of ovarian, cervical, oral, skin, pharyngeal, esophageal, bladder, stomach, colorectal, lung and pancreatic cancers. In fact, researchers in India gave 8 milligrams of pure lycopene to 40 men with high-grade precursors to prostate cancer. After one year, their blood levels of a marker for prostate cancer dropped by half, while those for the control group increased by a quarter. In a study at the University of Manchester in England, eating lycopene-rich tomatoes resulted in 33 percent more protection against sunburn. Lycopene may even enhance male fertility by improving sperm concentration and reduce the risk of age-related macular degeneration (AMD) as well.

WATERMELON

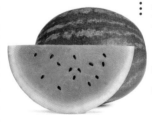

Lycopene

Top Dietary Sources	Quantity	mcg
Tomato Juice, canned	1 cup	21,960
Watermelon	1 wedge	12,962
Tomatoes, cooked	1 cup	7,298
Tomatoes, raw	1 medium	3,165
Ketchup	1 Tbsp	2,506

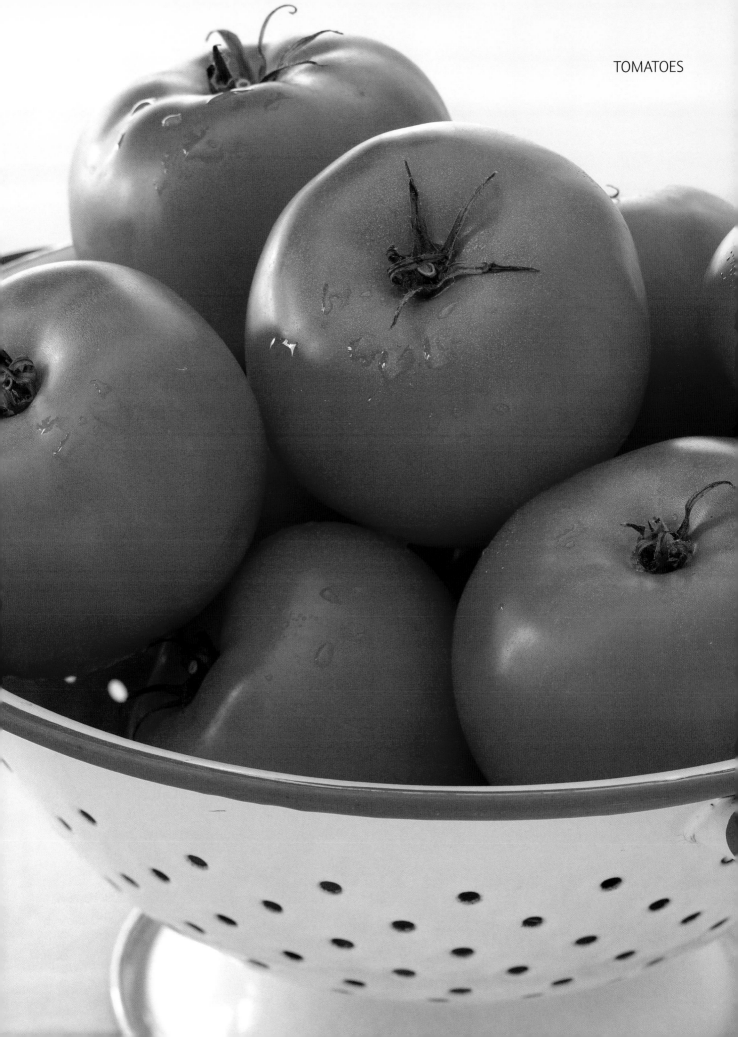

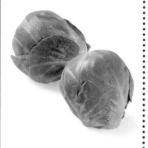

BRUSSELS SPROUTS

LUTEIN AND ZEAXANTHIN

Usually discussed together, these two carotenoids may help preserve eye health. Found naturally in the retina, they're believed to protect against damaging high-energy light beams, and studies suggest that diets rich in lutein and zeaxanthin may help slow the development of age-related macular degeneration (AMD) and cataracts. Researchers at the Massachusetts Eye and Ear Infirmary found that a high daily intake of lutein and zeaxanthin via dark green, leafy vegetables slashed the risk of AMD by 43 percent.

According to USDA researchers, zeaxanthin intake may also reduce the risk of certain types of cancer, particularly of the lung and breast.

Lutein and Zeaxanthin

Top Dietary Sources	Quantity	mcg
Kale, cooked	1 cup	23,720
Spinach, cooked	1 cup	20,354
Spinach, raw	1 cup	3,659
Zucchini, cooked	1 cup	2,070
Brussels Sprouts, cooked	1 cup	2,012
Corn, cooked	1 cup	1,486

Carotenoid Supplements

Compared with the benefits of dietary carotenoids, thus far, studies on carotenoid supplements have yielded mixed results. In fact, certain carotenoid supplements may actually be harmful. Although dietary-intake studies indicate that foods rich in beta-carotene and vitamin A may lower the risk of many types of cancer, when it comes to supplements, the findings are decidedly less promising: Not only have a number of studies found beta-carotene supplements ineffective in protecting against cancer, but in some studies they've actually been shown to exacerbate cancer. In the Alpha-Tocopherol, Beta-Carotene Cancer Prevention Study, more than 29,000 male smokers were randomized to receive 20 milligrams of beta-carotene, 50 milligrams of alpha-tocopherol (a form of vitamin E), supplements of both or a placebo for five to eight years. Lung cancer incidence was 18 percent higher among the beta-carotene-supplement takers, with 8 percent more deaths. The Carotene and Retinol Efficacy Trial had similar results when those researchers provided their subjects with supplements of 30 milligrams of beta-carotene and 25,000 IU of retinyl palmitate (a form of vitamin A) or a placebo. In fact, this study was stopped when researchers realized that the subjects receiving beta-carotene had a 46 percent higher risk of dying from lung cancer.

Although large doses of dietary carotenoids in humans results in a yellowing of the skin (hypercarotenemia), this condition is not thought to be harmful in normal, healthy people.

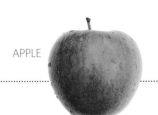
APPLE

Flavonoids

Group	Example	Dietary Source
Anthocyanins	Cyanidin	Raspberries
Flavanols	Catechin	Green Tea
Flavanones	Gingerol	Ginger
Flavonols	Quercetin	Apples
Flavones	Apigenin	Artichokes
Isoflavones	Genistein	Soybeans

Flavonoids

FUNCTION

Flavonoids, also known as polyphenols, are very powerful antioxidants. Their abundance of electrons allows them to neutralize the free radicals your body generates and encounters every day. Free radicals (essentially unstable oxygen molecules) are missing an electron and will rip an extra electron off anything they can—even from DNA—causing the kind of damage that can accelerate aging and lead to disease. Antioxidants sacrifice themselves to free radicals and thus protect other, more useful molecules.

By this process, they help reduce inflammation, oxidative stress and toxic metal poisoning (e.g., accumulation of excessive mercury), thereby defending against several neurodegenerative diseases, including Parkinson's and Alzheimer's. There is also evidence that polyphenols are players in the fight against cancer.

ANTIOXIDANT POWER

The more accepted method for measuring antioxidant "power" is the ORAC scale used by the USDA. *ORAC* stands for Oxygen Radical Absorbance Capacity—a complicated sounding name for something fairly simple: the ability of a food or other substance to absorb free radicals. The ORAC score is generally expressed per serving size (see page 133 for more on ORAC scores). Experts generally agree that you need a minimum of 3,000 ORAC units per day. For a scale of comparison, consider that a cup of blueberries has about 9,000 ORAC units and a tangerine has about 1,300.

NUTRITION TIP
The highest antioxidant rating per gram goes to ground cloves. Its ORAC score is 3,144 per gram. That's a bit higher than cinnamon (2,675 per gram), which is 43 times higher than blueberries. *The journal Diabetes Care* reported that cinnamon can lower cholesterol, glucose and trigylceride levels—important for type 2 diabetes sufferers as well as anyone struggling with high cholesterol. As little as half a teaspoon a day of cinnamon produced results.

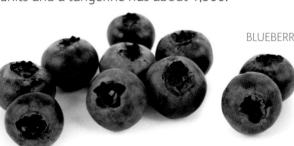
BLUEBERRIES

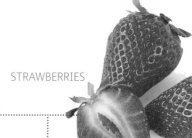

Top Antioxidant Fruits

Fruit	Serving	ORAC Score
Apples (Red Delicious)	1 large apple	10,346
Apples (Granny Smith)	1 large apple	9,346
Blueberries	1 cup	9,206
Cranberries	1 cup	8,983
Blackberries	1 cup	7,701
Prunes	½ cup	7,291
Raspberries	1 cup	6,058
Strawberries	1 cup	5,938

Anthocyanins

Also commonly referred to as bioflavonoids, anthocyanins are the red, blue and purple water-soluble pigments found in fruits and berries.

Anthocyanin

	Members of the Anthocyanin Family (distinguished by chemical structure)
Cyanidin	Elderberries, Sweet Cherries, Blueberries, Raspberries, Red Onions, Pomegranates, Strawberries
Delphinidin	Cranberries, Blueberries, Bilberries, Black Currants, Red Grapes, Pomegranates
Malvidin	Black Currants, Blueberries, Raspberries, Red Grapes, Bilberries
Pelargonidin	Sweet Cherries, Raspberries, Bilberries, Black Currants, Strawberries
Peonidin	Red Grapes, Blueberries, Sweet Cherries
Petunidin	Blueberries, Red Grapes, Bilberries

CHERRIES

POMEGRANATES

ANTICANCER BENEFITS

Anthocyanins are increasingly recognized for their anticancer effects. Scientists at Clemson University in South Carolina have used anthocyanins in raspberry, strawberry and muscadine grape extracts to cut the growth of cancer cell lines cultured from breast and cervical tumors by more than half. Blackberry and blueberry extracts weren't as effective against cervical cancer cells, but they did suppress the growth of breast cancer cells.

In addition, a University of Maryland study found that anthocyanin-rich extracts reduced several markers for colon cancer in animal studies. Whether these antioxidants could survive the harsh conditions of human digestion and similarly benefit humans has yet to be confirmed. Encouragingly, German scientists have shown that 85 percent of the anthocyanins in blueberries make it as far as the colon. And in a University of Georgia study, blueberry anthocyanins applied to human colon cancer cells reduced proliferation and increased apoptosis (programmed cell death), leading researchers to conclude that "blueberry intake may reduce colon cancer risk."

CARDIOVASCULAR HEALTH

Several animal studies have suggested that anthocyanins may also help promote heart health. Researchers at the Indiana University School of Medicine found that anthocyanins from chokeberries, bilberries and elderberries improved the vascular elasticity of blood vessels, even when they were exposed to free radicals, making them supple enough to function normally. Another study from the University of Maine demonstrated similar benefits, this time from wild blueberries, to the aortic blood vessels close to the heart.

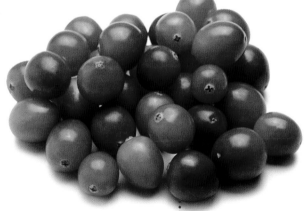

CRANBERRIES

Flavanols

FUNCTION

Flavanols give teas and cocoa their off-the-charts antioxidant power. The flavanols in baking chocolate, for example, weigh in with the very impressive ORAC value of 1,039 per gram. Compare this with wild blueberries' ORAC score of 92 per gram. One particular flavanol called epigallocatechin gallate (or EGCG) is considered the most powerful of them all and is believed to be 20 to 100 times more powerful than vitamins C or E. A study in the *Journal of the American Medical Association* reported that flavanol-rich chocolate raised the antioxidant activity of circulating blood within two hours of consumption. The same study noted a reduction in markers for free-radical damage.

HEALTH TIP

The anthocyanins in cranberries and blueberries are thought to inhibit bacteria from adhering to bladder walls, which would explain why these fruits seem to help ward off urinary-tract infections. Lab analysis suggests the same protective compounds may also help suppress herpes outbreaks.

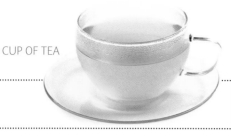

Flavanols

	Dietary Sources
Catechin	Green, White Tea
Epicatechin (EC)	Cocoa Beans
Epigallocatechin (EGC)	Green, White Tea
Epicatechin Gallate (ECG)	Green, White Tea
Epigallocatechin Gallate (EGCG)	Green, White Tea

DIET TIP

Why do the French, who consume far more saturated fat than Americans, have comparatively low cardiovascular disease rates? One possible explanation for the French paradox is that culture's penchant for flavanol-rich red wine, which is fermented with the grape skins that contain most of the fruit's flavanols.

CARDIOVASCULAR HEALTH

It's not just the antioxidant properties of cocoa flavanols that contribute to cardiovascular health. Flavanols also promote healthy blood flow by stimulating the production of nitric oxide, a naturally produced body chemical that dilates blood vessels. Additionally, flavanols may reduce blood clotting by moderating platelet function.

ALZHEIMER'S PREVENTION

In a 2006 Japanese study, those who drank two cups of green tea per day were 50 percent less likely to experience age-related cognitive decline. The authors did not study the effects of white tea, but there are in fact more milligrams of polyphenols in white tea than in green. Black tea contains less due to its additional processing.

CANCER PREVENTION

Green tea has been found to protect against a wide variety of cancers, including leukemia, lung, breast and prostate cancers. Asian men have a low incidence of prostate cancer in their native countries; but when living in the West, their cancer rates rise. Initially scientists blamed this on the bad Western diet (red meat,

The Kuna Indians of Panama

According to a study by Brigham and Women's Hospital and the Harvard Medical School, the Kuna Indians, islanders from Panama, typically drink five cups of flavanol-rich cocoa beverages a day—and they have a very low incidence of cardiovascular problems as they age. Those who have migrated to the Panamanian mainland, however, demonstrate a significant increase in age-related hypertension. Why? Researchers speculate that it's because they switch to processed cocoa drinks, the manufacturing process of which depletes the protective flavanol content.

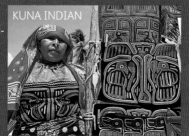

KUNA INDIAN

saturated fat, etc.), but eventually they began to suspect that it wasn't what had been added to the men's diet, but rather what had been *omitted* that was most significant. Chinese men drink large amounts of green tea in their native diets. Its importance to them is summed up in this Chinese proverb: "Better to be deprived of food for three days than tea for one."

OTHER BENEFITS

Green tea may help boost metabolism. Swiss research indicates that three cups per day can stimulate metabolism enough to spur fat oxidation. Other researchers have noted that black and green tea drinkers have better hip to waist ratios. Among other green tea benefits are lowered blood pressure, increased immunity and improved dental health.

Flavanones

FUNCTION

Flavanones are polyphenols found in citrus fruits. They are so bioavailable that they can appear in blood plasma as soon as 20 minutes after ingestion, though their concentrations aren't maximized until after about four hours. This makes flavanones a significant contributor to the antioxidant pool that circulates in your blood. However, since these flavanones are completely excreted after 24 hours, it's beneficial to consume foods that contain them, such as citrus fruits, on a daily basis.

> **NUTRITION TIP**
> The solid parts of citrus fruits (the skin and pith) are very high in flavanones. For this reason, the whole fruit may contain as much as five times the amount of flavanones as the juice from the fruit.

ORANGES

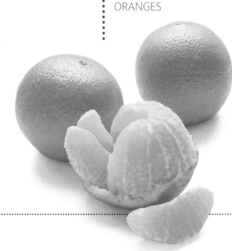

Flavanones	
	Dietary Sources
Naringenin, Hesperetin and Eriodictyol	Lemons, Grapefruits and Oranges

Grapefruit Juice

You may have heard that drinking grapefruit juice increases the concentration of certain medications in your blood. The reason? Naringenin, the main flavanone in grapefruit juice, inhibits the body's ability to metabolize these drugs.

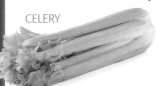

CELERY

Flavones

FUNCTION

Of this small category of antioxidants with potential chemo-protective benefits, luteolin and apigenin (found in celery and parsley) are the most common. Citrus peels also contain powerful flavones, such as tangeretin, nobiletin and sinensetin.

Flavones	
	Dietary Sources
Luteolin and Apigenin	Celery, Parsley, *Capsicum* Peppers

FOOD TIP

Though often dismissed as a nutrition zero, parsley packs the punch of a nutrition hero. A mere quarter cup contains 300 percent or your daily vitamin K (a nutrient that may help reduce the risk of fractures), while also providing an excellent source of vitamins A and C. It's also a top source of disease-fighting phytochemicals.

ANTICANCER BENEFITS

A study at Case Western Reserve University found that apigenin may be effective in slowing prostate tumor growth, and a 2008 Taiwanese study has shown that luteolin has the same potential. Apigenin has also shown promise in helping to reduce the risk of breast, colon, skin and thyroid cancers.

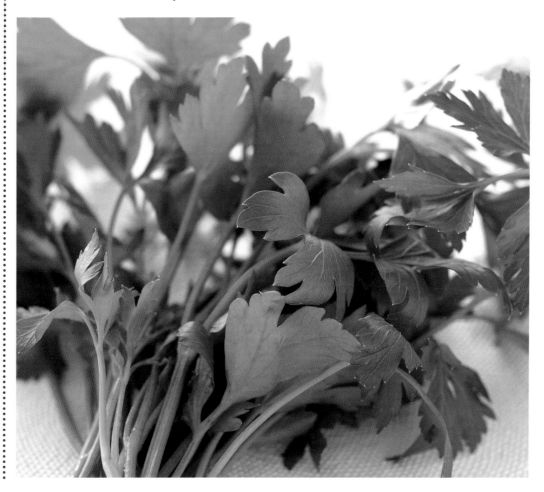

Isoflavones

FUNCTION

Isoflavones, another small group of antioxidant polyphenols, are sometimes referred to as phytoestrogens because of their similar structure to human estrogen. Scientists speculate that isoflavones may play a role in the balancing of hormones, but that has yet to be proven. They do, however, act as antioxidants, and a number of studies have shown that the isoflavone genistein can protect human cells from oxidative stress.

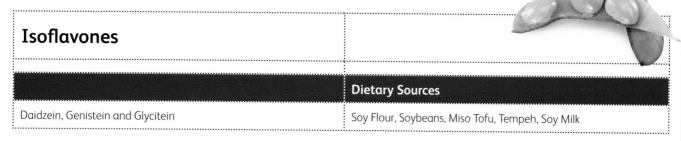

SOYBEANS

Isoflavones	
	Dietary Sources
Daidzein, Genistein and Glycitein	Soy Flour, Soybeans, Miso Tofu, Tempeh, Soy Milk

ANTICANCER BENEFITS

Researchers have had mixed results in studying the link between soy isoflavones and various cancers, particularly of the breast and prostate. While the evidence is not conclusive, a 2001 Chinese study published in *Cancer Epidemiology Biomarkers & Prevention* did find a correlation between soy intake early in life and the lower risk of breast cancer in adulthood. At the same time, a 2007 analysis of data from the Japan Collaborative Cohort Study, which looked at 30,454 women, ages 40 to 79, found that the consumption of soy-containing foods (tofu, boiled soybeans and miso soup) has no protective effects against breast cancer. In addition, there's currently concern that postmenopausal exposure to isoflavones may pose a risk to estrogen-sensitive breast-cancer patients and women at high risk of developing breast cancer.

Soy isoflavones show more promise when it comes to prostate cancer. After reviewing previously published studies on the subject, researchers concluded—in a 2009 *American Journal of Clinical Nutrition* report—that dietary isoflavones significantly decrease the risk of prostate cancer. A University of Minnesota study found that soy protein and soy isoflavone supplements decrease the markers of cancer development and progression—including prostate-specific antigen (PSA)—in the prostate cells of men with prostate cancer or at high risk for it. But a study in the *Journal of Urology* found that soy intake has no impact on blood levels of PSA in healthy middle-aged men—which indicates that the consumption of soy protein and isoflavones may have protective benefits only for men who already have or are at high risk for prostate cancer.

FITNESS TIP

Not only does vigorous exercise burn more calories, it may also alter your taste preferences postworkout. Japanese researchers believe working up a sweat may curb your cravings for sweets. Animal studies suggest the increased endorphin levels released by heavy exercise may be responsible.

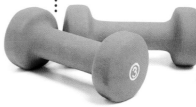

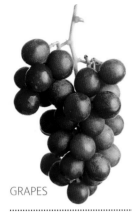

GRAPES

Flavonols

FUNCTION

Not to be confused with the flavanols, flavonols are a distinct subcategory of health-bolstering antioxidants found in fruits and vegetables.

The most-researched flavonol by far is quercetin. A search of scientific literature yields nearly 6,326 results for quercetin, whereas a search for another flavonol, kaempferol, yields only approximately 1,200 results. Onions are the top source of quercetin, but this flavonol is quite common in fruit as well. One study found it in 25 different types of berries.

Flavonols	Dietary Sources
Quercetin	Onions, Blueberries, Apples, Red Grapes, Celery, Cranberries
Kaempferol	Kale, Broccoli, Endive, Turnip Greens
Myricetin	Cranberries, Blueberries, Bananas
Isorhamnetin	Chives, Onions, Almonds
Rhamnetin	Cloves
Rutin	Buckwheat

NUTRITION TIP
High doses of quercetin combined with ultrasound treatment stopped 90 percent of skin and prostate tumor cells, in a study reported in the *British Journal of Cancer.*

HEART HEALTH

By scavenging free radicals in the blood, quercetin helps prevent oxidation of LDL, protecting against plaque deposits found in deteriorating arterial cell walls. And scientists have known for decades that quercetin can inhibit blood platelet aggregation, which impacts normal blood viscosity, or thickness, needed to maintain healthy blood pressure.

BRAIN HEALTH

Some of the most exciting studies on quercetin suggest that it may be even more powerful than vitamin C in protecting brain cells against the kind of oxidative stress that contributes to Alzheimer's disease. Cornell University scientists demonstrated that nerve cells treated with quercetin (versus with vitamin C) were more likely to survive the type of oxidative stress experienced in the brains of Alzheimer's sufferers. Since diets high in vitamin C are known to protect against Alzheimer's, it's likely that quercetin may be able to exert an even more powerful effect than this vitamin. Dr. James Joseph's 1999 landmark study at Tufts University indicated that age-related brain decline may even be reversible with diets rich in antioxidants. His experiments specifically highlighted blueberries, a known source of quercetin.

PROSTATE HEALTH

At some point in their lives, half of all men will experience prostatitis. This inflammation of the prostate gland is the number one urological disorder in men over the age of 50. Researchers at the Harbor-UCLA Medical Center discovered that high doses of quercetin reduced this painful condition in nearly two-thirds of their subjects.

CANCER PREVENTION

Though widely recognized for its prostate-cancer protective qualities, quercetin continues to prove beneficial in other ways. For example, a Finnish study found that men with the highest dietary intakes of quercetin had 60 percent less lung cancer (and 25 percent less asthma and 20 percent fewer deaths from diabetes and heart disease). Another large study, conducted in Italy on behalf of the American Association for Cancer Research, showed that people with the highest intakes of flavonols were 46 percent less likely to develop colorectal cancer—which the European School of Oncology estimates can be prevented 80 percent of the time by early detection and diet changes. In a 2005 study, Taiwanese scientists demonstrated that myricetin, another flavonol found in fruits and vegetables, is a powerful inhibitor of the aggressive growth of this type of cancer.

> **NUTRITION TIP**
> Did you think celery was a nutrition zero? It's actually a hero, containing quercetin, apigenin and luteolin, as well as a healthy supply of vitamin C, folate and potassium. Plus, just two stalks can fulfill 40 percent of your daily vitamin K needs.

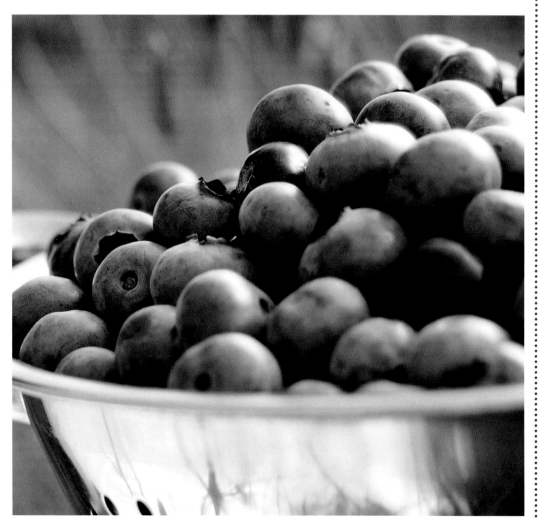

BLUEBERRIES, ALONG WITH ELDERBERRIES, APPLES AND ONIONS, ARE TOP SOURCES OF IMMUNITY-BOOSTING QUERCETIN.

HEALTH TIP

Eating just a half cup of broccoli or cauliflower per week could slash prostate cancer risk by nearly half, says a study published in the *Journal of the National Cancer Institute*. Scientists attribute these protective effects to the cruciferous vegetables' glucosinolates, which activate the body's detoxifying systems.

Glucosinolates

Top glucosinolate sources include cabbage, Brussels sprouts, broccoli, cauliflower, broccoli sprouts, kale and red cabbage

FUNCTION

Research suggests that glucosinolates can stimulate the body's own natural antioxidant systems, technically called Phase II enzymes. As such, glucosinolates act as indirect antioxidants triggering the liver to produce detoxifying enzymes that block free-radical attack on DNA. Once this process occurs, a cascade of antioxidant activity actually cycles over and over within the body, continuing to protect your system for up to four days after the glucosinolate-containing food was initially eaten—as opposed to the one-shot, finite benefit you get from most direct antioxidants.

ANTICANCER BENEFITS

In food-bearing plants, glucosinolates act as natural pesticides and are stored in the plant's cells, ready to be released upon tissue damage. Similarly, when consumed by humans, the action of chewing releases the glucosinolates into the body, where they are transformed into bioactive compounds believed to have anticancer properties. These anticancer compounds operate on several fronts: triggering the body's own detoxification systems, slowing cancer cell growth and supporting DNA repair. Chinese researchers have found lower levels of these compounds in people with lung cancer than in those who are cancer-free. Researchers at the University of Texas have found the same results among men in the United States.

The major dietary source of glucosinolates is cruciferous vegetables, the healing properties of which have been extolled for ages. In fact, ancient Roman healers believed that they could cure breast cancer by rubbing poultices made from cabbage on the chest. This may not be far from the truth. According to Jon Michnovicz, MD, PhD and president of the Foundation for Preventive Oncology, Inc. in New York City, "There are studies that show cabbage paste, when rubbed on animals, can prevent tumor development."

Cabbage is perhaps the most compelling example of how glucosinolate-containing vegetables can affect cancer. A review of 94 studies published in *Cancer, Epidemiology, Biomarkers & Prevention* showed that in 70 percent of the studies, cabbage consumption was associated with a decreased risk in cancer,

Storing the Glucosinolates

Ever wondered what happens to your veggies when you stick them in the fridge? Researchers at the University of Essex in the U.K. looked at the glucosinolate contents of broccoli, Brussels sprouts, cauliflower and green cabbage under different storage conditions. At ambient or refrigerated temperatures, minor losses were observed (9 to 26 percent) over seven days. Finely shredded vegetables, however, lost 75 percent of their glucosinolates after six hours.

especially of the lung, stomach and colon. By contrast, broccoli was linked to a reduced cancer risk in 56 percent of the studies, cauliflower in 67 percent of the studies and Brussels sprouts in 29 percent of the studies.

Fruit Enzymes

FUNCTION

Just as the human body contains enzymes, plants contain their own enzymes that catalyze various biochemical reactions. One enzyme class known as thiol proteases acts as a self-defense mechanism, a sort of natural pesticide. However, in humans these enzymes help metabolize protein. These enzymes are particularly averse to heat. For this reason, fresh or frozen food sources of these compounds are preferable to processed sources.

INFLAMMATION

Bromelain, found in pineapple, is in the same family of proteolytic, or protein-digesting, enzymes. Though researchers have only begun to study the therapeutic effects of bromelain, as far back as the late 15th century, Spanish explorers noted that the indigenous peoples of South and Central America used pineapples to reduce swelling and cure stomachaches.

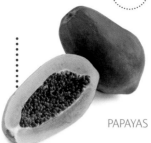

PAPAYAS

FOOD TIP

A variety of papaya from Chile has been found to contain such a large amount of papain that it can actually remove fingerprints. It's also full of vitamins C and A, potassium, fiber and folate.

KIWIFRUITS

Fruit Enzymes

Fruit	Enzyme
Pineapples	Bromelain
Kiwifruits	Actinidin
Figs	Ficin
Papayas	Papain

Bromelain Supplements

Money spent on bromelain supplements would be better spent on fresh pineapples, because the active enzyme content declines in potency over time. Fresh pineapples, by contrast, will always contain active bromelain. In addition, scientists at the Dole Nutrition Institute showed that one serving (112 grams) of fresh pineapple had at least as much, if not more, bromelain activity than the supplement used in a clinical study on knee pain done in the United Kingdom. Moreover, supplements provide nutrients in isolation, which means that you miss out on the synergistic nutrition provided by whole fruits and vegetables.

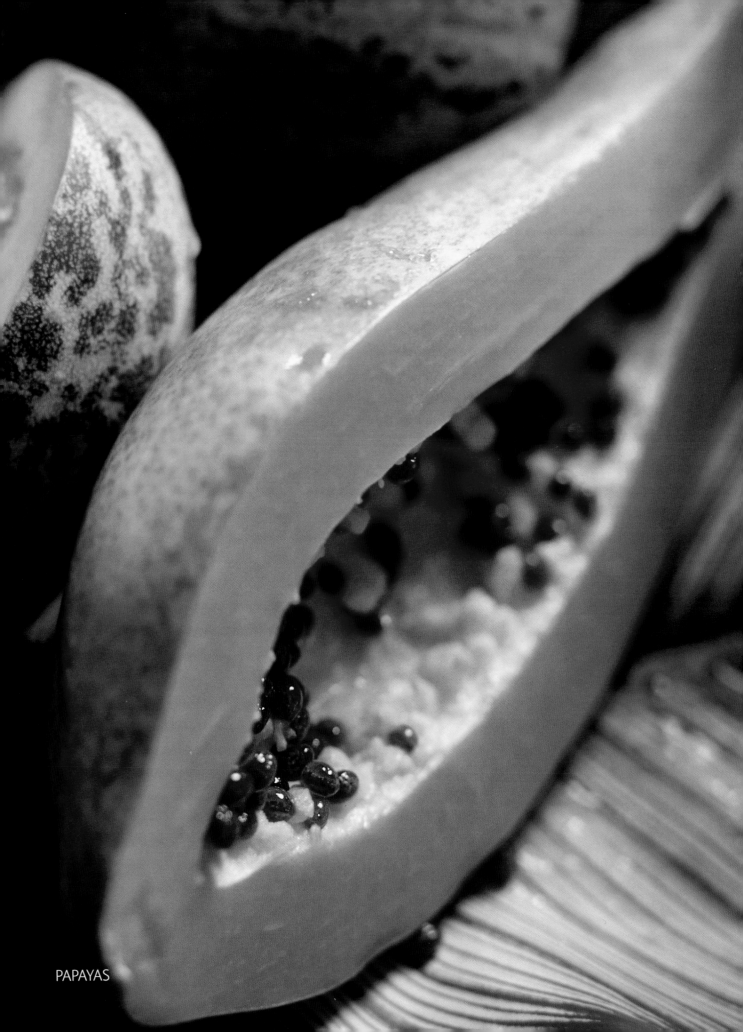

PAPAYAS

Cosmetics

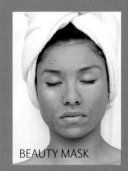

Unfortunately for consumers who buy high-priced pineapple and papaya enzyme masks and scrubs, it turns out that there's more bluffing than buffing going on. Sure, the skin-care manufacturers might be putting pineapple or papaya into their peels and potions, but the processing that makes these products shelf-stable also destroys their active enzymes. Bromelain (the active enzyme in pineapple) and papain (the active enzyme in papaya) are found only in fresh or frozen whole fruit—not in jars and tubes. If you're interested in letting these fruit enzymes invigorate your complexion, you're better off trying a do-it-yourself treatment made from the real thing.

BEAUTY MASK

Bromelain has seen an increase in interest of late, as it's shown promise as a remedy for a variety of conditions. A review of 10 studies by British scientists suggests that it can be an effective pain reliever and anti-inflammatory for osteoarthritis sufferers. Other research indicates that bromelain may be able to block the COX-2 enzymes that produce inflammation. Researchers at the University of Connecticut have found that it reduces asthma symptoms in rats, and they're now looking to extend this research to humans. Australian researchers believe that bromelain may help block the growth of cancer cells, providing a lead in the fight against cancer.

Research on other plant enzymes is still emerging, but since these enzymes have similar structures and functions, it wouldn't be surprising if they turn out to offer similar health benefits.

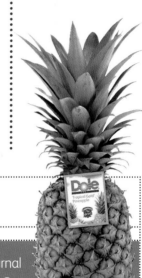

Post-Op Pineapple

According to a study published in *Plastic and Reconstructive Surgery* (the official medical journal of the American Society of Plastic Surgeons), a nutrient combo including bromelain, vitamin C, rutin and grape-seed extract cut down face-lift recovery time by 17 percent. Researchers say that bromelain can digest dead skin cells, acting as a "cleanup crew" and helping to improve the health of a wound site.

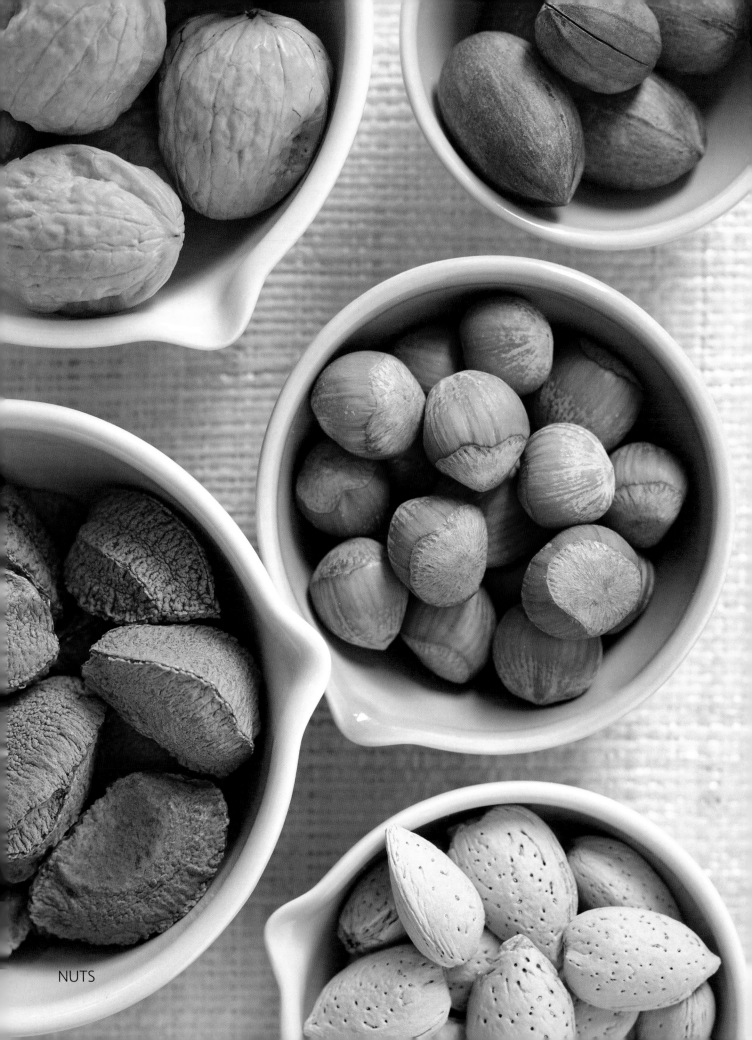

NUTS

CHAPTER 3

Superfoods

On an episode of *The Oprah Winfrey Show* dedicated to longevity, David H. Murdock, the 86-year-old chairman of Dole Food Company, revealed the secret to enjoying robust health, energy and mental sharpness throughout life: Eat large quantities of fruits and vegetables. As a pescatarian, Murdock also includes seafood, whole grains, beans and nuts in his diet.

Given his commitment to nutrition research, it's no coincidence that Murdock emphasizes those foods that clinical trials are now demonstrating have the most-potent health benefits. Many of their specific advantages are detailed in the pages that follow.

Fruits and vegetables not only taste great, but research also proves that they can help promote health and fight disease. Consider the following:

• Eating the USDA's recommended minimum of nine servings of fruits and veggies a day could possibly cut your stroke risk by half.

• Eating fruit and vegetables boosts bone-mineral content. A University of Tennessee study revealed that girls ages 8 to 12 who consumed more than three servings of fruit per day had greater bone mass (and less calcium excretion) than those who consumed fewer than three servings. Fruits and vegetables help the body hold on to calcium as well as supplying many other oft-overlooked nutrients, such as potassium, folate and vitamins K and C, which support bone health.

• Eating more fruit protects your heart. French researchers analyzed nine studies involving more than 220,000 individuals and found that the risk of cardiovascular problems declined as fruit intake increased.

• Eating more than four servings (that's 2 cups) of vegetables per day could yield a nearly 40 percent decrease in the rate of age-related mental deterioration.

• Eating more vegetables protects the prostate. Researchers followed 1,300 men for 11 years in a study published in the *International Journal of Cancer*. They found that those who consumed the most vegetables were 18 percent less likely to develop prostate cancer than those who ate the fewest veggies.

• Eating more vegetables protects reproductive health. Previous research has suggested that women who eat the most veggies are 50 percent less likely to have the kind of persistent infections that can lead to cervical cancer and infertility. Now, new data points to a 60 percent lower cervical-cancer risk among women with the highest produce intake. The same study found a nearly 70 percent increased risk among those with the highest intake of animal fat.

• Eating fruits and vegetables can also protect your health by keeping you trim. Fiber triples weight loss, filling you up and reducing fat absorption. In one study, low-fat dieters who were told to eat unlimited fruits and vegetables lost 21 percent more weight than those who simply reduced fat intake. It may sound like magic, but the fruit and veggie group actually consumed fewer calories—even though they were eating 25 percent more food by weight. By relying on fruits and vegetables, the dieters naturally felt fuller and cut back on other fattening foods.

Nutrient-dense produce may also curb deficiency-fueled cravings. Many fruits and vegetables contain resistant starch, which boosts fat metabolism.

While the rich vitamin, mineral and phytochemical content of fruits and vegetables is what makes them nature's top nutrition stars, plant-based protein also contributes significantly to health. British researchers found a strong inverse relationship between higher intakes of plant-based protein and lower rates of blood pressure. These results may help explain why a previous Mayo Clinic analysis found a 30 percent lower risk of death from heart disease

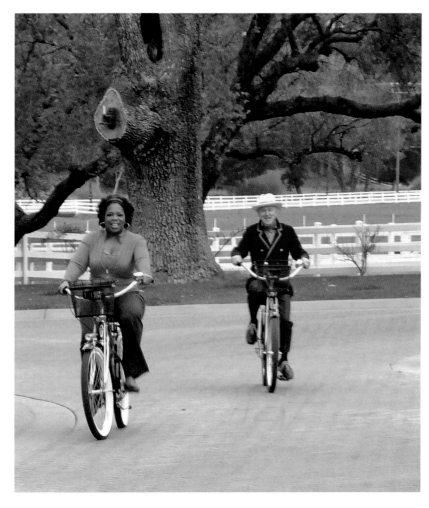

CHAIRMAN OF DOLE FOOD COMPANY DAVID H. MURDOCK BIKING WITH OPRAH WINFREY AT HIS ESTATE, VENTURA FARMS, IN CALIFORNIA.

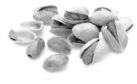

PISTACHIOS

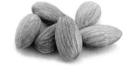

ALMONDS

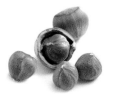

HAZELNUTS

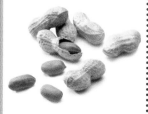

PEANUTS

among postmenopausal women who consumed high amounts of vegetarian protein sources.

Beans and nuts are the top vegetarian sources of protein, in addition to supplying many other key nutrients. That may be why the USDA Dietary Guidelines recommend Americans triple their bean consumption from the current average of 1 cup weekly to 3 cups. While beans are a well-known source of heart healthy fiber and high-quality protein, they're less famous for their off-the-charts antioxidant capacity. Most varieties provide half the folate you need, are an excellent source of phosphorus and a good source of potassium, and offer a decent dose of iron and zinc. The *B* in beans also stands for B vitamins: thiamin (B1), riboflavin (B2), niacin (B3), B5 and B6, which together help promote muscles and brain function as well as healthy skin and hair.

Nuts have also received a nod from the FDA, which found enough evidence to approve a qualified health claim to the effect that 1.5 ounces (a heaping handful) of nuts per day may reduce the risk of heart disease. Harvard researchers found that eating 5 ounces of nuts (including peanuts) weekly can lower the risk of gallstones by up to 34 percent. And the magnesium, fiber and phytosterols in nuts may help keep the gallbladder from overloading with cholesterol, which can crystallize into painful gallstones.

Are all nuts created equal? In some ways, yes: They're all cholesterol-free yet calorie-dense (ranging from 240 to 300 calories per 1.5 ounces, depending on the type of nut). But in other ways, they're strikingly different. Their top nutrition attributes are reviewed in the pages that follow.

Finally, when it comes to animal proteins, fish is the healthiest source by far. The American Heart Association recommends aiming for at least two 3-ounce servings of fish per week. Fish also contains important vitamins and minerals, in particular some of the

DRIs Versus RDAs

The information you see on food labels provides a quick way to assess how much of the various vitamins and minerals a serving of that food supplies. These daily value percentages are calculated from the recommended dietary allowances (RDA) for each vitamin and mineral originally developed during World War II. The RDAs reflect the minimum amount (in grams, milligrams, etc.) of each nutrient required to prevent a deficiency disease (i.e., vitamin C for scurvy and vitamin D for rickets).

In 1997 the Institute of Medicine (IOM) published new, expanded recommendations, called Dietary Reference Intakes (DRIs), based on population subgroups, such as sex, age, pregnancy, etc. There simply isn't enough room on food labels to include all the information for each subgroup, so for now food labels still only feature the older RDAs.

Consequently, the information on food labels is quite a bit out of date. That's why the daily values for the foods in the following section have been calculated from the newer RDA's outlined in the Dietary References Intake update. The percentages listed are for adults ages 19 and older. In ranges, the larger percentage is for females (the only exception is iron, where the opposite is true).

B vitamins, as well as iron, potassium, magnesium and phosphorus. Saltwater fish supply iodine. Canned salmon, sardines and herring, with their soft, mostly edible bones, are also a good source of calcium.

Plus, fish have a unique polyunsaturated fatty acid called omega-3 that protects your heart, combats arthritis and depression, and even fights wrinkles. A study found that older people who eat fish at least once a week might reduce their risk of Alzheimer's by more than half.

In addition, a study from the University of Georgia found that omega-3 fatty acids prevented the development of fat cells in laboratory tissue cultures. That's not the only way fish helps you maintain a healthy weight. In addition to having half the calories and a fraction of the saturated fat of red meat, fish helps you feel full longer, and thus reduces overall caloric intake.

Want to enjoy the health benefits of fish but worried about mercury contamination? Then eat more pineapple, bananas, mangoes, papayas and guavas! Researchers looked at the dietary habits in the Brazilian Amazon, where people eat fish up to 700 times a year, and found that those who ate tropical fruit at least once a day had 80 percent less mercury buildup in their systems.

Remember that a varied diet, drawn from many different nutritious sources—like the ones that follow—is your best bet for longevity, energy and optimum health.

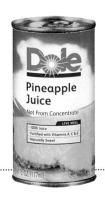

Serves You Right

A rose by any other name smells just as sweet—but a "serving size" may be larger than a single "serving" of a fruit or vegetable. Confused? Fortunately the difference is not as complicated as it sounds, and in fact, may make it easier to get your 9 to 13 daily recommended servings of produce, depending on your calorie intake and activity level.

You see, the serving size often printed on nutrition labels refers to the FDA's recommended amount of a particular food you would normally eat in one sitting. For example, one serving size of bananas is, you guessed it, one banana. While the serving size may vary depending on the food in question, a serving of a fruit or vegetable is typically a half cup and refers to your recommended daily intake of fruits and vegetables. To return to the example, since a large banana may contain a full cup (i.e., two half cups) of fruit, then one serving size (one banana) provides not one but nearly two servings of fruits and vegetables. Like a banana, a single large apple is a serving size, but it accounts for about four servings of fruit!

The same half-cup serving measurement holds true for vegetables. Thus, if you sit down to eat a serving size of broccoli (a cup and a half), you'll have consumed three of your daily recommended servings of fruits and vegetables.

And this is also true with fruit juice—8 ounces is a serving size, giving you two servings of fruit. That means you'll get nearly four servings in a 15.2 oz bottle of DOLE 100% juice.

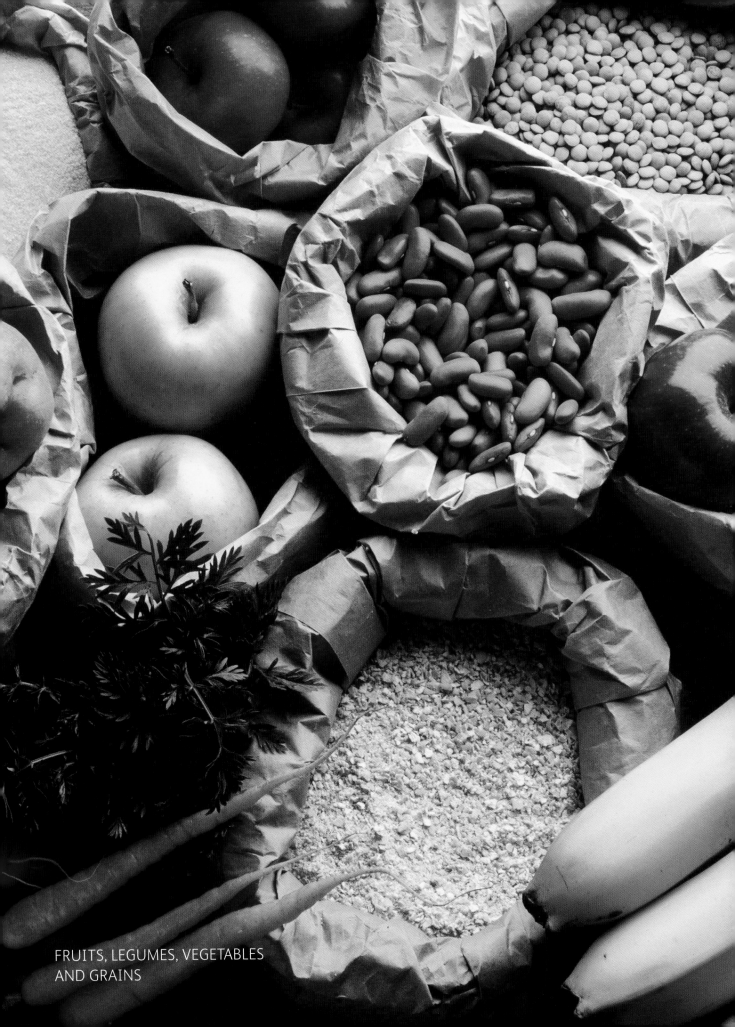

FRUITS, LEGUMES, VEGETABLES
AND GRAINS

Fruit Superfoods

Type	Quantity	Nutrients and % of Daily Value (DV)	Benefits
Bananas	1 7"–8" fruit (126g)	Vitamin B6, 36% Manganese, 15–19% Vitamin C, 12–15% Potassium, 10% Fiber, 9–13% Also: Resistant starch ORAC score = 1,108	The combination of nutrients in bananas makes them particularly heart healthy: Vitamin B6 reduces homocysteine levels, vitamin C prevents oxidation of LDL (bad) cholesterol, potassium helps control blood pressure and fiber helps lower LDL. In addition, banana consumption has been linked to a lower risk of leukemia, colorectal and kidney cancer. In fact, a study published in *Nutrition and Cancer* found that those who consumed bananas three or more times per week had a 72% lower risk of colorectal cancer than those who consumed them less than once a week. And British researchers report that children who ate just one banana a day reduced their asthmatic risk by 34%. Bananas also contain resistant starch, which acts as a prebiotic, selectively nourishing the "good gut" bacteria that line your intestinal tract and protect against foodborne viruses like E. coli. A University of Colorado study found that resistant starch may increase fat-burning metabolism as well.
Blueberries	1 cup (148g)	Vitamin K, 24% Manganese, 22–28% Vitamin C, 9–16% Fiber, 9–14% Also: High in anthocyanins (antioxidant phytochemicals) ORAC score = 9,206	In a USDA study, blueberries ranked fifth in total antioxidant capacity per serving out of more than 100 common foods. The highest levels were found in wild blueberries, however, which ranked second. Anthocyanins and flavonols are responsible for their antioxidant activity, allowing them to fight free-radical damage, strengthen tissues and blood vessels, protect eye health, and ward off varicose veins, ulcers, hemorrhoids, heart disease and cancer. Tufts University researchers have found that blueberries can also slow, and even reverse, age-related brain decline in animal studies. And, like their little red cranberry cousin, blueberries contain compounds that may reduce the risk of urinary-tract infections.

Fruit Superfoods

Type	Quantity	Nutrients and % of Daily Value (DV)	Benefits
Pineapple (extra-sweet variety)	1 slice, 4⅔" x ½" thick, or about ¾ cup of chunks (112g)	Vitamin C, 70–84% Manganese, 40–51% Also: Bromelain (protein-digesting plant enzyme) ORAC score = 990	Pineapple, whether fresh or frozen, is the only known source of bromelain—a protein-digesting enzyme that research shows to have anti-inflammatory properties that may alleviate symptoms of osteoarthritis, sinusitis and asthma; help heal injuries; and inhibit the growth of malignant lung and breast-cancer cells. A nutrient combo that included bromelain cut down plastic surgery recovery time by 17%, according to the American Society of Plastic Surgeons. Emerging research suggests that eating more fresh pineapple could counter colitis and thus play a role in preventing colon cancer. Duke University researcher Laura P. Hale, MD, PhD, has shown that bromelain can decrease some of the faulty immune responses that cause colitis.
Pomegranate	1 pomegranate (154g)	Manganese, 38–49% Vitamin B5, 18% Vitamin B6, 12% Vitamin C, 10–13%	UCLA researchers found that drinking 8 oz of pomegranate juice a day significantly reduces the levels of prostate-specific antigen in men following surgery or radiation treatment for prostate cancer. Another UCLA study suggests that consumption of a pomegranate extract may enhance protection of regular sunscreen up to 23%. And topical application of pomegranate extract has been found to inhibit the development of skin cancer in mice.

Type	Quantity	Nutrients and % of Daily Value (DV)	Benefits
Guava	1 cup, about 3–4 fruit (165g)	Vitamin C, 419–502% Copper, 42% Fiber, 23–36% Folate, 20% Potassium, 15% Manganese, 11–14% Also: 8,587mcg of lycopene (about twice that in a comparable serving of tomato or watermelon) and loaded with antioxidant phytochemicals ORAC score = 4,208	The white-fleshed guava is high in antioxidants, and the red-fleshed variety is even higher. Red- and pink-fleshed guavas, gram for gram, have more lycopene than even watermelon and tomato. A study from the Heart Research Laboratory in India found that people who ate five to nine guavas per day for three months reduced their cholesterol levels by 10%, their triglycerides by 8% and their blood pressure by 9.0/8.0mm Hg, while also boosting their HDL (good) cholesterol by 8%. Along with the antioxidant phytochemicals and vitamin C that prevent the oxidation of LDL, guava also offers fiber and potassium, which make it especially healthy for the heart.
Kiwifruits	2 medium-size kiwifruits (148g)	Vitamin C, 152–183% Vitamin K, 50% Copper, 21% Fiber, 12–18% Potassium, 10% Also: Actinidin (plant enzyme) ORAC score = 1,305	Norwegian researchers found that eating two kiwis per day can significantly lower blood-clot risk and reduce blood lipids. And Chinese researchers report that two kiwis a day counters chronic constipation, doubling the frequency of bowel movements. Kiwis contain the enzyme actinidin (related to bromelain in pineapple and papain in papaya), which suggests it may also help alleviate inflammation. And its vitamin C, fiber and potassium make the kiwi a particularly heart healthy fruit.
Prunes	½ cup, about 9 fruits (87g)	Vitamin K, 43% Copper, 27% Fiber, 16–25% Potassium, 14% Manganese, 11–14% Also: Full of antioxidant phytochemicals ORAC score = 7,300	Gram-for-gram, prunes were ranked the third highest in antioxidant activity compared with 100 other fruits and vegetables—beating out blueberries, blackberries and raspberries. A study from Oklahoma State University suggests that prunes may protect against postmenopausal bone loss, too.

Fruit Superfoods

Type	Quantity	Nutrients and % of Daily Value (DV)	Benefits
Plantains (cooked, mashed)	1 cup (200g)	Vitamin B6, 37 % Vitamin C, 24–29 % Potassium, 20 % Magnesium, 15–20 % Folate, 13 % Fiber, 12–18 % Vitamin A, 10–13 % Also: Resistant starch	Plantains, or cooking bananas, as they are often called, are longer, thicker-skinned and starchier in flavor than bananas. Unlike bananas, however, they're loaded with the carotenoid antioxidants alpha- and beta-carotene. British researchers found that the phytochemical leucocyanidin in unripe plantains may protect against ulcer formation. Plantains have a heart healthy combo of nutrients, including vitamin B6, vitamin C, potassium and fiber. They also contain resistant starch, which acts as a prebiotic, selectively nourishing the "good gut" bacteria that line the intestinal tract and protect against foodborne illness. The bacterial by-products of resistant starch, called butyrates, increase fat metabolism and boost calcium absorption.
Strawberries	1 cup, about 8 large fruits (147g)	Vitamin C, 96–115 % Manganese, 25–32 % Fiber, 8–12 % Also: Loaded with powerful antioxidants like anthocyanins and quercetin ORAC score = 5,258	UCLA researchers report that strawberries' anthocyanins may suppress colon, prostate and oral cancer cells. In animal studies, researchers at Tufts University found that strawberry-supplemented diets slowed, and even reversed, brain decline. Cornell University researchers also found that the quercetin in strawberries may help prevent Alzheimer's disease by protecting brain cells from oxidation. Another strawberry compound—cyanidin-3-glucoside, or C3G—is thought to help regulate appetite and increase fat-burning potential.

Type	Quantity	Nutrients and % of Daily Value (DV)	Benefits
Papaya	1 cup, cubes (140g)	Vitamin C, 96–115 % Folate, 13 % Vitamin A, 9–11 % Fiber, 7–10 % Also: Papain (protein-digesting plant enzyme) and beta-cryptoxanthin (a provitamin A carotenoid)	The papaya ranked first in a study that compared 40 different fruits for the Dietary Recommended Intake (DRI) of nine vitamins, potassium and fiber. It contains the proteolytic enzyme papain, which aids digestion. Plus, the combination of vitamins A and C, fiber and potassium make it super heart healthy. Also a top source of beta-cryptoxanthin, papayas may reduce the risk of lung cancer.
Oranges, navel	1 large fruit, about 1 cup, sections (154g)	Vitamin C, 101–121 % Folate, 13 % Fiber, 9–14 % Also: Naringenin and hesperetin (highly bioavailable antioxidant phytochemicals) ORAC score = 2,801	Citrus fruits' health benefits begin the moment you put them in your mouth. Australian researchers have linked high citrus consumption to a lower risk of developing cancers of the mouth, throat and stomach. In addition, regular consumption of oranges during the first two years of life has been associated with a reduced risk of childhood leukemia. The phytochemicals naringenin and hesperetin contribute significantly to the body's antioxidant pool, helping combat the damage caused by free radicals. Studies show they can reach the blood in as little as 20 minutes.
Blackberries	1 cup (144g)	Manganese, 40–52 % Vitamin C, 34–40 % Vitamin K, 24 % Fiber, 20–30 % Also: High amounts of anthocyanins ORAC score = 7,700	Blackberries are an antioxidant powerhouse, ranking seventh in total antioxidant capacity per gram out of more than 100 common foods. Their combination of fiber, vitamin C and polyphenolic antioxidants makes them good for the heart. And research suggests that their anthocyanins may have therapeutic potential in the prevention of obesity and diabetes.

Fruit Superfoods

Type	Quantity	Nutrients and % of Daily Value (DV)	Benefits
Raspberries	1 cup (123g)	Manganese, 36–46% Vitamin C, 36–43% Fiber, 21–32% Also: Loaded with antioxidant polyphenols ORAC score = 6,000	The USDA ranks raspberries eighth in total antioxidant capacity out of more than 100 common foods (per serving). Their combination of vitamin C, antioxidants and fiber make them super heart healthy. And UCLA researchers found that raspberry extract helps inhibit the growth of several kinds of cancers, including oral, breast, colon and prostate. In animal studies, black raspberries, a close cousin of the red variety, halved the incidence of cancerous throat tumors.
Dried Figs	½ cup (75g)	Copper, 24% Fiber, 19–30% Manganese, 17–21% Magnesium, 12–16% Potassium, 11% Also: Ficin (protein-digesting plant enzyme) and antioxidant phytochemicals ORAC score = 2,537	Figs contain a protein-digesting enzyme called ficin—rather like bromelain in pineapples and papain in papayas. They're also relatively high in antioxidants, ranking 13th among the USDA 100 common fruits and vegetables measured by the gram. Figs' antioxidant polyphenols help neutralize the free radicals that cause DNA damage and accelerate the aging process. And Chinese scientists have shown that some of the fig's antioxidant compounds are highly toxic toward certain human cancer cell lines in the brain and liver without being toxic to normal, healthy tissue. It's possible that these compounds signal cancer cells to self-destruct in a process called apoptosis.
Cantaloupe	About ⅓ small melon (134g)	Vitamin C, 55–66% Vitamin A, 25–32% ORAC score = 422	Cantaloupe provides more beta-carotene than any other melon. As such, its A-list benefits include preserving eyesight, supporting immunity, enhancing sun protection and reducing the risk of several types of cancer. Cantaloupe's rough surface makes it susceptible to bacterial contamination, but according to USDA scientists, placing a cantaloupe in hot water (172°F) for three minutes can significantly reduce levels of harmful bacteria without compromising fruit quality.

Type	Quantity	Nutrients and % of Daily Value (DV)	Benefits
Mangoes	1 cup slices, about ¾ fruit (164g)	Vitamin C, 51–61 % Vitamin E, 12 % Fiber, 8–12 % Also: Antioxidant polyphenols ORAC score = 1,600	Indian scientists found that mango pulp extract reduced free-radical damage to the prostate in animal studies. It also seemed to reactivate internal antioxidant enzymes needed to protect the prostate. Mangoes are good for the skin as well: Their vitamin C increases collagen formation, and beta-carotene may act as a gentle internal sunscreen. Those nutrients also help maintain a healthy immune system. And the vitamin C, vitamin E and fiber in mangoes help lower LDL cholesterol.
Grapefruit, pink or red	About ½ grapefruit (154g)	Vitamin C, 53–64 % Vitamin A, 10–13 % Fiber, 7–10 % Also: Lycopene, 2,185mcg, and other antioxidant phytochemicals ORAC score = 2,384	Grapefruit's low calorie count (60 calories per ½ grapefruit), combined with its high fiber and water content, helps support weight loss. While all grapefruit is high in vitamin C, the pink and red varieties are also an excellent source of vitamin A; and vitamins C and A support skin health and immunity. Red grapefruit also supplies a significant quantity of lycopene—a potent antioxidant thought to reduce the risk of heart disease and prostate cancer. In fact, grapefruit is loaded with anticancer phytochemicals, such as limonoids, which may reduce the risk of cancer by stimulating the body's natural detoxification enzymes. Be aware, though, that certain compounds in grapefruit (such as naringenin) can affect how some medications are absorbed in the intestine and may actually raise drug levels in the blood. Consult your physician if you're taking prescribed medications and frequently consume grapefruit or grapefruit juice.

Fruit Superfoods

Type	Quantity	Nutrients and % of Daily Value (DV)	Benefits
Dates (Deglet Noor)	½ cup (74g)	Copper, 17% Fiber, 16–24% Potassium, 10% Manganese, 8–11% Magnesium, 8–10% ORAC score = 3,500	While dates come in many varieties, the most common in the U.S. is the Deglet Noor, which is loaded with heart healthy nutrients that help lower bad cholesterol and regulate blood pressure. Researchers at the University of California, Davis, found Deglet Noor dates to have more antioxidant scavenging power than other varieties—and that a handful has about the same antioxidant capacity as half a glass of red wine.
Watermelon	About ¹⁄₁₆ of a melon, 1¾ cups, diced (280g)	Vitamin C, 25–30% Vitamin A, 9–11% Also: Over 12,690mcg of the antioxidant lycopene ORAC score = 398	Watermelon outperforms tomatoes in both content and bioavailability of lycopene—which is associated with lower risks of various cancers, including prostate, ovarian, cervical, oral, pharyngeal, esophageal, stomach, colorectal, lung and pancreatic. Eating 2½ cups of watermelon provides a dose of lycopene sufficient to increase sun protection by 33%. Studies also indicate that lycopene may enhance male fertility, while another watermelon compound—the amino acid citrulline, found mostly in the rind—may function as a natural alternative to Viagra. The combination of vitamins A and C and lycopene also make watermelon heart healthy.
Tangerines	½ cup sections, about 1 large fruit (109g)	Vitamin C, 32–39% Also: Antioxidant polyphenols ORAC score = 1,779	As the top citrus source of pectin, tangerines may make you feel fuller: Researchers at the State University of New York at Buffalo found that pectin consumption reduces caloric intake in the obese. Studies also show that this soluble fiber benefits your heart by helping lower blood cholesterol levels. Tangerines are a top source of beta-cryptoxanthin, which is linked to lower lung- and prostate-cancer risk. British researchers found that people in the top one-third of beta-cryptoxanthin intake were almost half as likely to develop polyarthritis (inflammation affecting two or more joint groups) as those in the lowest third.

Type	Quantity	Nutrients and % of Daily Value (DV)	Benefits
Cranberries	1 cup, whole (100g)	Manganese, 16–20% Vitamin C, 15–18% Fiber, 12–18% Also: Contain large amounts of anthocyanins ORAC score = 9,584	Cranberries rank first overall in antioxidant capacity (per gram) on the USDA list. Studies show that they may boost HDL levels, and scientists at Cornell University have isolated compounds in cranberries that have extremely potent antiproliferative effects on human liver and breast cancer cells. Scientists at the University of Massachusetts Dartmouth found these compounds to have similar potential for thwarting colon and leukemia cancer cells. One cranberry antioxidant—quercetin—may help reduce Alzheimer's risk and alleviate prostatitis (inflammation or infection of the prostate gland). Cranberry products have also been linked to the prevention and alleviation of urinary tract infections.
Plums	2 fruits, about 1 cup, slices (151g)	Vitamin C, 16–19% Vitamin A, 12–15% Copper, 10% Also: Antioxidant polyphenols ORAC score = 9,400	This fruit earns a "plum" spot on the USDA list, with the black variety ranking fourth and standard plums fifth in antioxidant activity per gram. French scientists found that one of the antioxidants in plums—chlorogenic acid—decreased anxiety-related behaviors in mice, possibly by combating the kind of oxidative stress that can induce anxiety and depression in humans. Note: Italian scientists have demonstrated that organically grown plums contain higher concentrations of the antioxidant vitamins A, C and E than conventionally grown varieties.

Fruit Superfoods

Type	Quantity	Nutrients and % of Daily Value (DV)	Benefits
Apples (Red Delicious, Granny Smith, Gala)	1 large fruit with skin (242g)	Fiber, 15–23% Vitamin C, 12–15% Also: One of the top sources of polyphenolic antioxidant compounds, including quercetin ORAC scores: Red Delicious = 10,346 Granny Smith = 9,433 Gala = 6,845	According to USDA researchers, three apple varieties—Red Delicious, Granny Smith and Gala—rank in the top 20 food sources for antioxidants per serving, with Red Delicious in the No. 1 slot. When eaten with the skin, Red Delicious apples have about twice as much fiber and 45% more antioxidants as they do when peeled. The apple antioxidant, quercetin, may boost immunity and reduce the risk of Alzheimer's as well as lung, prostate and liver cancers. In fact, Cornell University researchers found that treating liver-cancer cells with 50mg of apple extract slowed their growth by 57%. Apples also contain the fiber pectin, which can help you feel fuller; a State University of New York at Buffalo study found that the amount of pectin in one apple reduced caloric intake in obese participants.
Cherries (sweet)	1 cup (138g)	Vitamin C, 11–13% Fiber, 8–12% Also: Anthocyanins ORAC score = 4,644	Cherries came in 10th in antioxidant activity per serving on the USDA list. In addition, several studies have linked cherry consumption with the alleviation of inflammation, arthritic pain and gout, making cherries a superfood for the joints. Researchers at the USDA Agricultural Research Service found that five hours after eating about 45 Bing cherries, women's levels of plasma urate (which accumulates in the joints during a gout attack) decreased by 15%.
Nectarines	1 medium fruit, 2½" diameter (142g)	Vitamin A, 10–13% Vitamin C, 9–10% Also: Antioxidant polyphenols ORAC score = 1,065	Nectarines' antioxidant flavonoids help protect against free-radical damage. Their nutrient combo also supports healthy skin and immune function. Research suggests nectarines may have anticancer benefits, as well: National Cancer Institute studies found a 40% lower risk of cancers of the esophagus, head and neck among those with the highest intake of fruit from the *Rosaceae* family, which includes nectarines.

Vegetable Superfoods

Type	Quantity	Nutrients and % of Daily Value (DV)	Benefits
Kale (cooked)	⅔ cup, chopped (87g)	Vitamin K, 592% Vitamin A, 66–85% Vitamin C, 40–53% Manganese, 16–20% Also: "Indirect" antioxidants known as glucosinolates	As a top source of vitamin K, kale might help lower risk for fractures. Like other cruciferous vegetables, kale supplies an abundance of glucosinolates, one of which—indole-3-carbinol (I3C)—can reduce levels of harmful estrogens that may promote cancer growth in hormone-sensitive cells, such as breast cells. Kale is also a top source of eye-healthy carotenoids, such as beta-carotene, lutein and zeaxanthin.
Spinach (raw)	3 cups (90g)	Vitamin K, 362% Vitamin A, 47–60% Folate, 44% Manganese, 35–45% Iron, 31–14% Vitamin C, 28–34% Magnesium, 17–22% Potassium, 11% Also: 10,978mcg of lutein and zeaxanthin, and contains antioxidant phytochemicals ORAC score = 1,364	Spinach may be one of the healthiest foods on earth. It supplies large amounts of the eye-healthy carotenoids lutein and zeaxanthin, which have been shown to lower risk of cataract development. The folate, vitamin C, potassium, magnesium, and antioxidant phytonutrients in spinach promote heart health. In addition, Popeye's favorite veggie may help maintain mental sharpness and reduce the risk of cancers of the liver, ovaries, colon and prostate. A Dole Nutrition Institute study found spinach juice to be significantly more nutritious than wheatgrass juice. Although spinach is loaded with calcium, it's also high in oxalates—minerals that interfere with calcium's bioavailability—but there's evidence that cooking fruits and vegetables can significantly reduce oxalate content.
Collard Greens (cooked)	½ cup, chopped (95g)	Vitamin K, 348% Vitamin A, 43–55% Folate, 22% Vitamin C, 19–23% Manganese, 18–23% Calcium, 13% Fiber, 7–11% Also: Glucosinolates	Considered one of the milder greens, collards provide nearly four times the daily requirement of vitamin K, which along with their folate may help protect against osteoporosis. In addition, collards are loaded with beta-carotene, lutein and zeaxanthin, making them a superfood for the eyes.

Vegetable Superfoods

Type	Quantity	Nutrients and % of Daily Value (DV)	Benefits
Broccoli (raw)	1 medium stalk (148g)	Vitamin C, 147–176 % Vitamin K, 125 % Folate, 23 % Vitamin B6, 20 % Manganese, 14–17 % Phosphorus, 14 % Vitamin B2, 13–16 % Fiber, 10–15 % Potassium, 10 % Calcium, 7 % Also: Glucosinolates and antioxidant phytochemicals ORAC score = 2,016	Broccoli's glucosinolates show promise in protecting against prostate, bladder, colon, pancreatic, gastric, breast and other hormone-related cancers. Glucosinolates activate the liver's Phase II enzymes, which continue to scavenge damaging free radicals long after the food is eaten. Broccoli is also great for the bones: It's among the top calcium-containing vegetables, and it is high in vitamin K and folate—the upper intakes of which are linked to reduced risk of fracture. And researchers have found that consumption of broccoli strengthens the blood-brain barrier—a protective network of capillaries that protects the brain from infection after a head injury.
Swiss Chard (cooked)	½ cup, chopped (88g)	Vitamin K, 239 % Vitamin A, 30–38 % Iron, 25–11 % Magnesium, 18–23 % Vitamin C, 18–21 % Manganese, 13–16 % Potassium, 10 % Also: 9,638mcg of lutein and zeaxanthin	Swiss chard contains a unique combination of nutrients—vitamins C, K, magnesium, manganese and potassium—that help support bone health. The Framingham Heart Study found that elderly people who consumed approximately 250mcg per day of vitamin K (the amount in ½ cup Swiss chard) had a 35 % lower risk of hip fracture than those who consumed only 50mcg per day. Swiss chard also contains the carotenoids beta-carotene, lutein and zeaxanthin, which help protect the eyes from the sun's harmful rays. In fact, one study found a 60 % lower risk of age-related macular degeneration (the leading cause of blindness in the U.S.) in people whose intake of lutein and zeaxanthin was highest.

Type	Quantity	Nutrients and % of Daily Value (DV)	Benefits
Chicory (cooked)	3 cups, chopped (87g)	Vitamin K, 216% Vitamin A, 28–36% Folate, 24% Vitamin C, 23–28% Manganese, 16–21% Fiber, 9–14% Calcium, 9%	Chicory greens—the leaves of the chicory plant, often used as a salad green—are loaded with lutein and zeaxanthin, carotenoids that support eye health. The Nurses' Health Study (which followed more than 77,000 subjects) found that 22% fewer cataract surgeries were necessary among women over age 45 who had the most lutein and zeaxanthin in their diet. The combination of vitamins C, K, folate and manganese make chicory greens particularly healthy for your bones as well.
Sweet Potatoes (baked, with skin)	1 medium, 5" long (114g)	Vitamin A, 122–157% Manganese, 25–32% Vitamin C, 25–30% Potassium, 12% Fiber, 10–15% Magnesium, 7–10% Also: Antioxidant phytochemicals ORAC score = 2,750	This nutrient-rich tuber is often classified as a yam, but that's actually a different vegetable. Sweet potatoes are fairly common in the typical supermarket, while true yams are imported and less widely available. Sweet potatoes have orange-colored flesh and contain more than 100% of the daily value for vitamin A as beta-carotene—more than any other fruit or vegetable. Their unique combination of potassium, fiber, and vitamins A and C make them especially heart healthy. Plus, they supply a hearty dose of antioxidants, helping to neutralize free-radical damage.
Lettuce, green leaf	1½ cups, shredded (85g)	Vitamin K, 123% Vitamin A, 35–45% Vitamin C, 17–20% Manganese, 9–12% Also: Antioxidant phytochemicals ORAC score = 1,230	This lettuce variety contains vitamins A and C, which help support skin health and immune function. Green leaf lettuce also contains more than 100% of the daily value for bone-healthy vitamin K. The Framingham Heart Study found that elderly people who consumed approximately 250mcg per day of vitamin K (a single serving of green leaf lettuce supplies 148mcg) had a 35% lower risk of hip fracture than those who consumed only 50mcg per day. The beta-carotene in green leaf lettuce helps with vision in dim light, while lutein and zeaxanthin protect the eye from the sun's damaging rays, making this leafy vegetable super eye-healthy.

Vegetable Superfoods

Type	Quantity	Nutrients and % of Daily Value (DV)	Benefits
Red Bell Pepper	1 small (74g)	Vitamin C, 105–126% Vitamin B6, 17% Vitamin A, 13–17% Vitamin E, 8% ORAC score = 1,171	Extremely nutrient dense, red bell peppers are good for skin, immunity, bones and heart health. They might also help protect against cancer. Japanese scientists found that extracts from red bell peppers have the ability to selectively target human cancer tumors, while leaving normal, healthy tissue unharmed.
Cauliflower (raw)	1/6 medium head (99g)	Vitamin C, 51–61% Vitamin B6, 17% Folate, 14% Vitamin B5, 13% Vitamin K, 13% Fiber, 7–10% Also: Glucosinolates and some antioxidant phytochemicals ORAC score = 719	Cauliflower contains glucosinolates, which trigger the body's own antioxidant systems. Italian researchers found that cauliflower compounds suppressed breast-cancer cell growth and perhaps even promoted cancer-cell death. Canadian scientists report that men with prostate cancer who consumed cauliflower more than once a week cut their risk of the cancer becoming aggressive by more than 50%.
Arugula	3 cups (60g)	Vitamin K, 54% Folate, 15% Vitamin C, 10–12% Calcium, 10% Manganese, 8–11% Vitamin A, 8–10% Also: 2,133mcg of lutein and zeaxanthin	Arugula's combination of folate, vitamins C and K, calcium, magnesium and manganese helps prevent osteoporosis, lower the risk of fractures, and promote overall bone and cartilage health.

Type	Quantity	Nutrients and % of Daily Value (DV)	Benefits
Asparagus (cooked)	5 spears (93g)	Vitamin K, 39 % Folate, 35 % Thiamin, 13 % Vitamin C, 8–10 % Also: Antioxidant phytochemicals ORAC score = 1,529	Asparagus contains inulin, a prebiotic fiber that's indigestible by humans but can selectively nourish the "good" gut bacteria that line our intestinal tract and thereby protect us against "bad" bacteria, like E. coli. Asparagus tests highest among sources of glutathione, one of the most potent antioxidants, according to the National Cancer Institute.
Butternut Squash (cooked)	½ cup (103g)	Vitamin A, 64–82 % Vitamin C, 17–21 % Also: Some antioxidant phytochemicals ORAC score = 388	Butternut squash is an especially rich source of vitamin A as beta-carotene, which promotes healthy vision and has been shown to inhibit collagen breakdown and defend epithelial cells against the kind of ultraviolet radiation that can lead to wrinkles and age spots. Its vitamin C is also good for the skin, encouraging skin cell turnover and supporting the formation of collagen. Vitamins A and C boost the immune system: vitamin A, by helping to maintain the cells lining the airways, urinary and digestive tracts; and vitamin C, by facilitating white blood cell function. Butternut squash is also one of the best sources of beta-cryptoxanthin, a carotenoid linked to lower risks of lung and prostate cancer, as well as to improved joint health.

Vegetable Superfoods

Type	Quantity	Nutrients and % of Daily Value (DV)	Benefits
Carrots (raw)	1 medium, 7" long (78g)	Vitamin A, 72–93 % Also: Some antioxidant phytochemicals ORAC score = 519	Carrots support eye and skin health, bolster immune function and demonstrate cancer-prevention potential with their ability to neutralize free radicals and promote communication between cells. In an animal study, British and Danish researchers found that a carrot compound called falcarinol reduced the risk of developing cancerous tumors by a third. Note: Though raw carrots make a healthy and tasty snack, cooked carrots provide greater amounts of vitamin A because the cooking process breaks down the cell walls, enhancing nutrient availability.
Tomatoes (raw)	1 medium (148g)	Vitamin C, 21–25 % Also: 3,165mcg of lycopene and some antioxidant phytochemicals ORAC score = 543	Tomatoes are one of the best sources of lycopene, a potent antioxidant, which studies show may reduce the risk of heart disease and a range of cancers, including prostate, ovarian, cervical, oral, pharyngeal, esophageal, stomach, colorectal, lung and pancreatic. A University of Manchester study in the U.K. found that eating lycopene-rich tomatoes gave subjects 33 % more protection against sunburn. Note: Cooking tomatoes helps to maximize these benefits, because it releases lycopene from their cell walls, making it more available to the body.

Type	Quantity	Nutrients and % of Daily Value (DV)	Benefits
Russet Potatoes (baked with skin) Red Potatoes (baked with skin) White Potatoes (baked with skin)	1 medium potato (with skin) (148g)	**Russet** Vitamin B6, 40% Vitamin C, 21–25% Copper, 18% Potassium, 17% Manganese, 15–19% Phosphorus, 15% Vitamin B3, 12–14% Magnesium, 10–14% Folate, 10% Fiber, 9–14% ORAC score = 2,486 **Red** Copper, 29% Vitamin B6, 24% Vitamin C, 21–25% Potassium, 17% Vitamin B3, 15–17% Phosphorus, 15% Manganese, 11–14% Magnesium, 10–13% Folate, 10% Fiber, 7–11% ORAC score = 1,962 **White** Vitamin B6, 24% Vitamin C, 21–25% Copper, 21% Potassium, 17% Phosphorus, 16% Vitamin B3, 14–16% Folate, 14% Manganese, 12–16% Magnesium, 10–13% Fiber, 8–12% ORAC score = 1,684	Potatoes are the most widely consumed vegetable in the U.S., which wouldn't be so bad if they weren't primarily eaten deep-fried or mashed with added fat and sodium. Potatoes are naturally heart healthy, with all three of these varieties—russet, red and white—containing the same unique combination of potassium, vitamin B6, vitamin C and fiber. A British study discovered that potatoes also contain compounds called kukoamines, which lower blood pressure. And a small Swedish study found that boiled and mashed potatoes were more satiating than French fries when served as breakfast after overnight fasting. Potatoes also contain chlorogenic acid, a phytochemical that research shows may block the formation of carcinogenic nitrosamines and reduce the risk of liver and colon cancers. Korean scientists found that the potato peel can contain up to 20 times more chlorogenic acid than the pulp, while Indian researchers demonstrated that potato-peel extract can reduce the chemically induced oxidation of human red blood cell membranes by up to 85%—two good reasons to leave the skins on!

Vegetable Superfoods

Type	Quantity	Nutrients and % of Daily Value (DV)	Benefits
Brussels Sprouts (cooked)	½ cup (78g)	Vitamin K, 91% Vitamin C, 54–65% Folate, 12% Vitamin B6, 11% Manganese, 8–10% Also: Glucosinolates and antioxidant phytochemicals ORAC score = 2,016	Austrian researchers have shown that consumption of Brussels sprouts can reduce oxidative DNA damage by nearly 40%. Brussels sprouts appear to fight free radicals with double barrels, using both direct and indirect antioxidants. The same researchers found that consumption of the vegetable increased blood vitamin C levels by 37%. Brussels sprouts also contain lutein and zeaxanthin carotenoids (which protect eye health), high concentrations of glucosinolates (which help with detoxification), and nearly all of your vitamin K needs for the day (which makes them bone-healthy, too).
Lettuce, romaine	2 cups, shredded (85g)	Vitamin K, 73% Vitamin A, 41–53% Folate, 29% Vitamin C, 23–27% Also: 1,965mcg of lutein and zeaxanthin ORAC score = 818	Like green and red leaf lettuces, romaine also contains the eye-healthy antioxidant carotenoids beta-carotene, lutein and zeaxanthin—which studies have linked to reduced risk of cataracts and age-related macular degeneration.
Lettuce, red leaf	3 cups, shredded (85g)	Vitamin K, 100% Vitamin A, 35–46% Also: Anthocyanins and other antioxidant phytochemicals ORAC score = 2,030	Like the green leaf variety, red leaf lettuce contains high amounts of vitamins A (as beta-carotene) and K, as well as lutein and zeaxanthin, making it extremely healthy for the eyes.

Type	Quantity	Nutrients and % of Daily Value (DV)	Benefits
Green Cabbage (cooked)	1/12 medium head, about 1/2 cup, shredded (84g)	Vitamin K, 76% Vitamin C, 35–42% Also: Glucosinolates and some antioxidant phytochemicals ORAC score = 719	Green cabbage provides the highest levels of two anticancer glucosinolates, which are converted upon consumption into compounds that may inhibit tumor growth. Research shows that one compound, allyl isothiocyanate, disrupts the cell division of colon cancer, while the other, indole-3-carbinol, may lower the risk of developing estrogen-related cancers, such as breast and ovarian cancer. Yet a third compound released with cabbage consumption may inhibit the growth of human prostate cancer cells, according to research from the University of California, Berkeley.
Red Cabbage (cooked)	About 1/2 cup, shredded (84g)	Vitamin K, 33% Vitamin C, 32–39% Also: Glucosinolates and anthocyanins ORAC score = 2,642	Red cabbage contains glucosinolates, which stimulate the body's natural detoxification systems and may reduce the risk of developing several cancers. But, unlike its greener cousin, red cabbage also contains anthocyanins. Both types of antioxidants can reduce the damage caused by free radicals and protect against DNA damage.
Artichokes (cooked)	1/2 cup (84g)	Folate, 25% Fiber, 10–16% Manganese, 10–13% Also: Antioxidant phytochemicals ORAC score = 7,909	Artichokes ranked second overall and first among vegetables in the USDA study's per gram category. The fiber in artichokes, along with the phytochemicals luteolin and cynarin, is thought to help lower cholesterol levels. Artichokes also contain inulin, the prebiotic fiber that can selectively nourish the "good" bacteria that line your intestinal tract and ward off E. coli and other foodborne viruses. Amazingly, California produces virtually 100% of the artichokes in the U.S.—and consumes almost half of them!
Parsnips (cooked)	1 parsnip, 1/2 cup	Vitamin C, 11–13% Folate, 11% Manganese, 10–13% Fiber, 7–11%	Parsnips are a pale brown root vegetable, similar in shape to the carrot. Their combination of vitamin C, fiber and folate make them super heart healthy.

Vegetable Superfoods

Type	Quantity	Nutrients and % of Daily Value (DV)	Benefits
Yams (cooked)	$^2/_3$ cup (91g)	Vitamin B6, 16% Potassium, 13% Vitamin C, 12–15% Fiber, 9–14%	While orange sweet potatoes are often sold in the grocery store as yams, true yams are lighter in color and are rarely sold in the U.S. (Their size—they can grow up to 7 ft long and weigh up to 150 lbs—makes them difficult to import from their subtropical environs). Yams contain a unique combination of heart healthy nutrients: potassium, fiber, and vitamins C and B6.
Pumpkin (cooked)	$^1/_3$ cup, mashed (82g)	Vitamin A, 23–29% Also: 828mcg of lutein and zeaxanthin and some antioxidant phytochemicals ORAC score = 396	In addition to a healthy dose of vitamin A as beta-carotene, pumpkin also provides the eye-healthy phytochemicals lutein and zeaxanthin. It's also one of the best sources of beta-cryptoxanthin, a carotenoid linked to lower risks of lung and prostate cancer, as well as to improved joint health. A British study found that people with the highest intake of beta-cryptoxanthin had half the risk of developing polyarthritis (inflammation affecting two or more joint groups) than those with lower consumption levels.

Fish Superfoods

Type	Quantity	Nutrients and % of Daily Value (DV)	Benefits
Atlantic Salmon (cooked)	6 oz (170g)	Vitamin B12, 198% Selenium, 128% Vitamin B3, 85–98% Vitamin B6, 85% Phosphorus, 61% Vitamin B5, 50% Vitamin B1, 48% Vitamin B2, 18–21% Potassium, 14% Magnesium, 12–16% Also: High amount of omega-3 fatty acids	Salmon is one of the only foods that supplies the entire spectrum of B vitamins, supporting energy conversion and mood stability. This "oily" fish is a particularly rich source of the two most important omega-3 fatty acids, DHA and EPA, which are both linked to protection against Alzheimer's disease and cancer. A Tufts University study linked a twice-weekly intake of fatty fish to a 41% reduction in Alzheimer's incidence compared with an intake of once per month. Wild versus fresh: USDA data shows that farmed Atlantic salmon actually has slightly higher combined amounts of omega-3 fatty acids. Testing shows that the levels of PCBs in farmed salmon continue to drop and are now comparable to those found in wild salmon.
Yellowfin Tuna (cooked)	6 oz (170g)	Selenium, 145% Vitamin B6, 136% Vitamin B3, 127–145% Vitamin B1, 71% Phosphorus, 59% Vitamin B12, 43% Vitamin B5, 29% Magnesium, 26–34% Potassium, 21%	Tuna has many of the nutrient benefits of salmon, but with less omega-3 fatty acids. It's a lean fish with a low overall fat content. Its spate of B vitamins makes it heart healthy, but the possibility of heavy metal contamination (mercury) means that tuna consumption should be limited to 2–3 times per month.
Atlantic/Pacific Halibut (cooked)	6 oz (170g)	Selenium, 145% Vitamin B12, 97% Vitamin B3, 76–86% Phosphorus, 69% Vitamin B6, 52% Magnesium, 43–57% Potassium, 21% Vitamin B5, 13% Vitamin B2, 12–14% Vitamin B1, 10%	Halibut is one of the safest fish to eat as far as mercury contamination is concerned. It contains some fat, but mostly the heart healthy monounsaturated and polyunsaturated kind. It's also very high in selenium, which is needed for the proper functioning of some of the body's detoxification enzymes that prevent DNA damage from free radicals and toxins.

Fish Superfoods

Type	Quantity	Nutrients and % of Daily Value (DV)	Benefits
Sardines	6 oz (170g)	Vitamin B12, 633 % Vitamin D, 231 % Selenium, 163 % Phosphorus, 119 % Vitamin B3, 105–120 % Calcium, 65 % Iron, 62–28 % Sodium, 37 % Copper, 35 % Vitamin B2, 30–35 % Choline, 26–34 % Vitamin E, 23 % Vitamin B6, 22 % Vitamin B5, 22 % Zinc, 20–28 % Magnesium, 17–21 % Potassium, 14 % Vitamin B1, 11–12 % Also: Contains omega-3 fatty acids	Usually sold canned, sardines are loaded with omega-3s, which protect your heart, combat arthritis and depression, fortify against cancer and even fight wrinkles. Sardines also contain the highest amount of calcium of any fish. Just two tiny sardines give you as much calcium as $\frac{1}{3}$ cup of milk, as well as a full day's supply of B12.
Flounder (cooked)	6 oz (170g)	Selenium, 180 % Vitamin B12, 177 % Vitamin B3, 71–81 % Phosphorus, 70 % Vitamin B6, 31 % Choline, 25–32 % Magnesium, 25–32 % Vitamin B5, 20 % Vitamin B2, 15–18 % Potassium, 12 % Vitamin B1, 11–12 % Also: Contains omega-3 fatty acids	Like sardines, salmon and black cod, flounder contains a high level of omega-3s and selenium. Flounder is also known for being a low-calorie, low-mercury fish.

Type	Quantity	Nutrients and % of Daily Value (DV)	Benefits
Shrimp (cooked)	6 oz (170g)	Selenium, 122% Vitamin B12, 106% Vitamin B3, 79–90% Iron, 66–29% Copper 36% Phosphorus, 33% Choline, 25–32% Zinc, 24–33% Vitamin B6, 17% Sodium, 17% Vitamin E, 16% Magnesium, 14–19% Vitamin A, 13% Vitamin B5, 12%	Shrimp are the most widely consumed seafood worldwide and are renowned for their sweet, mild taste, similar to that of lobster—but for a fraction of the cost. A fairly low-mercury option, shrimp are also low in fat and calories. Despite containing dietary cholesterol, they are considerably lower in saturated fat than other kinds of animal protein. Shrimp can also help meet your daily iron requirements.
Black Cod (cooked)	6 oz (170g)	Selenium, 145% Vitamin B12, 102% Vitamin B3, 87–101% Phosphorus, 52% Vitamin B6, 45% Iron, 35–15% Magnesium, 30–39% Vitamin B5, 29% Vitamin A, 19–25% Vitamin B1, 17–19% Potassium, 17% Vitamin B2, 15–18% Also: High amounts of omega-3 fatty acids	Black cod, or sablefish, can contain as much omega-3 (EPA and DHA) as salmon. (It also has three times more saturated fat than salmon.) Sablefish has many of the other nutrients found in salmon as well, such as vitamin B12. Its rich, succulent taste and texture are often compared to sea bass.
Catfish, wild (cooked)	6 oz (170g)	Vitamin B12, 205% Phosphorus, 74% Vitamin B3, 62–71% Selenium, 44% Vitamin B1, 32–35% Vitamin B5, 31% Potassium, 15% Vitamin B6, 14% Magnesium, 12–15%	Long served as a Southern delicacy, catfish is a very lean fish (89 calories per serving), containing more than 100% of your daily vitamin B12 needs. It also is an excellent source of phosphorus and selenium. Though sometimes shunned as a so-called bottom-feeder, catfish is actually quite low in mercury and PCBs, making it a safe and healthy choice.

Nut Superfoods

Type	Quantity	Nutrients and % of Daily Value (DV)	Benefits
Almonds	1 oz (28g)	Vitamin E, 49% Vitamin B2, 22–26% Copper, 31% Manganese, 28–36% Magnesium, 18–23% Fiber, 9–14% Also: Mono- and poly-unsaturated fats ORAC score = 1,247	Almonds are the top nut source of alpha-tocopherol, a potent form of vitamin E that's thought to protect the heart. Purdue University researchers found that overweight women who added 2 oz of almonds to their daily diet for 10 weeks—an extra 21,000 calories—didn't gain weight! Instead, they effortlessly ate less of other foods, maintaining a calorie balance.
Brazil Nuts	1 oz (28g)	Selenium, 988% Copper, 55% Phosphorus, 29% Magnesium, 27–34% Manganese, 15–19% Vitamin B1, 15–16% Vitamin E, 11% Zinc, 10–14%	Brazil nuts are perhaps the best source of selenium, a mineral needed for proper thyroid and immune function. Selenium may also protect against cancers of the prostate, liver and lungs. But keep in mind that just one Brazil nut provides 160% of the RDA for selenium, and anything above eight times the RDA could be harmful (leading, eventually, to selenosis, the symptoms of which include brittle hair and nails). How many Brazil nuts are in 1.5 oz? Ten, which provide 15 times the RDA, or twice the upper tolerable level of selenium.
Cashews	1 oz (28g)	Copper, 68% Phosphorus, 24% Iron, 23–10% Magnesium, 20–26% Manganese, 20–26% Zinc, 15–20% Thiamin, 10–11% Selenium, 10% Also: Mono- and poly-unsaturated fats ORAC score = 545	Cashews supply a host of minerals in high amounts, including some that are hard to get, like zinc, which helps maintain healthy vision and support the immune system. Cashews also contain a class of compounds called phytosterols, compounds similar in structure to cholesterol that can reduce the absorption sites for dietary cholesterol in the gut and thus inhibit the body's absorption of LDL.

Type	Quantity	Nutrients and % of Daily Value (DV)	Benefits
Hazelnuts	1 oz (28g)	Manganese, 76% Biotin, 72% Copper, 54% Vitamin E, 28% Iron, 17–7% Vitamin B1, 15–16% Magnesium, 12–15% Vitamin B6, 12% Phosphorus, 12%	Hazelnuts, also referred to as filberts or cobnuts, are the top nut source of those heart healthy monounsaturated fats, which may raise levels of HDL and reduce the risk of clogged arteries. They are also excellent sources of manganese, copper and vitamin E.
Macadamia Nuts	1 oz (28g)	Manganese, 51% Vitamin B1, 28–31% Copper, 24% Iron, 13–6%	Macadamias are the highest nuts in total fats and calories, so they should only be eaten in moderation. They are, however, an excellent source of vitamin B1 (thiamin). Though their saturated-fat content excludes them from the FDA's qualified heart-health claim, Pennsylvania State University researchers found that a handful of macadamia nuts a day reduced total cholesterol and LDL by about 9%. The effect may be due to the increased monounsaturated fat from a daily macadamia diet.
Peanuts	1 oz (28g)	Biotin, 68% Copper, 36% Vitamin B3, 29–33% Manganese, 24% Folate, 17% Vitamin E, 16% Iron, 16–7% Vitamin B1, 15–16% Phosphorus, 15% Magnesium, 12–15% Vitamin B5, 10%	Though not strictly a nut (they are, in fact, a legume), peanuts contain more protein than tree nuts. They also contain resveratrol—a potent antioxidant with potential cancer-fighting properties. Though high in healthy unsaturated fats, some peanuts have been cultivated for even higher levels of monounsaturated fat, which may raise levels of HDL and reduce the risk of clogged arteries.

Nut Superfoods

Type	Quantity	Nutrients and % of Daily Value (DV)	Benefits
Pecans	1 oz (28g)	Manganese, 55–70% Copper, 38% Thiamin, 15% Zinc, 11–16% Phosphorus, 11% Magnesium, 8–11% Fiber, 7–11% Also: Mono- and poly-unsaturated fats ORAC score = 5,023	Pecans are tops in terms of antioxidant activity, ranking highest among all nuts on the USDA's ORAC scale. They also have up to 70% of the daily value of manganese, which supports bone health and wound healing. Pecans' healthy fats aid in the absorption of other fat-soluble nutrients, like vitamins A, D, E and K.
Pine Nuts	1 oz (28g)	Manganese, 108–139% Copper, 42% Phosphorus, 23% Iron, 20–9% Magnesium, 18–23% Vitamin E, 18% Zinc, 17–23% Vitamin K, 13% Vitamin B3, 11–12%	Pine nuts pack a powerful punch when it comes to manganese. In fact, they're the only nut that can meet your recommended daily value of this mineral, which is essential for bone health and wound healing.
Pistachios	1 oz (28g)	Copper, 41% Vitamin B6, 37% Vitamin B1, 21–22% Phosphorus, 20% Vitamin K, 17% Manganese, 15–19% Iron, 15–6% Vitamin B3, 10–12%	Pistachios contain phytosterols, compounds similar in structure to cholesterol that can inhibit cholesterol absorption by the body. They are also an excellent source of hearth healthy vitamin B6.

Type	Quantity	Nutrients and % of Daily Value (DV)	Benefits
Walnuts	1 oz (28g)	Copper, 49% Manganese, 42–53% Iron, 15–10% Phosphorus, 14% Vitamin B6, 12% Magnesium, 10–14% Also: Mono- and poly-unsaturated fats ORAC score = 3,791	Walnuts meet the recommended daily value for heart healthy, brain-boosting omega-3 oils in one 1.5-oz serving. Like pistachios, they also contain phytosterols, compounds similar in structure to cholesterol that can inhibit cholesterol absorption by the body. Plus, they're a source of gamma-tocopherol, a unique form of vitamin E thought to inhibit prostate- and lung-cancer cell division. Walnuts may also help calm and moisten dry, irritated skin. An ounce of walnuts contains *twice* the amount of omega-3 and omega-6 fatty acids found in the flaxseed and borage oils used by German and French scientists to reduce skin redness and dry, flaky skin. A study of 45 women, ages 18 to 65, found that skin redness was reduced by 44% after 12 weeks, and the skin also retained 17% to 19% more water.

Bean Superfoods

Type	Quantity	Nutrients and % of Daily Value (DV)	Benefits
Black Beans	1 cup, cooked (172g)	Folate, 64% Iron, 45–20% Copper, 40% Fiber, 39–60% Vitamin B1, 35–38% Phosphorus, 34% Manganese, 33–42% Magnesium, 30–39% Vitamin B3, 24–28% Zinc, 18–24% Potassium, 13%	Black beans are loaded with antioxidants, ranking fourth among bean sources of antioxidants per gram. They're also the top bean source of magnesium—a mighty mineral lacking in the diets of 64% of men and 67% of women that has been shown to help lower the risk of colon cancer, diabetes and high blood pressure.
Red Kidney Beans	1 cup, cooked (177g)	Iron, 65–29% Folate, 58% Fiber, 34–52% Magnesium, 18–25% Zinc, 17–24% Vitamin B6, 16% Potassium, 15%	Red kidney beans rank second-highest in antioxidants among all beans. They also provide nearly 60% of daily folate needs, helping to maintain heart health and guard against colorectal cancer. Note: If you're among the 50% of Americans who fail to get enough fiber, keep some kidney beans on hand; 1 cup (cooked) provides about half the daily fiber needs for women and one third for men.
Navy Beans	1 cup, cooked (182g)	Folate, 64% Iron, 54–24% Fiber, 50–76% Copper, 42% Phosphorus, 37% Thiamin, 36% Magnesium, 23–30% Zinc, 17–23% Potassium, 15%	Sometimes known as great northern beans, navy beans are the top bean source of fiber. Just 1 cup provides half the daily requirement to help control cholesterol levels. They're also the top bean source of phosphorus, a mineral needed for healthy bones and teeth—especially important for women ages 9 to 18, 40% of whom do not get adequate phosphorus.

Type	Quantity	Nutrients and % of Daily Value (DV)	Benefits
Lima Beans	1 cup, cooked (188g)	Iron, 56–25% Manganese, 42–54% Folate, 39% Fiber, 34–52% Phosphorus, 30% Vitamin B1, 25–28% Vitamin B3, 23–26% Vitamin B6, 23% Magnesium, 20–26% Potassium, 20% Zinc, 16–22% Vitamin B5, 16% Selenium, 15% Choline, 11–14%	Limas are the top bean source of potassium, a mineral needed for blood pressure regulation. Of men, 90% don't get enough potassium, and nearly 100% of women. Lima beans also contain the phytochemicals coumestrol and saponin, compounds that may impart anticancer benefits.
Pinto Beans	1 cup, cooked (171g)	Folate, 74% Iron, 45–20% Fiber, 39–60% Phosphorus, 36% Manganese, 34–43% Vitamin B6, 30% Vitamin B1, 28–30% Vitamin B3, 23–26% Magnesium, 21–28% Selenium, 19% Potassium, 16% Zinc, 15–21% Choline, 11–14% Vitamin E, 11%	Pinto beans are a top bean source of selenium—a trace mineral linked to lower prostate-cancer risk. Pintos are also ranked higher than blueberries in antioxidant power.

Whole-Grain Superfoods

Type	Quantity	Nutrients and % of Daily Value (DV)	Benefits
Oatmeal	1 cup, cooked (234g)	Manganese, 59–75% Phosphorus, 26% Iron, 26–12% Selenium, 23% Zinc, 21–29% Copper, 19% Magnesium, 16–20% Vitamin B1, 15–16% Vitamin B5, 15% Vitamin B3, 12–14% Fiber, 11–16%	Oats are most famous for their soluble fiber. They are an excellent source of iron, zinc, phosphorus and selenium, as well as being a good source of copper. They also have plenty of B vitamins, which help convert food to energy and promote muscles, brain function, and healthy skin and hair.
Quinoa	1 cup, cooked (185g)	Manganese, 51–65% Phosphorus, 40% Copper, 39% Iron, 35–15% Magnesium, 30–38% Folate, 19% Zinc, 18–25% Vitamin B6, 18% Vitamin B1, 17–18% Vitamin B2, 16–19% Vitamin B3, 15–17% Fiber, 13–20%	Quinoa incorporates quite a lot of nutrients into tiny seeds. It contains more protein than most grains and offers a more evenly balanced array of amino acids, the building blocks of protein. Quinoa is also higher in phosphorus, magnesium, copper, zinc and iron than most grains.

Type	Quantity	Nutrients and % of Daily Value (DV)	Benefits
Whole Wheat Bread	2 slices (56g)	Manganese, 52–66% Selenium, 41% Copper, 23% Vitamin B3, 21–24% Iron, 17–8% Vitamin B1, 16–18% Phosphorus, 16% Fiber, 11–16% Magnesium, 11–15% Biotin, 11% Sodium, 11%	Whole wheat products are the most nutritious of wheat products because they have not been milled as extensively as more refined items have been. Whole wheat products are high in manganese, selenium and copper.
Brown Rice, (medium-grain)	1 cup, cooked (195g)	Manganese, 93–119% Selenium, 25% Vitamin B3, 22–26% Vitamin B6, 22% Magnesium, 21–28% Phosphorus, 21% Vitamin B1, 17–18% Vitamin B5, 15% Iron, 13–6% Fiber, 11–16% Zinc, 11–15%	Because brown rice only has its tough hull removed during processing, it retains most of the nutrients that more refined products are missing. Brown rice is a good source of fiber, potassium, phosphorus and selenium.

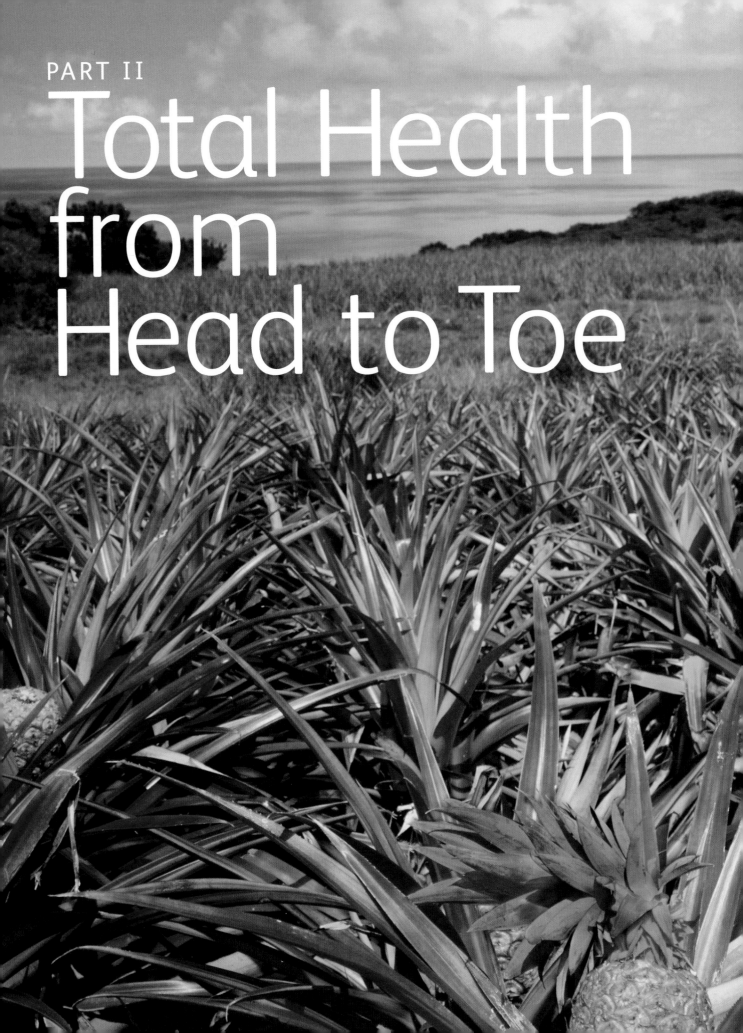

PART II

Total Health from Head to Toe

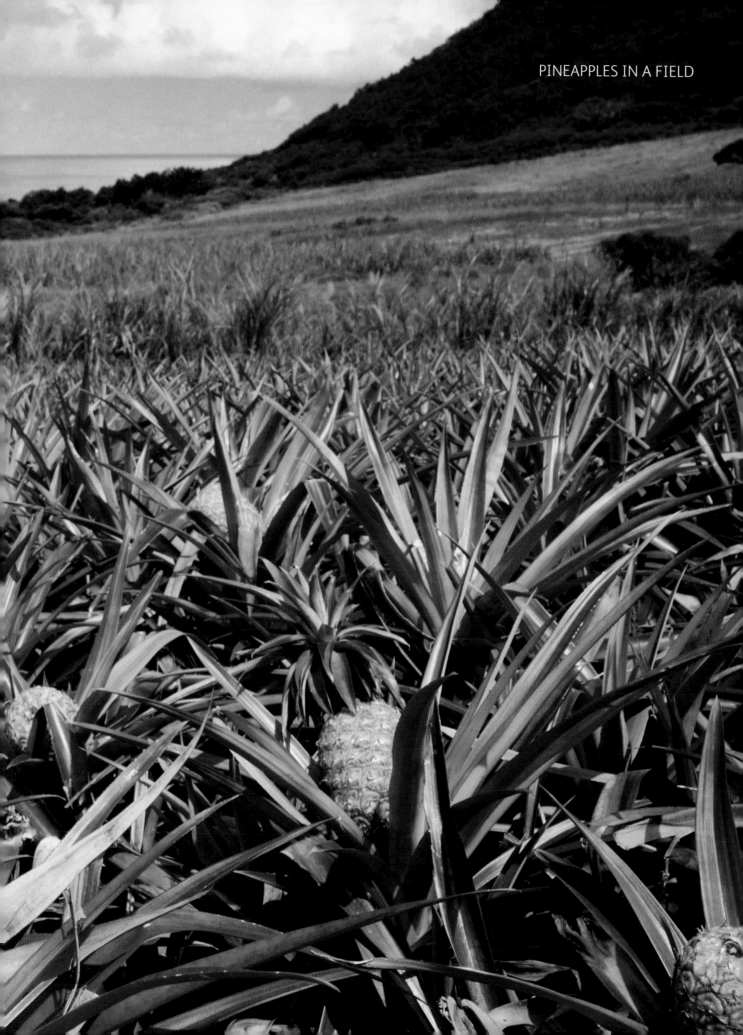

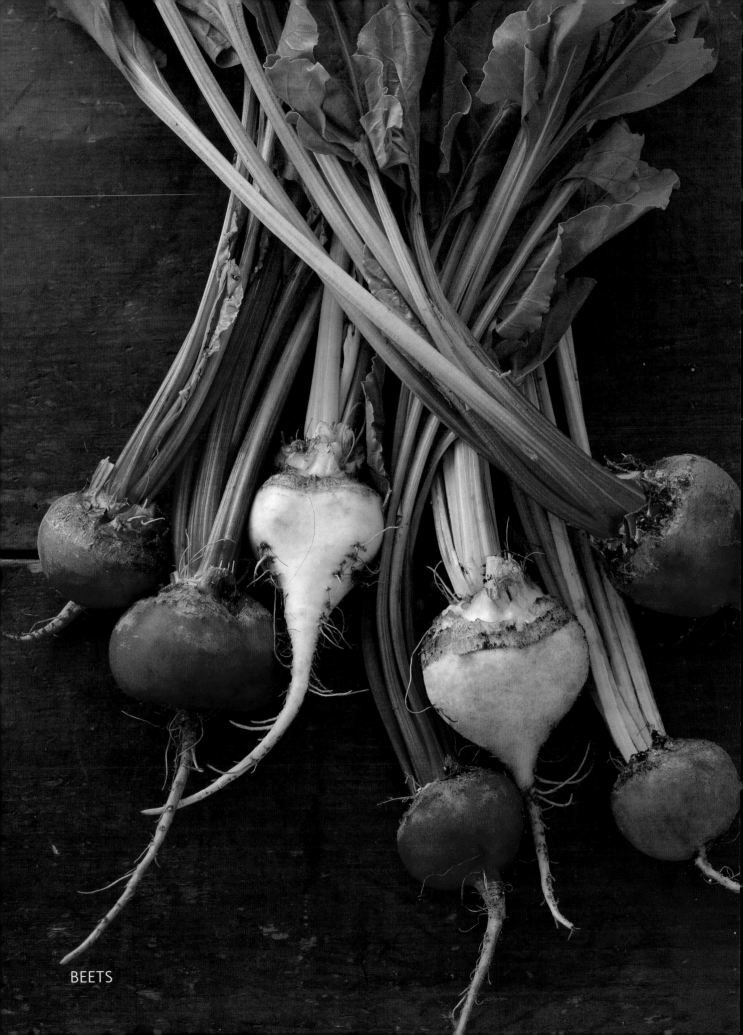

BEETS

CHAPTER 4

You Are What You Eat

Gaining a better understanding of the link between food and health will be one of the biggest challenges—and opportunities—of the 21st century. What you eat should enhance your health, not undermine it, and yet the American diet—high in refined sugar, processed carbohydrates, saturated and trans fats—adds up to too many calories and too few nutrients. For the first time in the history of the United States, according to the Centers for Disease Control and Prevention (CDC), poor diet and inactivity are threatening to overtake smoking as the leading cause of preventable death.

At the same time, scientists are rapidly discovering new compounds in fruits and vegetables that have the potential to prevent disease and lengthen life. What's more, while fad diets come and go, countless studies confirm that diets rich in fruits and vegetables are the key to losing weight. In this chapter, some of the leading experts from Dole's North Carolina Research Campus—Steven Leath, PhD, of the University of North Carolina; Mary Ann Lila, PhD, of North Carolina State University; and Keith Erikson, PhD, of the University of North Carolina at Greensboro—explain how and why fruits and vegetables are so good for us, how the plants themselves evolve to bear nutrients and antioxidants, and how humans metabolize and utilize nutrients for optimal health.

▶ Steven Leath

Steven Leath, PhD, is currently vice president for research of the University of North Carolina (UNC) system, promoting research at UNC's 16 university campuses. Previously affiliated with North Carolina State University for more than two decades, he holds a bachelor's degree in plant science from the Pennsylvania State University, a master's degree in the field from the University of Delaware, and a doctorate in plant pathology from the University of Illinois.

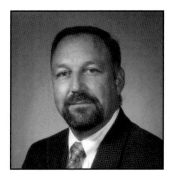

Much of this book is devoted to explanations of how components of our food affect the brain, heart, overall health and many other facets of our well-being—which begs the questions: Where do these nutrients come from, why do they exist in our food and what was their role before they got to us?

Plants and humans have the same basic biological processes, and thus need many of the same nutrients. But we diverge in our abilities to ingest minerals and transform them into usable forms. Plants can extract minerals from the soil or water, whereas humans rely on plants to take up minerals for them. We get seven essential minerals from plants—nitrogen, phosphorus, sulfur, potassium, calcium, magnesium and iron—all of which play a critical role in our health and survival.

When you see a sequence of three numbers, such as 20-10-10, on a bag of fertilizer, it represents the breakdown of nitrogen, phosphorus and potassium. Most important biochemical processes in plants and animals require potassium. In humans, potassium is involved with nerve function, muscle control and blood pressure, possibly through regulating water balance—which is similar to its role in water balance in plants.

In addition to fertilizer, we often put lime on our gardens, because the calcium it contains is essential to both plants and humans. In plants, calcium plays a critical role in membrane structuring and pollen growth and development. Calcium can move only from the roots to the shoots of plants, but not back down, so this mineral accumulates in excess levels of a plant's needs. In humans, calcium is the most abundant mineral in the body and is critical to our growth, development and maintenance of health. Calcium's role in strengthening the cell walls of plants is similar to its structural role in our bones and teeth.

In the popular press, the role of minerals is often overshadowed by other plant components that figure into human health—for instance, pigments, such as the carotenoids, lycopene and flavonoids. Chlorophyll, which gives plants their green color, is perhaps the most important pigment. Although it doesn't have a direct nutrition benefit to humans, it's responsible for the transformation of light energy into chemical energy—essentially turning light into food.

There's an entire spectrum of pigments, thought to have protective properties in plants, that function as nutraceuticals in humans, with documented effects on cancer, heart disease, vision problems and other disorders. The carotenoids, responsible for the great fall-colored pigments in carrots, squash, apricots and other fruits and vegetables, enable plants to absorb and utilize light energy over a broader range of wavelengths and protect chlorophyll from sun damage. Plants can produce carotenoids in response to environmental stresses and thereby protect themselves, not unlike how they protect us. The orange and red pigments have broad antioxidant properties as well as more specific roles, such as combating prostate cancer,

> We get seven essential minerals from plants, all of which are key to health and survival.

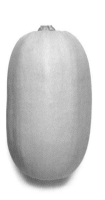

SPAGHETTI SQUASH

delaying macular degeneration, improving immune system efficiency, and protecting against heart disease and cancer.

Similarly the flavonoid compounds, which include the red, blue and purple pigments, contribute to a wide array of human functions. Their antioxidant activity helps protect plants from harmful ultraviolet radiation, and in humans, they're thought to help improve night vision, combat age-related neurological disorders and reduce the incidence of heart disease.

The role of plant pigments is not fully understood due to the way they function in complex interactions rather than alone—which is why eating whole fruits and vegetables is often more effective in maintaining a healthy diet than taking supplements. When you consider the array of vibrant colors in fruits and vegetables, from tomatoes and peppers to watermelon and blueberries, it's easy to imagine that plant pigments are nature's way of attracting us to the most healthful fruits and vegetables.

Mary Ann Lila

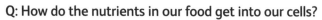

Professor Mary Ann Lila, PhD, is the director of the Plants for Human Health Institute, North Carolina State University, North Carolina Research Campus. She holds the endowed David H. Murdock Chair, and is a professor in the Department of Food, Bioprocessing and Nutrition Science. She develops and promotes fruits and vegetables with enhanced health benefits, utilizing plant breeding and biochemical analysis. Previously, Dr. Lila was a faculty member at the University of Illinois for more than 24 years.

Q: How do the nutrients in our food get into our cells?

MAL: First, I think it may be important to differentiate between nutrients and nutraceuticals, both of which come from our food and play important roles in health maintenance.

Nutrients are compounds from plant or animal food sources that are essential for the human body to grow and function properly. Proteins, vitamins, minerals and carbohydrates are included in this group.

Nutraceuticals are not integral to growth and development, but they're highly beneficial as part of our diet because of their specific roles in prevention or therapy against chronic human diseases. For example, some of the pigments produced by plants can impede the development of cardiovascular disease, various cancers, diabetes, infections and more.

Phytochemicals are an important category of nutraceuticals. Once ingested, they can contribute to a variety of physiological functions, whether by inhibiting an enzyme that would otherwise lead to disease symptoms, favoring a pathway that leads to lower blood sugar levels or helping to bolster the immune response. Fruits and vegetables are particularly concentrated, rich sources of nutraceutical phytochemicals, which is why they're so important in proactively maintaining optimal health.

Q: Aren't nutraceuticals supplements made from nutrients that are extracted from foods?

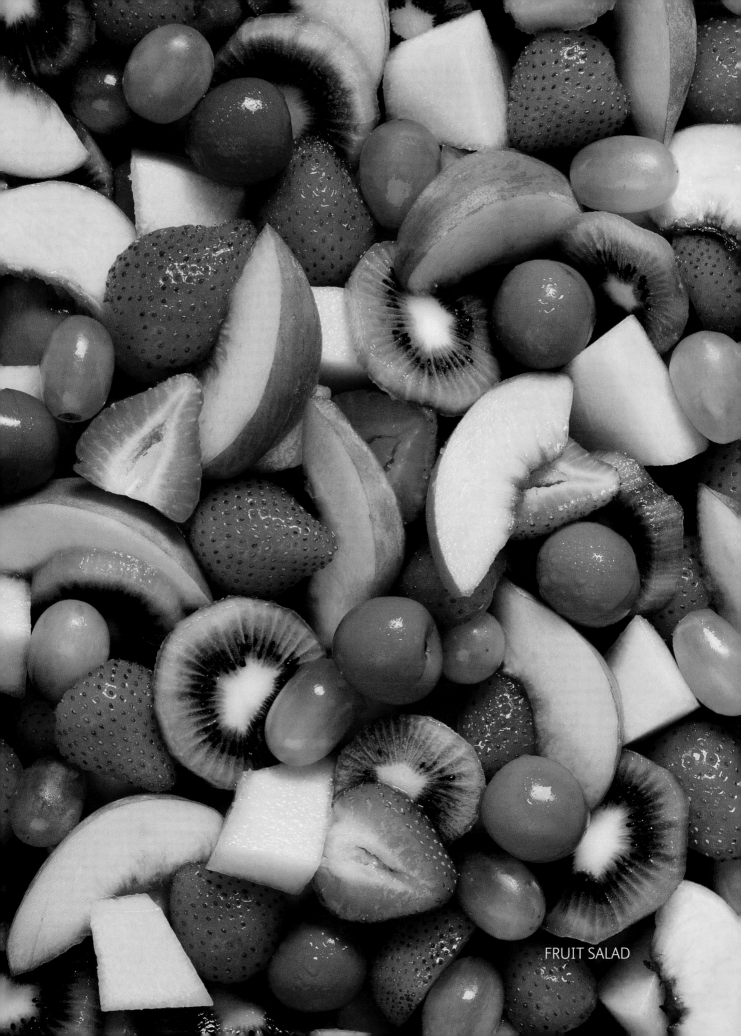

FRUIT SALAD

We've now shown that compounds from fruit do in fact penetrate, and benefit, the brain.

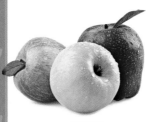

APPLES

FOOD TIP
Give your peeler a rest—Red Delicious apples with the skin have 45 percent more antioxidants than naked ones. Among these antioxidants is quercetin, which is thought to protect against Alzheimer's, boost bone health, ease prostate pain and support immunity.

MAL: Nutraceuticals are also the foods themselves—and many of us believe that it's more effective to receive their benefits from whole foods than supplements. Digestion is key. For the human body to benefit from nutrients or nutraceuticals, foods must be broken down into components. The digestion process begins as soon as food is eaten. First, enzymes in the mouth begin breaking structures into smaller components, which enter the esophagus when we swallow. Then, gastric enzymes and acids in the stomach further break down those structures until they become liquid and can pass into the small intestine. There, digestion and absorption continue in earnest, as enzymes and secretions break down what remains into component nutrients and nutraceuticals that can be readily absorbed.

The extent to which a food component can be absorbed during digestion and then distributed into tissues and fluids of the body is what's considered its bioavailability. The components released from the food during digestion may be immediately bioavailable, or they may need to be further broken down before the body can make use of them.

Q: What determines how bioavailable a food constituent is?

MAL: This is an interesting puzzle. Consider the anthocyanin pigments, which provide the red to blue colors in many fruits, vegetables and flowers. They're very stable, but only at highly acidic pHs. Hydrangea plants, which shift in flower color from blue to pink and white depending on the pH of the soil, provide a graphic example of how pH influences the stability of anthocyanins. Humans consume a significant amount of anthocyanins in wine and various fruits and vegetables—and the vast majority disappear from the gastrointestinal tract within a few hours of consumption—but it's unclear how much of the intake is degraded in the body and how much is modified to another, more active or available form of the molecule. Anthocyanin consumption has been linked to protection against cardiovascular disease, diabetes, some cancers and infections, but we still don't know exactly how anthocyanins work.

Q: Is there progress in coming to a better understanding?

MAL: Research has shown that after ingestion, anthocyanins are absorbed intact and then transported in the blood to organs throughout the body. But for a long time, many scientists doubted that anthocyanins from fruits could be transported to the brain or have a role in moderating cognitive health. There was anecdotal evidence that, for example, red wines or fruits in the diet benefited cognitive function, but these observations were disputed because the molecules were assumed to be too large to pass through the blood-brain barrier. Only recently were we able to conclusively show that compounds from fruit cells do indeed get into the brain—where they may have a role in the prevention of Alzheimer's disease and other brain disorders.

Q: What are your recommendations for maximizing the health benefits available through food?

MAL: Your dietary choices should be based on a diversity of health-protective foods—not on meals that are quick, easy and convenient. Variety is really the key. The human body is a highly complex organism that requires constant, consistent and multiple nutrients and nutraceuticals from different foods—especially the nutrient and nutraceutical-rich fruit and vegetable groups—in order to most efficiently work on multiple therapeutic targets and tissues at once, while maximizing performance, health and life span.

▶ Keith Erikson

Keith Erikson, PhD, is an associate professor in the Department of Nutrition at the University of North Carolina at Greensboro, who has published numerous papers on oxidative stress. Currently, his laboratory is focusing on understanding how trace element imbalances (iron and manganese) in the brain can leave the central nervous system vulnerable to toxicity and disease. His work could improve the lives of people suffering from Parkinson's and other diseases that impact the central nervous system.

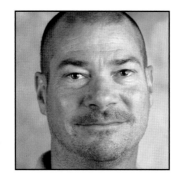

Q: What is an antioxidant and why do plants have them?

KE: An antioxidant is a compound that fights the oxygen-containing molecules—called free radicals—that naturally occur in our cells. Examples of these antioxidants are vitamins C and E, carotenoids and flavonoids. Fruits and vegetables are rich sources for each of these antioxidants because the plants that produce these foods use these compounds to protect themselves from pests (flavonoids) and to attract insects and birds for pollination purposes (carotenoids). Recent scientific studies suggest that the flavonoids and carotenoids found in fruits and vegetables may provide health benefits in addition to their antioxidant roles.

Q: How do the antioxidants in food help the body?

KE: High levels of cellular free radicals are linked to diseases such as cancer and heart disease, as well as to aging. When we eat foods rich in antioxidants, we provide our cells with the compounds they need to "neutralize" the harmful effects of free radicals, and this greatly reduces the risk of several chronic diseases.

Q: How do we know which foods are high in antioxidants?

KE: The National Cancer Institute recommends that people eat a colorful variety of fruits, vegetables and whole grains everyday. This ensures that you not only get the antioxidants found naturally in plants, but also consume other compounds that support antioxidant function and provide healthful benefits.

Q: What is ORAC and how can a food's ORAC score translate into helping us live healthier lives?

KE: Oxygen Radical Absorbance Capacity (ORAC) is a method for assessing a food or supplement's antioxidant abilities. The United States Department of Agriculture (USDA) recently compiled a list of the ORAC scores for more than 200 foods, and many nutritionists use these scores to strategically plan a more healthful diet. Because the ORAC method measures only one aspect of a food's nutrition value, there's not necessarily a direct correlation between a high ORAC score and increased health benefits. For example, dry cocoa powder has one of the highest ORAC scores reported on the USDA list, but is it healthier than a handful of blueberries? The answer, of course, is no: The blueberries provide much more than antioxidant abilities; they're high in fiber and nutrients, while the cocoa powder isn't. Thus, choosing foods that are nutrient dense coupled with a high ORAC score would be an excellent strategy for healthy dietary planning.

Foods rich in anti-oxidants help offset damage caused by free radicals.

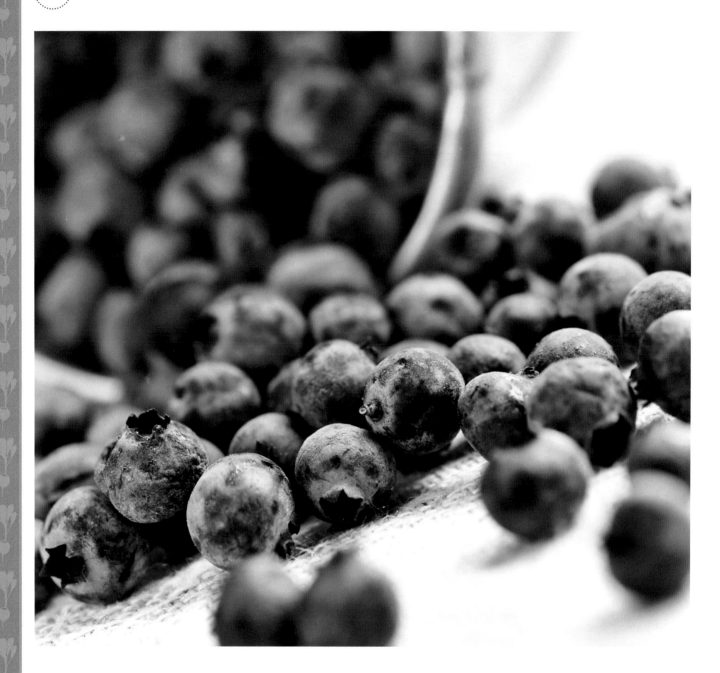

ALL-AROUND HEALTHY,
BLUEBERRIES ARE
PACKED WITH
ANTIOXIDANTS, FIBER
AND OTHER NUTRIENTS.

Q: What's your opinion of the effectiveness of the antioxidants contained in foods versus those in supplements?

KE: To date, no scientific study has demonstrated that receiving antioxidants in supplement form provides health advantages over receiving them from food. In fact, the studies that have looked at the health benefits from antioxidants contained in supplements showed that there was no benefit, and in some cases, there were even negative health effects associated with supplement intake. When you eat fruits and vegetables that are loaded with antioxidants, you're also ingesting other compounds that likely have health properties and/or may assist the antioxidants with their disease-fighting roles. Therefore, in my opinion, antioxidants in food are superior to those in supplements.

Antioxidants

Most people tend to think of oxygen as life-giving—and it can be. You breathe it into your lungs, and it travels via your blood to every cell of your being, revitalizing and reenergizing your organs and muscles. Who would suspect that oxygen has a dark side too? Well, it does. Because of its molecular structure, oxygen causes the oxidation (the rust, if you will) of organic life, and oxidative stress contributes to disease risk. But antioxidants help counteract oxygen's destructive potential, sacrificing electrons to neutralize, or rebalance, molecules that have destabilized due to oxidative influence.

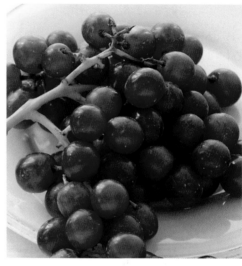

While not as well-known as common vitamins and minerals, antioxidants are gaining attention for their power to slow aging and protect against disease. They neutralize free radicals, which are harmful, unstable molecules generated by your body in response to environmental stresses, such as smoke, pollution, poor diet and overexposure to the sun.

Metabolizing rich foods, in particular, tends to produce an overload of free radicals, which drain the body's antioxidant reserves. A study suggests a simple solution. USDA researchers found that eating certain fruits almost instantly replenishes any drop in antioxidant levels experienced after eating a caloric meal. Thus, their recommendation: Consume high-antioxidant foods—such as blueberries, grapes, cherries, kiwifruits and strawberries—with each meal to prevent postprandial damage.

GO FOR THE GRAPES FOR A RICH DOSE OF ANTIOXIDANTS, MANGANESE, AND VITAMINS C, B1 AND B6.

Certain organs, certain cells and certain aspects of your physiology may be more vulnerable to one particular free radical or another, just as certain antioxidants found in different fruits and vegetables may be more effective in combating one particular free radical than another. Still, antioxidants are just one measure of a food's nutrition power: Foods that are high in antioxidant activity aren't necessarily healthier, overall, than foods that are lower in antioxidant activity. For example, apples rank near the top of the antioxidant charts, but bananas, which rank lower in antioxidants, are, in fact, gram per

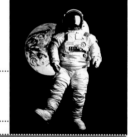

Berries in Space

Cutting-edge research by James Joseph, PhD, and Barbara Shukitt-Hale, PhD, suggests that the antioxidants in berries and other foods could someday protect astronauts against the radiation-induced free-radical damage experienced during extended space flight. Given the similarities between the effects of aging and of radiation on the brain, researchers fed strawberry and blueberry extracts—which have proven effective in ameliorating the consequences of aging—to rats and then simulated the radioactive conditions of space travel. The berry-fed rats weathered irradiation without experiencing the ill effects observed in the control group: tumor development, rapid aging, hair loss and a severely shortened life span. In fact, the berry-fed irradiated rats fared as well as those that had not been irradiated at all.

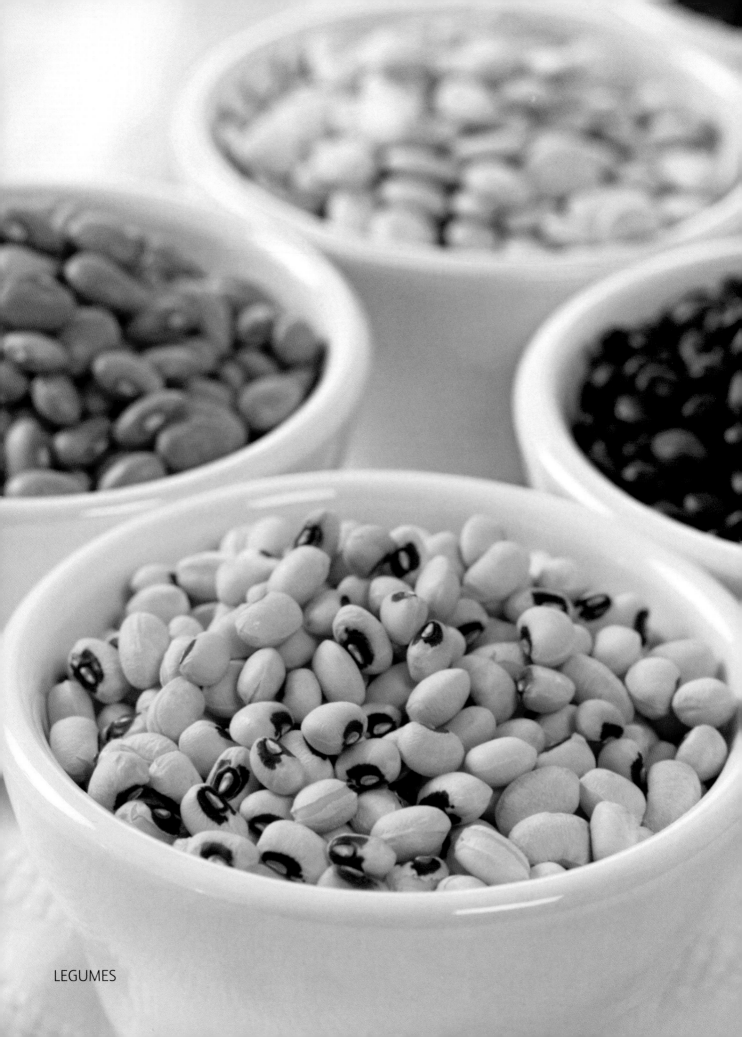

LEGUMES

gram much higher in important nutrients like vitamin C (twice as high), vitamin B6 (nearly 10 times higher), and potassium (more than three times higher) compared with apples.

Another thing to keep in mind: Antioxidant rankings are not set in stone. For example, just when you thought blueberries were No.1 in antioxidants, a *Life* magazine article featured a different ranking, demoting blueberries to No. 5, behind blackberries, strawberries, cranberries and raspberries. Then, there is the Mayo Clinic newsletter, which gave the top three antioxidant slots to three varieties of dried beans: red, kidney and pinto.

Why the variation? Who's right? They all are. A number of factors affect a food's placement within a given antioxidant list. These factors include: (a) which antioxidant test is being used; (b) what's being ranked—e.g., all foods, or just fruits and vegetables; (c) whether serving size or gram for gram is being compared; and (d) whether serving-size rankings take into account USDA portion-size revisions.

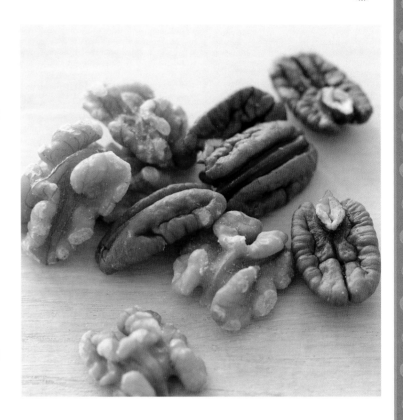

Consider blueberries, which were crowned antioxidant king using the Oxygen Radical Absorbance Capacity (ORAC) assay. The latest, most comprehensive ORAC ranking was published before the latest round of USDA serving size revisions, which upgraded the standard apple serving portion from 154 to 242 grams—and catapulted Red Delicious apples above blueberries.

Despite its ubiquity, ORAC is not the only antioxidant game in town. The Norwegian researchers who published the ranking that places blackberries first used a different method. But regardless of which measurement is used, rankings get reshuffled again when foods are compared gram for gram rather than by serving size. For example, artichokes and cranberries come out ahead of blueberries when measured in terms of grams—but not when measured by serving size.

The picture can shift yet again depending on whether the antioxidant ranking is limited to fruits and vegetables or broadened to include legumes, nuts and spices. For instance, while dried beans rank high when legumes are included, if you add nuts to the mix—particularly, pecans and walnuts—then beans suffer a significant drop in status. When spices are also included, ground cloves blow the roof off the rankings entirely—but keep in mind, that's in a gram-for-gram comparison (as opposed to serving size).

Furthermore, most antioxidant rankings reflect only the free radical scavenging power of direct antioxidants—those contained within the plants themselves—and not indirect antioxidants, which activate your body's own detoxification processes. Most of the antioxidants you read about, such as lycopene, lutein, beta-carotene and

GRAM FOR GRAM, PECANS AND WALNUTS ARE AMONG THE TOP FOOD SOURCES FOR ANTIOXIDANTS.

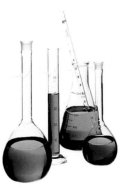

BEAKERS

An-Tea-Oxidants

Green, white and black teas get their antioxidant powers from flavanols called catechins. They all come from the same plant, with the differences between them having to do with how the leaves are treated after harvesting. White tea is made from steamed and dried new buds and leaves, while green tea involves a light steaming of the mature leaves. The steaming process prevents naturally occurring tea enzymes from oxidizing the plant. Left unchecked, the enzymes naturally produce black tea. Although not as high in antioxidants as its lighter colored counterparts, black tea retains powerful health benefits. An Indian study showed that black-tea extract significantly reduced the oxidative stress that can lead to prostate cancer.

FOOD TIP

Red cabbage combines the detox power of cruciferous vegetables with anthocyanins, a type of antioxidant that's usually associated with berries. The glucosinolates in red cabbage trigger the body's own natural detoxification enzymes while the anthocyanins directly neutralize harmful free radicals.

RED CABBAGE

quercetin, act as direct antioxidants. When you consume fruits and vegetables that contain these compounds, they work directly to neutralize free radicals by absorbing their negative energy, rendering them harmless and allowing them to be flushed out of your system.

While you get a one-shot, finite amount of direct antioxidants from eating a particular fruit or vegetable, indirect antioxidant activity—kicked off by consumption of cruciferous veggies—actually cycles over and over within the physiology and continues to offer protective benefits for as many as three to four days after the glucosinolate-containing food has been consumed. Despite this extremely powerful—and extended—antioxidant cascade, none of the glucosinolate-rich, cruciferous vegetables made it into the USDA's ORAC rankings.

Researchers at the Johns Hopkins University School of Medicine estimate that broccoli sprouts have the highest indirect antioxidant power (from glucosinolates) of all cruciferous vegetables, providing 20 to 50 times that of a mature broccoli. Just 2 or 3 tablespoons of broccoli sprouts per day provide a powerful dose. After broccoli sprouts, cauliflower sprouts are second highest in terms of glucosinolates. Sprouts that aren't in the cruciferous family, such as alfalfa sprouts, aren't as high in these compounds.

Researchers speculate that indirect antioxidants are most concentrated in the budding plant because the organism needs a high concentration of protective phytochemicals to shield it from predators, pollution and the elements. As plants grow, their phytonutrients become somewhat diluted in concentration, although they're still present and retain their health benefits when eaten. The chewing process sets off the effect, mixing glucosinolates with plant enzymes (they're normally separated by the plant's cell walls), which converts them into their active form and then triggers the detoxification process.

Glucosinolates are a hot topic in phytochemical research right now. Some studies suggest that they help lower blood pressure; other studies are focusing on their potential preventative benefits for various cancers, such as those of the stomach, colon, esophagus, lung and breast.

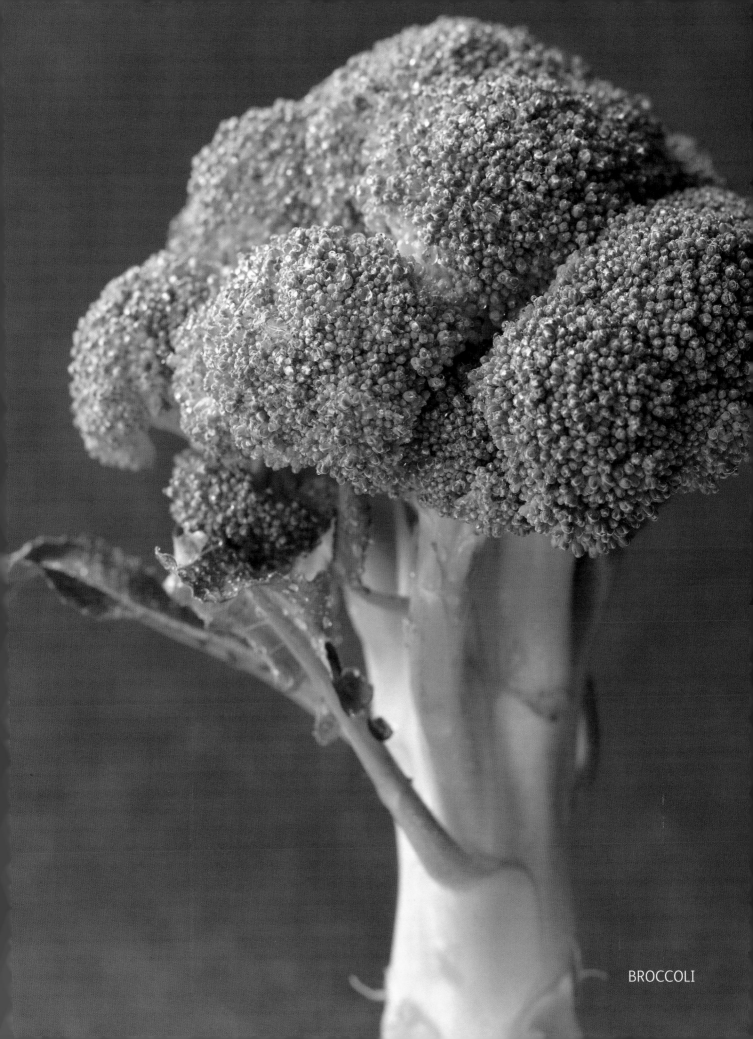

BROCCOLI

DIET TIP

An easy way to increase your intake of fruits and vegetables is by adding them to what you already eat. Slice bananas onto your cereal, add extra lettuce to your sandwiches, slice bell peppers onto your pizza, toss mushrooms into your pasta or give antioxidant-rich berries a starring role in your desserts.

Get Antioxidants from Food, Not Supplements

Whether antioxidants are as beneficial when taken in supplement form as they are in whole foods has been the topic of much debate. While clinical studies have found some conflicting information, a growing number of meta-analyses (reviews of previous studies) are reporting some disconcerting discoveries. A 2008 review by the Cochrane Collaboration of 67 large, randomized controlled trials involving more than 200,000 participants came to the conclusion that antioxidant supplements are largely ineffective when it comes to preventing disease and prolonging life. It even found evidence that some supplements—including vitamin A, beta-carotene and vitamin E—may actually increase mortality.

These findings echo those of a watershed study, published in 2004 in the *Lancet*, which reviewed 14 randomized trials with more than 170,000 participants to establish whether antioxidant pills reduce the risk of gastrointestinal cancer. Far from finding any protective benefits of such supplements, it reports, "on the contrary, they seem to increase overall mortality." Similarly, the Alpha-Tocopherol Beta-Carotene (ATBC) Cancer Prevention Study, which involved more than 29,000 male smokers and was completed in 1996 in Finland, found that lung cancer incidence was 18 percent higher (and the death rate 8 percent higher) among those who took a beta-carotene supplement over a period of five to eight years, compared with those who received a placebo or other treatment. And, more recently, a 2009 study found that longer use of beta-carotene, retinol and lutein supplements in the general population (as opposed to just smokers) was associated with a higher risk for lung cancer.

British Paradox

In the French paradox, red wine polyphenols are credited with countering the negative effects of saturated fat, which is so abundant in French cuisine. Along similar lines, researchers have wondered why the U.K.'s tea consumption doesn't translate into the protective effects that drinking tea has in Asia. In the British paradox, milk gets the blame. The assumption has been that milk proteins bind with and neutralize tea's polyphenol activity, but findings suggest that that may not be the case: In a small study at the University of Aberdeen in Scotland, nine male volunteers, ages 24 to 37, had their blood tested for antioxidant presence after drinking tea with and without milk. A brewing time of seven minutes yielded the maximum antioxidant activity—regardless of whether milk was added or not. On the other hand, another recent study raises the possibility that milk may act in a different way to blunt tea's cardiovascular benefits. German researchers had 16 female volunteers consume either freshly brewed black tea, black tea with 10 percent skimmed milk, or boiled water (as a control). The black tea drinkers showed significantly improved blood flow and vessel dilation compared with the water drinkers, whereas the addition of milk completely blunted the effects of tea. The researchers speculated that the inhibiting effect was caused by the interaction between caseins (the predominant protein in milk) and catechins (the antioxidants in tea).

When it comes to heart disease, the findings suggest supplements are a waste of money at best. A 2007 *Archives of Internal Medicine* report analyzing the effects of beta-carotene and vitamins C and E on cardiovascular disease in more than 8,000 high-risk women over age 40 concluded that the supplements "had no overall effect." Along similar lines, the Physicians' Health Study-II, which has been tracking 14,641 doctors (over 50-years-old at the start) for nearly a decade, concluded in 2007 that neither vitamin E nor vitamin C supplements were effective in reducing the risk of major cardiovascular events. In an even more troubling report, which appeared in the May 2004 issue of the *Journal of Clinical Investigation,* researchers at Mount Sinai School of Medicine in New York came to the conclusion that vitamin E pills were actually responsible for increasing LDL (bad) cholesterol in animal studies.

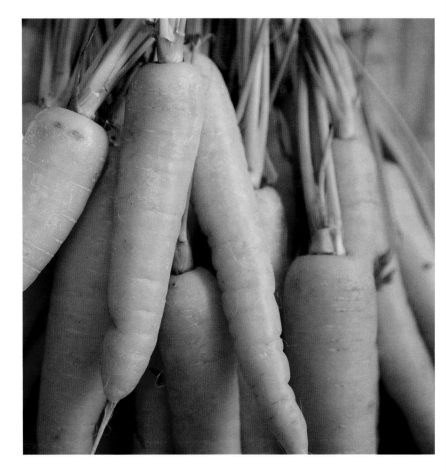

If antioxidant-rich fruits and veggies are associated with decreased risk of cancer and cardiovascular disease, why would antioxidant supplements on their own show little benefit, or even potential risk? As mentioned in Chapter 1, a likely possibility is that the many different nutrients—vitamins, minerals and phytochemical antioxidants—within whole foods work in synergy, so when they're isolated from their natural matrix, the body may process them differently, making their effect different as well.

Conclusion

There's still much to learn about the manifold, seemingly miraculous properties of antioxidants and other health-supporting compounds in fruit and vegetables, but the known universe is rapidly expanding. Case in point: More than 4,000 flavonoids have been identified —which sounds like a lot until you consider that flavonoids are just one small subcategory of antioxidants. As researchers report findings from all over the globe, it's become increasingly clear that Mother Nature has done much to provide an abundance of nutritive sources to counter the molecular wear and tear that occurs as you breathe, eat, exercise and age. It's left to us to continue the process of discovery.

RESEARCH INDICATES WHOLE FOOD SOURCES, SUCH AS CARROTS, ARE PREFERABLE TO SUPPLEMENTS FOR ANTIOXIDANTS.

FOOD TIP
When you wash your fruits and vegetables before eating or preparing, make sure they get a shower— not a bath. Just give fresh produce a quick dip and scrub, as vitamins can leach out the longer they sit in water.

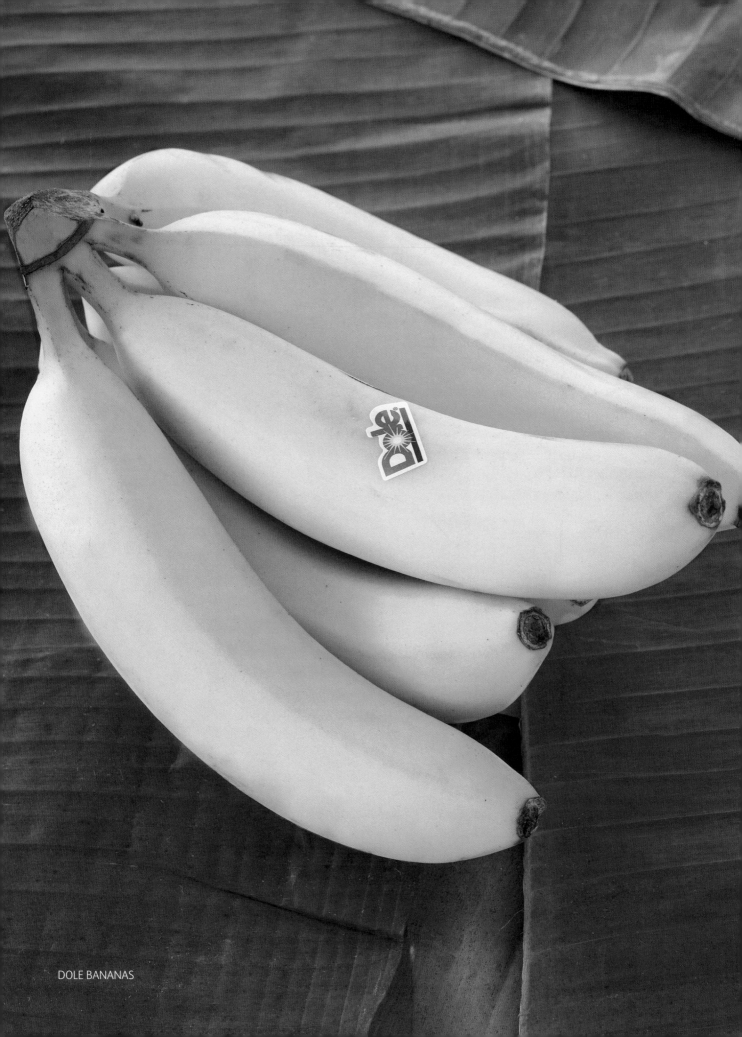

DOLE BANANAS

CHAPTER 5

Heart Health

You Need: FIBER, POTASSIUM, FOLATE, VITAMIN B6, MAGNESIUM, VITAMIN C, ANTIOXIDANTS

Eat These:

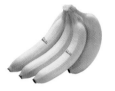

BANANAS

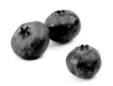

BLUEBERRIES

GUAVA

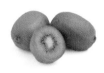

KIWIFRUITS

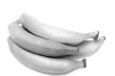

PLANTAINS

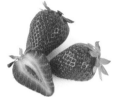

STRAWBERRIES

ORANGES

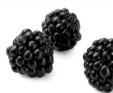

BLACKBERRIES

RASPBERRIES

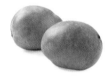

MANGOES

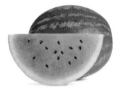

WATERMELON

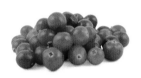

CRANBERRIES

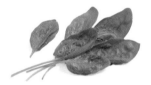

SPINACH

BROCCOLI

SWISS CHARD

RED BELL PEPPER

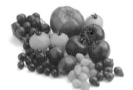

TOMATOES

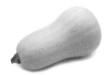

BUTTERNUT SQUASH

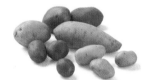

POTATOES

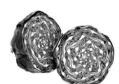

RED CABBAGE

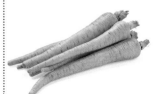

PARSNIPS

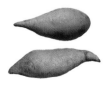

YAMS

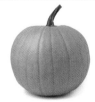

PUMPKIN

ACORN SQUASH

▶ L. Kristin Newby

She is an associate professor of Cardiology at Duke University Medical Center. Dr. Newby's general research interests include risk assessment and treatment of patients with acute and chronic coronary artery disease and ways to improve delivery of care to patients with these illnesses. L. Kristin Newby, MD, MHSc, serves as principal investigator on the MURDOCK Study cardiovascular disease project.

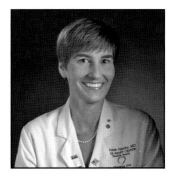

Q: What is cholesterol and how does it contribute to heart disease risk?

LKN: Cholesterol is a type of blood lipid. It has a number of subfractions. High-density lipoprotein cholesterol (sometimes called HDL, or "good" cholesterol) protects against atherosclerosis, while low-density lipoprotein cholesterol (LDL, or "bad" cholesterol) leads to the development of atherosclerosis. As the body tries to eliminate cholesterol, it becomes oxidized and is taken up by macrophages (scavenger cells) that, in an attempt to remove the cholesterol from the blood, move it into the walls of arteries, creating atherosclerotic plaques (or coronary disease). The more cholesterol and active macrophages in an artery, the more unstable it becomes; and the more unstable the plaque in an artery, the greater the likelihood of a heart attack.

Q: How does diet affect cholesterol levels?

LKN: Diets that are high in saturated and trans fats, fried foods, and high-fat meats and cheeses can raise cholesterol levels, especially the atherogenic (or plaque-causing) LDL cholesterol. Intake of some foods and beverages has been associated with higher HDL levels—as is the case with modest wine consumption.

Q: What specific nutrients are especially heart healthy, and why?

LKN: In general, a well-balanced diet that limits fats and carbohydrates—meaning a diet of fruits and vegetables (due to their natural minerals and antioxidants) and lean meats and fish that are high in omega-3 fatty acids—is important for heart health. Most randomized trials that have looked at specific nutrient supplementation (in excess of what would be obtained from a prudent diet) have found either no benefit or potential harm to heart health.

Q: Which fruits and vegetables are the healthiest for your heart?

LKN: Green, leafy vegetables and fruits with high natural-antioxidant levels, such as tomatoes, citrus fruits and strawberries.

Q: What foods should we avoid, and why?

LKN: Foods that are high in saturated fats and trans fats, fried foods and the like, which are associated with hypercholesterolemia.

Q: What is homocysteine, and what can it tell us about our risk of developing heart disease?

LKN: Homocysteine is an amino acid that's manufactured in the body from methionine. Deficiencies of vitamin B12, folate and vitamin B6 may lead to high levels of homocysteine, but there may be genetic

> A well-balanced diet that limits fats and carbs is important for heart health.

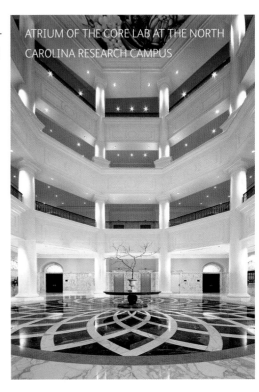

ATRIUM OF THE CORE LAB AT THE NORTH CAROLINA RESEARCH CAMPUS

Omega-3 fatty acids from food sources help ward off atherosclerosis.

predispositions to higher homocysteine levels as well. High levels of homocysteine have been associated with increased risk for coronary disease and myocardial infarction. These high levels degrade key structural proteins in arterial walls, making them prone to atherosclerosis. Also, it's possible that homocysteine participates in DNA methylation in vascular cells, which may also promote atherosclerosis. While increased levels of homocysteine have been associated with increased risk for coronary disease and myocardial infarction, randomized trials of therapy to reduce homocysteine (predominantly from folate and vitamin B6 supplementation) have been neutral or have shown harm from treatment with these supplements.

Q: How are omega-3 fatty acids beneficial?

LKN: These are essential nutrients that the body can't make without precursors from food. They appear to help reduce triglycerides and increase HDL cholesterol, and both effects are beneficial in warding off atherosclerosis. Interestingly, however, in some randomized clinical trials, supplementation with omega-3s beyond what you'd get in a prudent diet has not led to improved cardiovascular outcomes.

Q: The American Heart Association (AHA) came out with a statement regarding the ineffectiveness of antioxidant supplements on heart health. Why is a whole food diet so much more effective than receiving nutrients through supplements?

LKN: No one knows for sure, but it's probably because these components of food are only one part of the complex balance of nutrients, chemicals and the interactions between them in the human body. Overwhelming part of that system with large doses of one component likely leads to actions and adjustments that are unintended and/or counterproductive within these systems.

More than 80 million adults in the United States are afflicted by heart disease, the country's leading cause of death. It takes more than 800,000 lives each year. Just under 500,000 of those fatalities result from a heart attack; nearly 150,000 from a stroke; and the remainder are from cardiac arrhythmia, high blood pressure, congestive heart failure, congenital defects and other heart disorders.

A tragic aspect of these figures is that 80 percent of heart disease cases are preventable. Smoking, for instance, is a major contributor, raising blood pressure, generating free-radical damage and aggravating other risk factors, such as diabetes, hypertension and high cholesterol. Smoking more than doubles the risk for sudden cardiac death; and yet just one year after someone quits, their risk of having a heart attack is cut in half. Obesity, poor nutrition and chronic stress are other high-risk factors that could be mitigated by diet and exercise. Even for those who are born with heart disease (congenital heart disease) or are genetically predisposed to it, lifestyle choices can make the difference between keeping the condition manageable and letting it become debilitating.

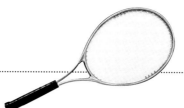

Antistress Activity

Aerobic exercise of any kind has the power to transform a bad mood, ease anxiety and tension, and calm rattled nerves. As soon as you start to exercise, more than 40 types of endorphins are released into the bloodstream. Levels of mood-enhancing neurotransmitters—such as serotonin, dopamine and norepinephrine—increase, and stress hormones begin to calm the brain and relieve stress. Over time, regular exercise helps the brain better cope with stress and stimulates the birth of new brain cells, which helps the brain adapt to changing life circumstances and counteract the corrosive effect of stress.

A 2005 study in the *Journal of the American Medical Association* reported that heart disease patients who received aerobic-exercise training for 35 minutes three times a week for 16 weeks, in addition to standard medical care, showed greater improvement in markers of cardiovascular risk than those who received only standard medical care. While vigorous exercise tends to be associated with stress relief, any type of activity—from strength training to tai chi and tennis—can be beneficial. In fact, studies show that a brisk 20-minute walk can deliver the same palliative effects as a mild tranquilizer.

Obesity

Excessive weight gain elevates the risk for high blood pressure, high cholesterol and atherosclerosis—all major factors in heart disease. Researchers with the Framingham Heart Study found that "obesity was associated with an approximately 50 percent increased risk of developing atrial fibrillation" (an abnormal heartbeat that can lead to stroke and cardiac arrest). "Once you get atrial fibrillation, it may be very difficult for doctors to get you back into the normal rhythm," warns study author Dr. Thomas Wang, "and what that means ... is that the patient may be stuck with a lifetime of taking medications to protect against stroke and other complications."

Being overweight or obese also increases the risk for diabetes and, according to the American Diabetes Association, an obese person with diabetes is two to four times more likely to develop heart disease and suffer a stroke or heart failure than someone who maintains a healthy body weight.

Cholesterol

About one in five Americans has high blood cholesterol (more than 240 milligrams per deciliter), according to the American Heart Association, which doubles their risk of heart attack compared with those whose cholesterol levels are below 200 milligrams per deciliter. Reducing your cholesterol by a mere 10 percent at age 40 can lower your heart attack risk by 50 percent; at age 50, by 40 percent; at age 60, by 30 percent; and at age 70, by 20 percent.

Before tackling how to lower cholesterol, it's important to understand what it is and how it works in the body. To begin with, cholesterol is a structural component in every cell membrane throughout the body; it maintains nerve integrity, facilitates hormone production and keeps cell walls strong. The body produces the amount of

HEALTH TIP

Four more reasons to stop smoking *now*: (1) Cigarette smokers are two to four times more likely to develop coronary heart disease and twice as likely to suffer a stroke; (2) Smoking doubles your risk of breast cancer; (3) Cigarettes are a ticket to early menopause; and (4) Smoking raises your risk of osteoporosis.

DIET TIP
Successful dieters know to bulk up on fiber-rich foods to combat hunger. Fiber also plays an important role in reducing the risk of heart disease (by lowering LDL levels), cancer and diabetes. It's easy to get the recommended 25 to 38 grams daily through raspberries, figs, artichokes, pears, and other fruits and veggies.

cholesterol it needs, but dietary factors can heavily increase its production, and of course, too much cholesterol circulating in the blood (serum cholesterol) can clog the arteries, elevating the risk of both heart attack and stroke. Cholesterol is transported to and from the cells by specific "carrier" proteins, referred to as low-density lipoproteins (LDL) and high-density lipoproteins (HDL). Cholesterol is carried by LDL *to* the blood and tissues, and carried by HDL out of the blood and back to the liver to be broken down, which is why moderate increases in HDL are seen as healthy.

While some dietary fats can raise blood-cholesterol levels, there does not seem to be a simple relationship between dietary cholesterol and blood cholesterol. *Dietary Guidelines for Americans, 2005* recommends keeping cholesterol obtained from food to less than 300 milligrams per day (the amount found in two small eggs). Findings from a University of Connecticut study published in *Metabolism* suggest that while egg cholesterol raises levels of certain less dangerous LDL molecules, it has virtually no effect on those smallest, densest LDL particles most closely linked with heart damage.

The Skinny on Fats

Saturated fats, so-called because they are "saturated" with hydrogen atoms, raise cholesterol levels and are found in animal products like meat, butter and cheese. Yet there are some exceptions: Coconut oil, for instance, although technically more saturated than butter, not only doesn't raise LDL levels, but may also actually help to increase HDL.

Many medical experts believe that trans fats have even stronger adverse effects than saturated fats. Typically found in processed, fried and fast food, trans fats are primarily produced through hydrogenation—a process that turns liquid vegetable oils into solids, such as the shortening and margarine often used in baked goods and snack foods. Trans fats are thought to increase insulin resistance and thus raise the risk of developing type 2 diabetes. They also raise levels of LDL and lower HDL levels. In fact, their effects are so pernicious that replacing just 2 percent of calories from trans fats with calories from unsaturated fats (for instance, using canola or olive oil instead of hydrogenated or partially hydrogenated vegetable oil) is associated with an astonishing 53 percent lower risk of coronary heart disease, according to a report from Harvard's ongoing Nurses' Health Study.

What's remained somewhat murky, until now, is an understanding of the precise mechanism by which trans fats send blood levels of cholesterol and triglycerides soaring. Scientists at the Dana-Farber Cancer Institute discovered that trans fat consumption triggers a biochemical switch in the liver, which "turns on" the genes that push cholesterol production into overdrive. (Unsaturated fats do not activate gene activity to the same degree, which is why they don't raise cholesterol as saturated and trans fats do.)

DIET TIP
When dining out, ask the waiter if it's possible to steam, roast or dry-broil your food rather than having it fried. Deep-frying foods can double the calorie content. For example, 4 ounces of baked fish is 135 calories and 1 gram of fat, while 4 ounces of fried fish is 265 calories and 13 grams of fat.

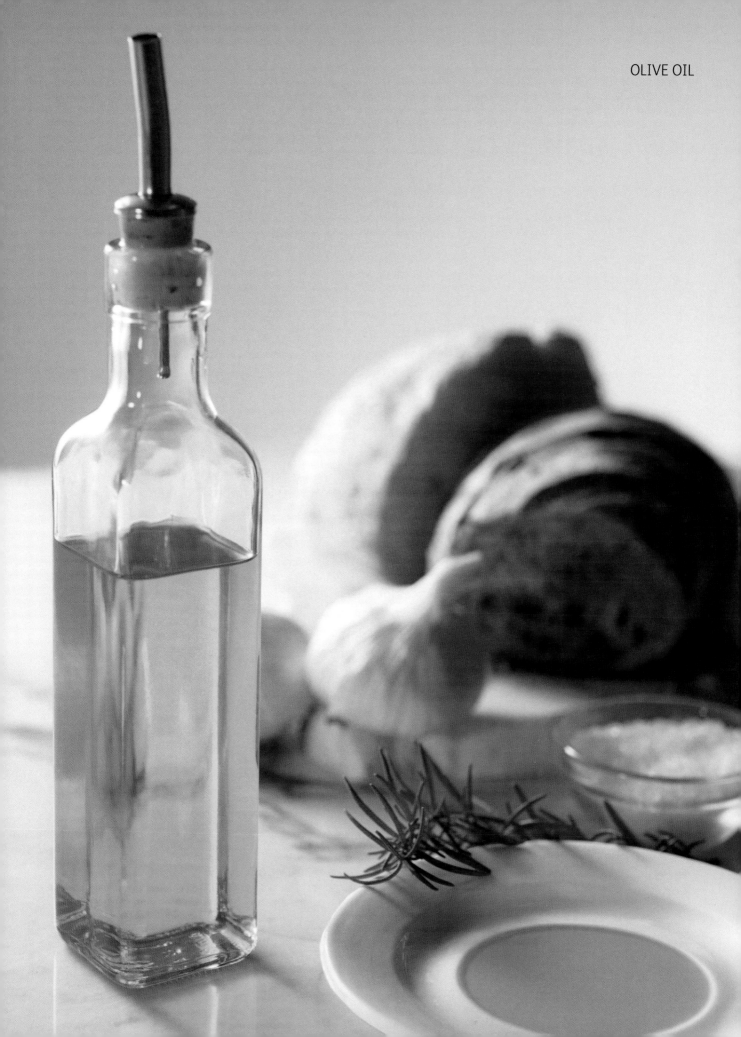

Omega-3 Fatty Acids

WALNUTS

Omega-3s are a type of polyunsaturated fat that can be found in soybean oil, canola oil, walnuts, flaxseeds, salmon and trout. Several studies point to the likelihood that higher dietary intakes of these particular fatty acids can reduce the risk of cardiovascular disease and even heart attack. In fact, the evidence is so strong that the American Heart Association recommends eating fish (particularly oily types like salmon, sardines and halibut) at least twice a week.

LDL-Lowering Strategies

Managing cholesterol levels isn't just about avoiding unhealthy foods; it's also about maintaining a fiber- and nutrient-rich diet with plenty of fruits and vegetables, particularly those shown to have LDL-lowering properties.

DIET TIP
Eating antioxidant-rich fruits—like blueberries, grapes, cherries, kiwifruits and strawberries—after an overindulgent meal helps offset the damage caused by the drop in antioxidant levels that occurs when the body is metabolizing fats and carbohydrates.

FIBER
Scores of studies show that fiber helps lower LDL and also link it to a significant reduction in coronary heart disease (CHD) risk. Most fiber-rich foods contain both soluble and insoluble fiber, both of which you need, so the following are only loosely categorized.
• Soluble fiber (also known as beta-glucan) lowers cholesterol and increases the feeling of fullness.
Top soluble fiber sources include fruits, oats, wild rice, quinoa and other whole grains
• Insoluble fiber helps keep blood cholesterol in check and prevents plaque buildup on artery walls.
Top insoluble fiber sources include all kinds of beans, peas, lentils and artichokes

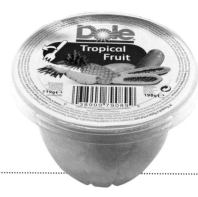

A Fruitful Strategy

DOLE FRUIT BOWLS

French researchers analyzed nine studies involving more than 220,000 individuals and found that the risk of cardiovascular problems declines as fruit intake increases. They also found an 11 percent drop in stroke risk for each extra fruit serving consumed daily.

Another study found that each extra (½ cup) serving of fruit you eat per day reduces your risk of heart disease by 7 percent. Consider how many servings you get with some of your favorite fruits, and you'll see how easy it is to lower your risk. Three large bananas, for example, would provide 42 percent more heart disease protection and slash your risk for stroke by 66 percent!

ANTIOXIDANTS

Antioxidants help prevent the oxidation of LDL, keeping it from clogging the arteries and thus reducing the risk of heart attacks and strokes.

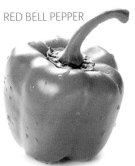

RED BELL PEPPER

- Vitamin C is a potent, water-soluble antioxidant.

Top vitamin C sources include pineapples, kiwifruits, red bell peppers and broccoli

- Anthocyanins and carotenoids, the free radical–fighting pigments found in colorful produce, have been shown to help prevent the oxidation of LDL and improve the elasticity of blood vessels.

Top anthocyanin and carotenoid sources include blueberries, tomatoes, grapes and cantaloupes

- Betanin is the antioxidant pigment that gives beets their rich red color.

Top betanin sources include beets and Swiss chard

Note: Beets are also a good source of folate, which helps lower homocysteine levels in the blood (high levels of homocysteine are linked to an increased risk of cardiovascular disease).

HEALTHY FATS

When used in place of saturated fat, monounsaturated fats help keep cholesterol levels in a healthy range.

Top sources of healthy fats include nuts, avocados and olive oil

FITNESS TIP

Sedentary women who become active in middle age have a lower risk of heart attacks than those who remain inactive. According to a study in the *New England Journal of Medicine*, women ages 40 to 65 years who walked the equivalent of three or four hours a week at a brisk pace reduced their risk of heart disease by 35 percent as opposed to sedentary women.

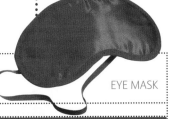

EYE MASK

Don't Ignore a Heavy Snore

Heavy snoring may be more than just a nightly nuisance. A 2008 study in the journal *Sleep* found that heavy snorers have a 34 percent higher risk of heart attack, a 40 percent increased risk of high blood pressure and a 67 percent increased risk of stroke than non-snorers.

The Hungarian researchers involved in the study surveyed nearly 13,000 people—of which a third of the men and a fifth of the women reported that they snore loudly—and found a significant correlation between loud snoring and heart disease. The link between the two held true even after adjustments were made for body mass index and alcohol consumption, both of which can aggravate snoring.

The sound of snoring is caused by breath vibrating through partially obstructed throat and nasal passageways. While the normal aging process can contribute to sagging throat muscles, the biggest contributor of all is excess weight. In fact, 60 to 90 percent of adults with obstructive sleep apnea are overweight: Fat compresses their air passages and weakens their upper-airway muscles. Not only can weight problems worsen snoring, but snoring can also hamper efforts to control your weight. By interrupting your sleep, it can deprive you of much-needed shut-eye, raising levels of cortisol (linked to increased abdominal fat), lowering levels of appetite-regulating leptin and sapping your energy for exercise. Fortunately, you can stop the vicious cycle of dwindling sleep and rising weight by exercising more and changing your diet.

Blood Pressure

At least 65 million American adults have high blood pressure, or hypertension, and this figure is up from 50 million a decade ago. If left untreated, hypertension can lead to stroke and heart failure, as well as to damage of the kidneys, blood vessels, eyes and brain (indeed, a Mayo Clinic study found that people with high blood pressure are more likely to lose mental ability as they age). In addition to lifestyle and genetic factors, the aging process also plays a role: Even a healthy individual with normal blood pressure at age 55 has a 90 percent risk of eventually developing hypertension.

But the concern among health experts isn't just limited to the adult population. According to a study published in the *Journal of the American Medical Association*, blood pressure levels are rising among American youths as well. The fact that kids in the United States are growing fatter by the year is partly to blame, as are lack of exercise and proper nutrition. While these blood pressure increases are occurring across racial groups, Mexican-American and African-American children are disproportionately affected, with average levels about two to three points above their Caucasian peers.

Fortunately, diet and lifestyle changes can help protect both adults and children from high blood pressure and its associated conditions.

Consider sodium. Children in the United States (ages 1 to 18) typically consume two to three times the 1 to 1.5 grams needed daily to maintain health—and high sodium intake is a known contributor to high blood pressure. In fact, a large-scale analysis of 23 countries implicated salt in 81 percent of preventable heart disease deaths and found that a mere 15 percent reduction in salt consumption could translate into nearly 9 million fewer deaths caused by the complications brought on by hypertension.

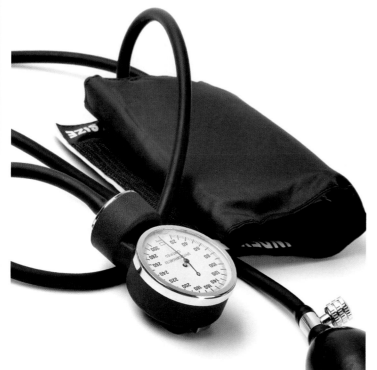

Processed food—not the salt shaker—accounts for at least 75 percent of salt intake, so opting for whole foods, or at least reaching for lower-sodium versions of prepared products, can make a big difference. *Dietary Guidelines for Americans, 2005* advises adults to consume less than 2.3 grams (approximately 1 teaspoon) of salt per day, while middle-aged and older adults, as well as African-Americans and those with hypertension, should consume no more than 1.5 grams a day.

Here are some additional ways to reduce hypertensive risk:

DRINK TEA

Taiwanese researchers found that folks who drink two and a half cups of tea per day have lower blood pressure than non-tea drinkers. Benefits accrue with both black and green tea consumption (but not with herbal varieties), lowering the risk for hypertension by nearly 50 percent.

INCREASE POTASSIUM CONSUMPTION

Potassium is essential for maintaining normal blood pressure and regulating the fluid balance in your cells. It also blunts the effects of excess sodium.

Top potassium sources include bananas, cooked spinach, sweet potatoes, cooked beets and lima beans

GET MORE MAGNESIUM

Magnesium has been shown to be effective in lowering some types of blood pressure by affecting the dilation of blood vessels.

Top magnesium sources include soybeans, seeds, nuts, wheat germ and seafood

GET SUFFICIENT VITAMIN C

This antioxidant vitamin helps prevent high blood pressure by combating the oxidation of LDL, thus preventing deposits, decreasing arterial blockage and allowing blood to flow with less impediment.

Top vitamin C sources include pineapples, red bell peppers, papayas, citrus fruits, kiwifruits, broccoli, Brussels sprouts, cantaloupes and strawberries

VARY YOUR PROTEIN SOURCES

When British researchers matched dietary intake data against blood pressure measurements for 4,680 subjects over a six-week period, they found that those who ate the most plant-based protein had lower blood pressure.

Top plant-based protein sources include beans and soy nuts

EXERCISE

Regular exercise can help you shed excess pounds, manage stress and strengthen your heart so that it can pump more efficiently—all of which can translate into lower blood pressure. The AHA recommends at least 30 minutes of moderate-to-vigorous exercise (e.g., brisk walking, bike riding and light weight training) at least five times a week.

BUNDLE UP WHEN IT'S COLD

If you're prone to high blood pressure, exposure to chilly temperatures, which constricts blood flow, can increase your vulnerability to heart attacks. French scientists have documented a correlation between dips in temperature and spikes in heart attack rates among those with high blood pressure. In fact, when the thermometer sank below 32.9°F, they found that hypertensives doubled their risk for heart attack.

FITNESS TIP

Don't let cold weather get in the way of keeping active. Winter offers lots of fun, calorie-burning activities to choose from:

* Build a snowman
  – 250 calories/hour
* Walk in the snow
  – 270 calories/hour
* Dance at a party
  – 350 calories/hour
* Shovel snow
  – 405 calories/hour
* Hit the ski slopes
  – 450 calories/hour

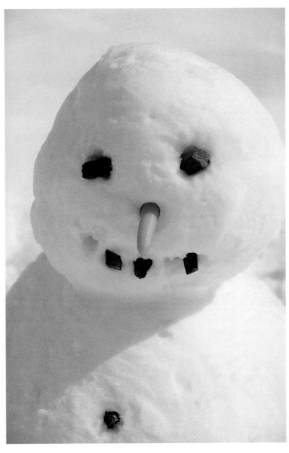

Heart-Healthy Hot Chocolate

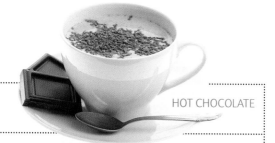

HOT CHOCOLATE

Research on cocoa's cardiovascular benefits suggests that it can, in moderation, be beneficial.
Here are some reasons that a little cocoa can go a long way in helping your heart:

• Cocoa powder is high in flavanols—potent antioxidants.

• In numerous studies, consumption of cocoa powder and dark chocolate has helped lower the oxidation of LDL and raise HDL.

• British researchers report that cocoa powder inhibits the platelet activity that causes clotting.

• German researchers report that chocolate can help control blood pressure. In their study, participants with mild hypertension were given 3 ounces of either dark chocolate or white chocolate (which some do not technically consider chocolate, as it contains only cocoa butter and cocoa liquor) daily. After two weeks, blood pressure levels dropped in the dark-chocolate group and remained unchanged in the white chocolate group.

• Greek researchers report that dark chocolate may alleviate arterial stiffness. Their study found that it improves the flexibility of blood vessels in the hours immediately after consumption. It's possible that by improving the function of the cells lining blood vessel walls, cocoa compounds may play a part in preventing the hardening of arteries that can lead to heart attacks.

Note: Keep in mind that when cocoa is incorporated into chocolate candy, the end product is high in calories, half of which come from fat—and most of it is of the saturated kind.

So, should you eat chocolate for your health? Penny Kris-Etherton, PhD, RD, distinguished professor of nutrition at Pennsylvania State University and author of several chocolate studies, observes: "It's okay to eat dark chocolate in small amounts, as long as you eat an otherwise healthy diet and can afford the calories. Try eating it with nuts or fruit for more good fats and even more antioxidants."

FITNESS TIP

Heal faster by keeping fit! An Ohio State University study found that exercise accelerates wound healing by as much as 25 percent. Why? Because it enhances immune function and blood circulation. So rather than being sidelined by minor scrapes and bruises, regenerate more rapidly by staying in the game.

Inflammation

Chronic inflammation can put your heart out of commission for good. Inflammation is basically an immune response to infection or injury. Externally, it's recognized as redness, elevated temperature and swelling—symptoms that are evidence of immune cell activity working to break down injured and dying tissues so that new, healthy ones can replace them. In proper proportion, this serves as part of the healing cycle. But certain factors can force this delicate balance out of whack, leading to inflammatory overkill that can cause damage over time to otherwise healthy tissue.

One of the most accurate predictors of future cardiovascular disease is the level of C-reactive protein (CRP) in the blood, which indicates the extent of inflammation in the body. A 2002 study in the *New England Journal of Medicine* found the CRP blood test to be twice as effective as a standard cholesterol test in predicting heart attacks and strokes—which isn't all that surprising when you consider that half of all heart attack and stroke victims have normal cholesterol levels. Other well-established cardiac risk factors for heart disease, such as obesity, smoking, hypertension and chronic periodontal disease, are all associated with elevated levels of CRP.

Water Your Heart

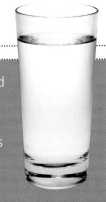

Fluid intake may also help support heart health, by affecting factors such as the thickness of blood and plasma. In fact, a study in the *American Journal of Epidemiology* found that subjects who drink five or more glasses of water per day have half the risk of fatal coronary heart disease compared with those who drink less than two glasses of water each day. A diet that is rich in fruits and vegetables provides additional hydration help, as produce can provide roughly 20 percent of your water needs. Cucumbers, celery, zucchini, tomatoes, watermelon, strawberries, spinach, grapefruit and broccoli are all more than 90 percent water.

A study published in the July 2003 issue of *Circulation: Journal of the American Heart Association* found that seniors with the highest CRP levels had a 60 percent increased risk of stroke. In addition, the Women's Health Study, which involved 39,876 healthy, postmenopausal women, found that those who had the highest CRP levels had five times the risk of developing cardiovascular disease and seven times the risk of having a heart attack compared with subjects who had the lowest levels. This is key: CRP levels predicted risk even in women who appeared to have no other pertinent risk factors.

LOWERING CRP LEVELS

What should you do if your CRP levels are high? The first place to turn may be the produce aisle of your local grocery store. A study published in the *Journal of the American Medical Association* found that those who maintained a diet high in vegetables, fruits, soy foods and nuts for one month lowered their CRP levels by an average of 28.2 percent.

The following nutrients are thought to be effective in keeping CRP protein levels in check:

- **Top vitamin C sources include** pineapples, red bell peppers, mangoes, citrus fruits, kiwis and broccoli
- **Top alpha-carotene sources include** carrots, butternut squash, pumpkins and persimmons
- **Top beta-carotene sources include** butternut squash, cantaloupes, carrots and apricots
- **Top beta-cryptoxanthin sources include** butternut squash, pumpkins, red peppers and tangerines
- **Top lycopene sources include** watermelons, tomatoes, pink grapefruit and pink-fleshed guavas
- **Top selenium sources include** Brazil nuts, rye bread, salmon and brown rice

When it comes to reducing inflammation, avoiding unhealthy foods is just as important as eating healthy foods. Researchers at the State University of New York at Buffalo tested subjects after they ate a McDonald's Egg McMuffin, a Sausage McMuffin and hash browns, and found that a big, fatty breakfast sent their levels

FOOD TIP

Help your heart by going meatless one day each week. According to research done at Johns Hopkins Medical Center, this can reduce your saturated fat intake by 15 percent. Legumes, nuts and even certain grains like quinoa can serve as healthy nonmeat protein sources.

WHEAT

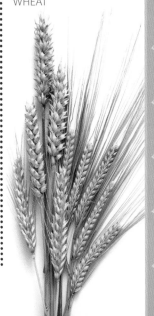

DIET TIP
The urge will ebb. If you're hankering for treats you've recently cut from your diet, don't give in to temptation. Research suggests cravings subside over time. Test subjects who eliminated sweets, saturated fat and fast food desired them significantly less after five weeks.

GET THE HEALTH BENEFITS OF WINE WITHOUT THE ASSOCIATED RISKS BY OPTING FOR CONCORD GRAPES.

of free radicals and CRP through the roof. The subjects' levels were still high several hours after breakfast, when most people begin thinking about lunch.

What else can you do to keep your CRP levels in check? Get active. Research presented at the 52nd annual meeting of the American College of Cardiology in 2003 found that people who exercised four or more times a week had CRP levels that were 34.6 percent lower than people who exercised less than once per week.

Stroke

Every year, 780,000 Americans suffer a stroke, and for more than 150,000 of them, it's fatal. A stroke occurs when a blood clot blocks the arteries and blood vessels that carry oxygen to the brain. A healthy diet that promotes vascular health can help lower your risk of having a stroke. For example, according to a 2004 report from the University of Oslo in Norway, eating two to three kiwis a day can significantly lower the risk for blood clots and reduce blood lipids.

RAISE A GLASS TO HEART HEALTH?

Enthusiasm over the heart-health benefits of moderate alcohol consumption makes it easy to lose sight of the fact that heavy drinking poses significant health risks—among them, elevated blood pressure, abnormal heart rhythm and a dramatically increased likelihood of stroke. In fact, Harvard researchers found that men who consume an average of three or more alcoholic beverages a day were nearly 43 percent more likely to suffer a stroke compared with abstainers and men who had one to two drinks a day.

Until recently, many researchers have attributed the potential health benefits—an increase in HDL, decrease in blood pressure and lower risk of death by cardiovascular disease—to ethanol, the intoxicating agent in alcoholic beverages. But findings suggest that other compounds—polyphenols, B vitamins, resveratrol, and nonalcoholic by-products of fermentation—might play a more significant role.

A small German study in the May 2004 issue of *Alcoholism: Clinical and Experimental Research* reported that alcohol-free beer had the same cardiovascular benefits on 12 healthy male volunteers as alcoholic beer does—and without the risks. Excessive alcohol consumption actually increases the risk of thrombosis, or blood vessel clotting, and the nonalcoholic beer caused a significant decrease in clot creation.

In addition, a 2004 Boston University study found that Concord grape juice increased HDL and significantly lowered two markers for inflammation, just as wine has been shown to do. French researchers have found that Concord grape juice helps relax cells lining the blood vessels in

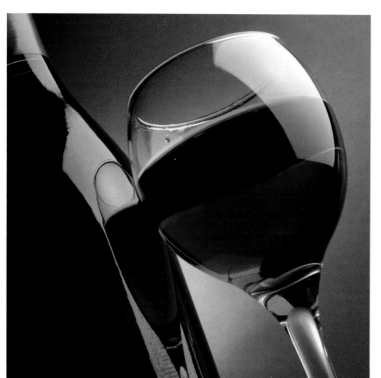

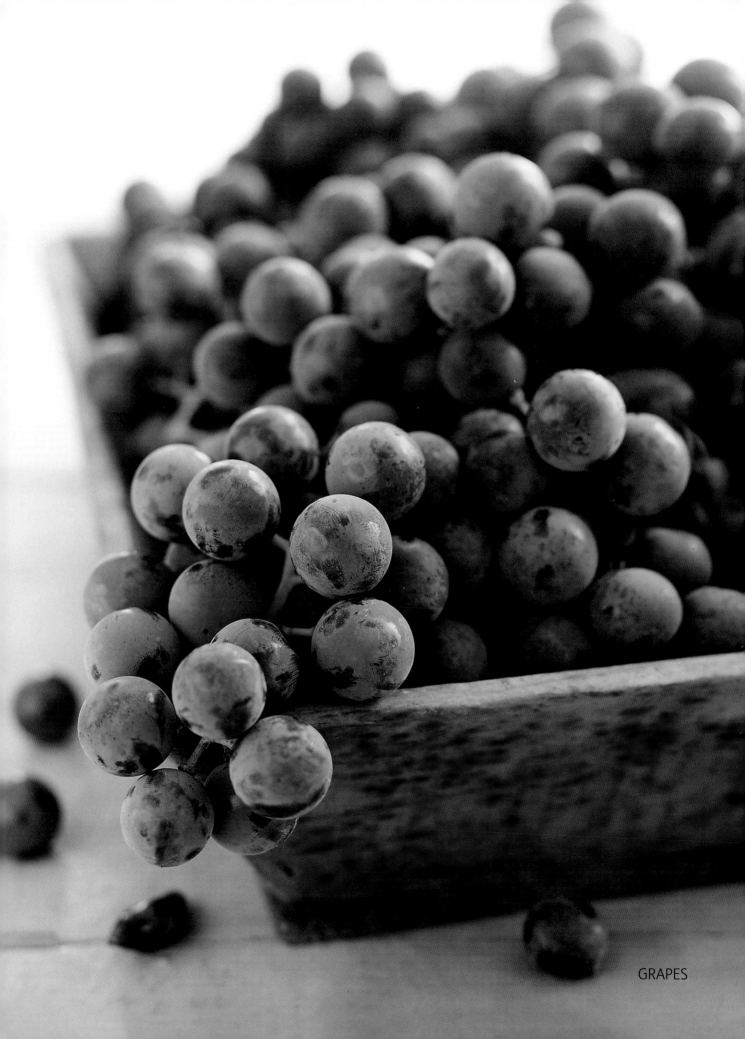

GRAPES

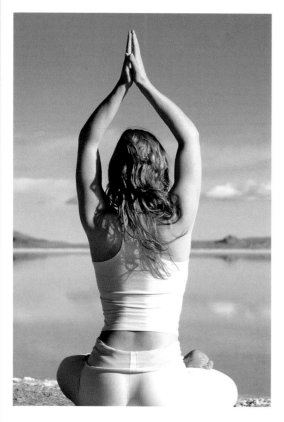

YOGA IS A GREAT
WAY TO RELAX AND
REDUCE STRESS.

NUTRITION TIP
Manage your stroke
risk with foods that
are rich in vitamins
C and E. A six-year
Dutch study of 5,200
men and women
found that those
with the highest
vitamin C intake were
30 percent less likely
to have a stroke than
those with the lowest
intake. And diets high
in vitamin E reduced
stroke risk by more
than 20 percent.

animal lab cultures as well. And when German researchers compared the relative bioavailability of anthocyanins in red grape juice to that in red wine, they found that the urine of grape-juice drinkers had 28 percent higher anthocyanin levels than that of red wine drinkers. In addition, antioxidant activity was higher—and remained so—in the blood of the grape-juice drinkers than in that of the wine drinkers.

The Stress Factor

The INTERHEART study, a global endeavor involving 29,972 heart attack survivors from 52 countries, evaluated risk factors that had affected subjects during the year preceding their cardiac event. INTERHEART researchers reported in a 2004 issue of the *Lancet* that psychosocial factors—including financial stress, job stress, a stressful life event and stress at home—increased the odds of having a heart attack approximately threefold, a magnitude similar to that for standard risk factors, such as obesity and hypertension. They point out that previous studies have found links between psychosocial stress and vascular function, inflammation, increased blood clotting and more.

Researchers in one study found that those rated as having a dominant personality had a 47 percent higher risk of heart disease, while those with the highest scores of irritability had a 27 percent higher risk compared with their more patient, passive and unperturbed peers. Among women, the increased risk was associated with more restrained displays of anger, such as sarcasm and making faces, whereas men's risk rose relative to more full-blown expressions of ire. Irritability was a cardiac risk factor for both sexes.

Duke University researchers found that people who are physically healthy but prone to anger, hostility and mild depression have levels of inflammation as much as two or three times higher than their calmer counterparts. Their study, published in the September 2004 issue of *Psychosomatic Medicine*, observes that "50 percent of all heart attacks occur among people without any traditional risk factors (obesity, smoking, diabetes, hypertension, high cholesterol and sedentary lifestyle), so it is critical to identify other factors"—like stress.

The good news is that there are countless ways to reduce stress, including meditation, counseling, relaxation techniques and exercise.

Exercise

Physical inactivity is a major risk factor for heart disease, and according to the American Heart Association, the majority of Americans aren't nearly active enough. Healthy adults, ages 18 to 65, can satisfy the minimal AHA guidelines with just 30 minutes of a moderate intensity activity five days a week—e.g., brisk walking, bike riding and light weight training.

Although the benefits increase with the frequency, intensity and duration of physical activity, some studies indicate that even less exertion is still beneficial. A 2001 Harvard study found that walking just 60 to 90 minutes per week cut the risk of coronary artery disease in half among nearly 40,000 women over 45-years-old. And Duke University researchers report that adults who began walking 12 miles a week showed significant improvements in cardiovascular fitness and lowered their risk of death from heart disease by 8.1 percent.

Joggers in the Duke University study saw even greater health gains than the walkers, with a 14.5 percent drop in risk of death from heart disease. Jogging and other aerobic exercise—anything that gets your heart rate up, such as swimming, biking and skiing—strengthen the heart, increase the flexibility of the blood vessels, lower blood pressure and improve the heart's ability to recover after a heart attack or other cardiac event.

In fact, in an Italian study, heart patients who took up ballroom dancing experienced greater gains in cardiac function and quality of life than those who relied on traditional exercise for rehabilitation. The researchers assigned 110 male and female seniors to either waltzing classes, exercise training (cycling, treadmill) or a control (no exercise) group. Eight weeks into the regimen, they found that the dancers had a slight edge on the exercisers in terms of cardiopulmonary fitness, including aerobic capacity and arterial flexibility. But where the waltzers really came out ahead of the exercisers (not to mention the nonexercisers) was in enhancing their quality of life—especially the emotional aspects, such as having reduced anxiety and decreased depression.

A total heart-healthy exercise program should include muscle-strengthening activities about twice a week, according to the AHA, in addition to aerobic activity. Anything that involves resistance, lifting and the repetitive use of large muscle groups qualifies as muscle-strengthening—from weight lifting to exercises like deep knee bends, lunges and push-ups.

Conclusion

At the end of the day, your heart is in your hands. Even though you can't control the genetic factors that affect your chances of heart disease, you can take control of your diet and lifestyle to dramatically reduce your risks for it.

While most people who die from heart attacks are over the age of 75, prevention can never begin too early. A study from the University of Missouri–Kansas City found that obese adolescents have circulatory systems comparable with those of normal 45-year-old adults. Fortunately, fruit and vegetables are the best weapons against obesity at any age; they fill you up, help you meet nutrient requirements, and supply the fiber and potassium needed to keep your cholesterol and blood pressure levels normal. Whether you're young, or simply young at heart, it's never too late to reap the rewards of a healthier diet and lifestyle. With the right choices, many adverse heart-healthy conditions can be halted—and even reversed.

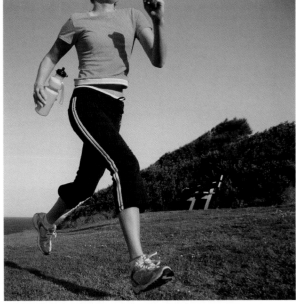

FITNESS TIP
Turn ad time into ab time by exercising during TV ad breaks. Many don't have time for exercise, yet the average American manages to fit in nearly four hours of TV-watching per day. With an average of six three-minute commercial breaks per broadcasting hour, you can get in 18 minutes of push-ups, sit-ups, lunges or squats between segments.

REGULAR EXERCISE, EVEN AT MODERATE LEVELS, SIGNIFICANTLY BENEFITS THE HEART.

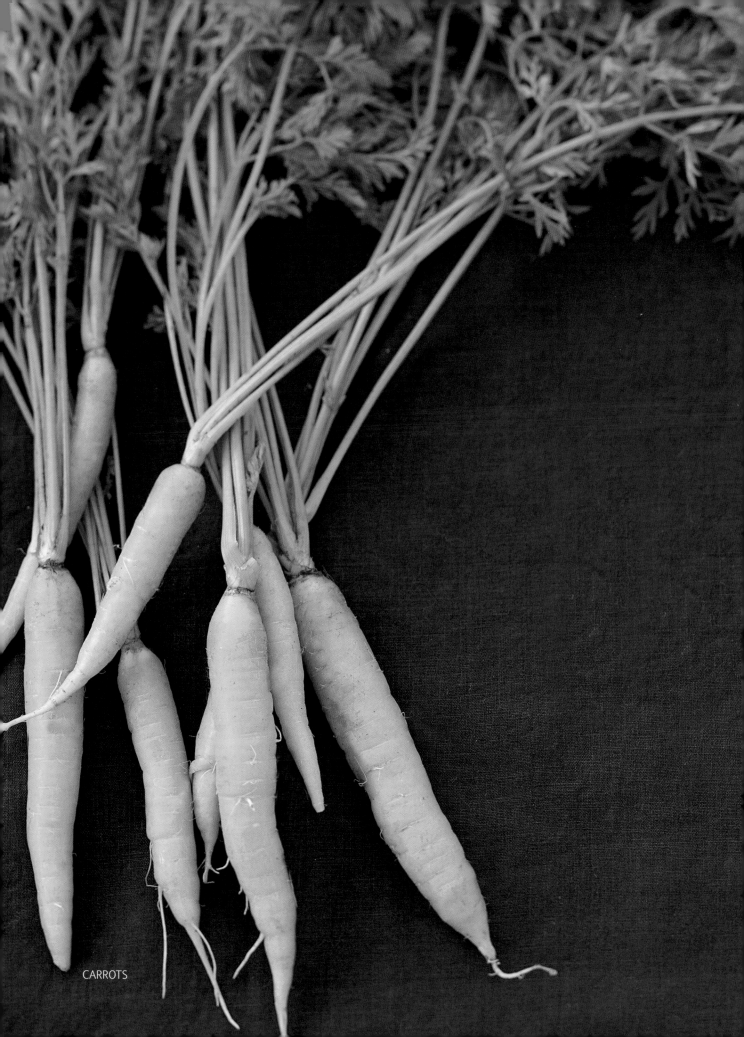

CARROTS

CHAPTER 6

Eye
Health

You Need: BETA-CAROTENE, ALPHA-CAROTENE, BETA-CRYPTOXANTHIN, LUTEIN, ZEAXANTHIN

Eat These:

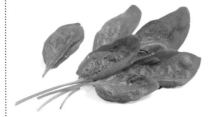

SPINACH

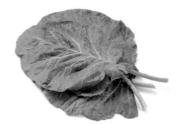

COLLARD GREENS

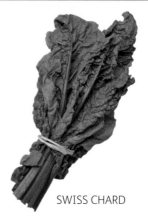

SWISS CHARD

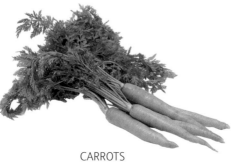

CHICORY

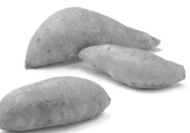

SWEET POTATOES

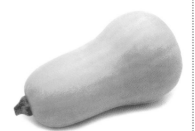

BUTTERNUT SQUASH

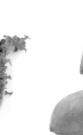

CARROTS

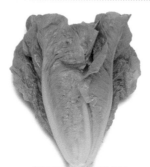

ROMAINE LETTUCE

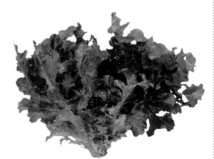

RED LEAF LETTUCE

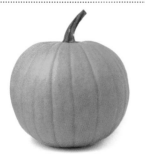

PUMPKIN

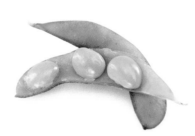

SOYBEANS

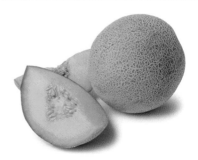

CANTALOUPES

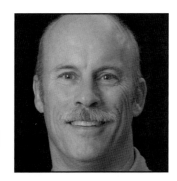

Michael McIntosh

Michael McIntosh, PhD, RD, is the Lucy S. Keker Excellence Professor in the Department of Nutrition at the University of North Carolina at Greensboro. He received his PhD in Nutrition from the University of Georgia and his RD from the University of Wisconsin. His current research focuses on bioactive food components that prevent inflammation or insulin resistance associated with obesity.

Q: Why do we need vitamin A for healthy vision?

MM: Vitamin A is essential for healthy vision because it maintains the integrity of cells in mucous membranes, including those in the eye. It is also needed for the synthesis of rhodopsin and other light receptor pigments in the eye. Without these, a number of vision problems occur, including poor dark adaptation (night blindness), xeropthalmia (abnormal dryness of the eye), keratomalacia (softening and necrosis of the cornea) and Bitot's spots (foamy gray, triangular spots of keratinized epithelium on the conjunctiva).

Q: What's the difference between vitamin A and beta-carotene?

MM: Vitamin A is a fat-soluble vitamin, generally referred to as a group of compounds that have the biological activity of all-trans retinol, the alcohol form of vitamin A. Many carotenoids, including beta-carotene, are termed pro-vitamin A, because they can be enzymatically converted to vitamin A. Carotenoids like beta-carotene also have antioxidant properties, which are thought to contribute to their ability to neutralize free radicals that damage tissues, including those in the eye. The carotenoid family includes alpha and beta-carotene, lutein, zeaxanthin, cryptoxanthin and lycopene.

VITAMIN A, ABUNDANT IN SWEET POTATOES, HELPS PROTECT THE LENSES AGAINST OXIDATIVE DAMAGE.

Q: There's scientific evidence to support that higher dietary intake of lutein and zeaxanthin can reduce the risk of developing age-related macular degeneration (AMD), the leading cause of blindness in people over 65-years-old. What's your view of the research concerning this observation?

MM: AMD involves the degeneration of the central part of the retina—or the macula—the portion of the eye that acts like the film in the camera, capturing the image. The macula helps us identify colors and see fine details of objects directly in front of us. Loss of function in the macula makes it difficult to read, drive, recognize people and perform detailed tasks. Long-term exposure to sunlight, cigarette smoke and pollution, along with low blood levels of antioxidant vitamins (i.e., carotenoids and vitamins A, C and E) and minerals (i.e., zinc and selenium) may contribute to the disease. The intake of two carotenoids in particular, lutein and zeaxanthin, which concentrate in the macula, were shown recently to have an inverse relationship to AMD. These two carotenoids are found in the retina, and have been coined macular xanthophylls. These and other

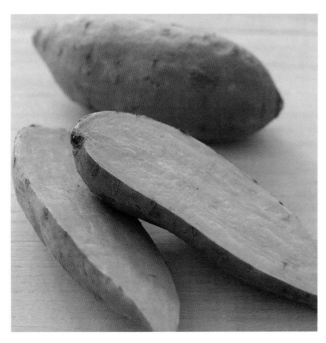

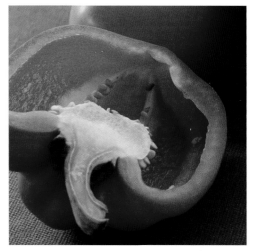

RED BELL PEPPERS
ARE LOADED WITH
VITAMIN C, WHICH
HELPS ACTIVATE
DEFENSES AGAINST
LENS DAMAGE.

FOOD TIP

When it comes to
superfoods, romaine
lettuce earns a triple
crown, benefitting
the eyes, skin and
immune function.
It's an excellent
source for vitamin C
and contains the eye-
healthy antioxidant
carotenoids lutein
and zeaxanthin.
Two cups provide
100 percent of
your daily vitamin
A requirement—at
only 14 calories!

carotenoids may help protect the eye against oxidative damage that contributes to the development of AMD.

Q: What foods contain the most lutein and zeaxanthin?

MM: Egg yolks, corn, pumpkin, squash, red peppers, Brussels sprouts and leafy greens like collards, turnip greens and spinach contain lutein and zeaxanthin. In general, consuming five or more servings of fruits and vegetables daily ensures adequate intake of carotenoids and vitamins A, C and E. Deep green and dark yellow or orange fruits and vegetables, such as Swiss chard, bok choy, spinach, cantaloupe, mango, sweet potatoes, and acorn or butternut squash are packed with carotenoids. Vegetables from the cabbage family, such as cauliflower, sprouts and broccoli also are good sources of carotenoids.

Q: What are the most important things you can do to protect your eyesight?

MM: Getting regular eye exams, wearing sunglasses that block out UV light, controlling blood pressure, quitting smoking, staying active and consuming foods such as fruits and vegetables rich in antioxidants may decrease the progression of AMD and cataracts.

Q: What's your opinion on the controversy surrounding the benefits of supplements versus whole foods in the area of eye health?

MM: Studies have shown that whole foods like fruits and vegetables offer greater protection than the consumption of individual nutrients or phytochemicals. This could be due to several things, including better absorption or metabolism from whole foods and additional, enhanced or synergistic effects of the multiple phytochemicals found in foods, as opposed to individual phytochemicals in supplements.

Q: How much of a role does genetics play in the development of these diseases as we age? And how important is a healthy diet—containing foods rich in antioxidants, particularly lutein and zeaxanthin, as well as omega-3 fatty acids—in reducing the risk of developing AMD and possibly cataracts as we age?

MM: About 30 percent of white adults over the age of 75 suffer from AMD. Nonwhites are not as prone to AMD. Clearly, having a genetic propensity for diseases like AMD and cataracts increases the risk of early onset of these diseases when superimposed on an environment that initiates, promotes or progresses their development. Although no food will directly improve your vision, consuming certain foods on a regular basis promotes optimal vision and can help prevent or slow the progression of AMD and cataracts, the two leading causes of vision loss. For example, a study published in 2002 in the *American Journal of Clinical Nutrition* found that the odds for getting cataracts among nonsmoking women decreased as the level of dietary antioxidants, including vitamin C and carotenoids, increased. Thus, consuming carotenoid-rich foods may help protect against AMD and cataracts. Concerning omega-3 fatty acids and eye disease, a recent meta-analysis concluded that a high intake of omega-3 fatty acids was linked to a 38 percent reduction in late AMD. Consuming fish twice per week reduced the risk of developing early and late AMD. However, these authors cautioned that without more rigid prospective or clinical trials, these findings are premature.

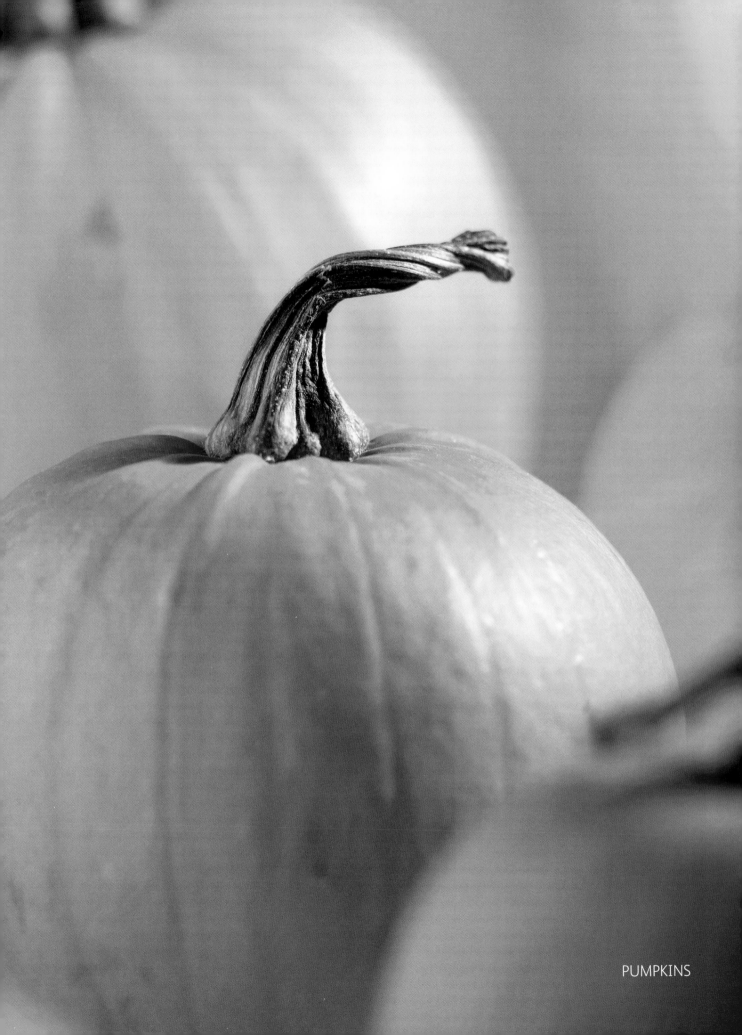

PUMPKINS

More than a million Americans over the age of 40 are blind as a result of eye disease. An additional 2.3 million are visually impaired. Even more—over 20 million Americans age 40 and older—have age-related cataracts, the world's leading cause of blindness, and by the year 2020 that number will reach 30.1 million. In addition, age-related macular degeneration (AMD), the leading cause of severe vision loss in Americans age 50 or older, affects an estimated 12 million people.

Because most Americans are unaware of just how pervasive eye disease is, efforts to prevent, detect and treat these ailments before they progress to debilitating levels of vision loss aren't as effective as they might be. Because AMD is barely perceptible in its early stages, it's often left untreated until after vision loss sets in.

ANTIOXIDANTS IN SPINACH PROTECT THE EYES FROM DAMAGING LIGHT WAVES.

Obesity is a factor in the growing rate of eye disease—as is the simple fact that people are living longer. Most serious eye ailments have a genetic component as well. But still, there's plenty you can do to protect your eyesight, including being vigilant about proper nutrition. The American Optometric Association (AOA) lists vitamins B2, C and E, as well as beta-carotene, omega-3 fatty acids, zinc, lutein and zeaxanthin among the most essential eye-healthy nutrients.

Inflammation also has an impact on eye health. Harvard Medical School researchers found that C-reactive protein levels were significantly higher among people with advanced AMD than among those without AMD. Whether or not the inflammation is a co-factor of age-related macular degeneration—or its result—needs to be further investigated.

What to Choose
SPINACH FOR LUTEIN

According to the AOA, dark, leafy greens are the healthiest food for eyes overall. When researchers at Brigham Young University analyzed dietary data for more than 35,000 women, they found that those who consumed the most

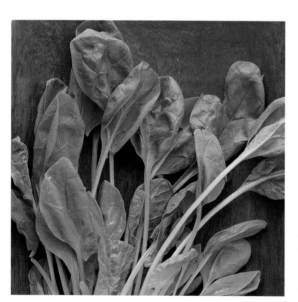

lutein and zeaxanthin—6,700 micrograms per day—enjoyed an 18 percent lower risk of developing cataracts. Spinach is loaded with these potent antioxidants, believed to filter the high-energy light waves that cause free-radical damage to the eyes and skin. They've also been found to cut the risk of age-related macular degeneration (AMD), which women are more prone to than are men. Research suggests that daily intake of the amount available in one cup of cooked spinach is enough to realize the benefits.

Other lutein sources include colorful fruits and vegetables such as broccoli, kale, collard greens, turnip greens, corn, green beans, peas, summer squash, oranges and tangerines

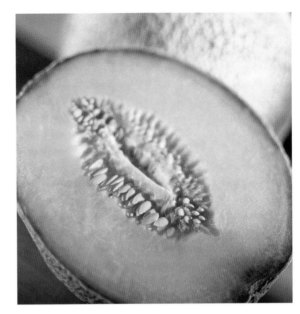

CANTALOUPES FOR BETA-CAROTENE

According to Harvard researchers, eating fruits and vegetables can reduce the risk of cataracts by 10 to 15 percent. The body converts beta-carotene into vitamin A, making cantaloupes and other foods that are high in this carotenoid essential for night vision and overall eye function. Vitamin A deficiency has been associated with a higher incidence of macular degeneration.

Other beta-carotene sources include carrots, kale, spinach and apricots

CANTALOUPE IS RICH IN BETA-CAROTENE, WHICH IS ESSENTIAL FOR OVERALL EYE FUNCTION.

BROCCOLI FOR RIBOFLAVIN

Broccoli is a top source for riboflavin (also known as vitamin B2), which is found in the pigment of the retina and helps your eyes adapt to changes in light. Riboflavin deficiency can make the eyes overly sensitive to light, leading to inflammation, blurred vision and ocular fatigue. Animal research suggests that adequate B2 may help prevent cataracts or delay their progress.

Other riboflavin sources include beans, spinach, mushrooms, mangoes, asparagus, Brussels sprouts and nuts

DIET TIP
If your salad is looking a bit bland, toss in some color! Dice bell peppers, shred carrots, chop tomatoes, and sprinkle dried fruit and nuts, creating a salad that tempts the palate while pleasing and protecting the eyes.

SELENIUM AND VITAMINS C AND E TO REGULATE GLUTATHIONE

Glutathione is a powerful antioxidant enzyme, manufactured in the body, that functions as part of the defense system for the lenses of your eyes. When glutathione levels are deficient, the eyes are more vulnerable to oxidative damage. Nutrients required to increase glutathione levels include selenium and vitamins C and E.

Top vitamin C sources include oranges, grapefruits, strawberries, papayas, kiwis, green peppers, red bell peppers and tomatoes

Top vitamin E sources include almonds, pecans, sweet potatoes, sunflower seeds, dark, leafy greens and vegetable oils (e.g., safflower and corn)

Top selenium sources include Brazil nuts (with a whopping 95.8 micrograms per nut), snapper and shrimp

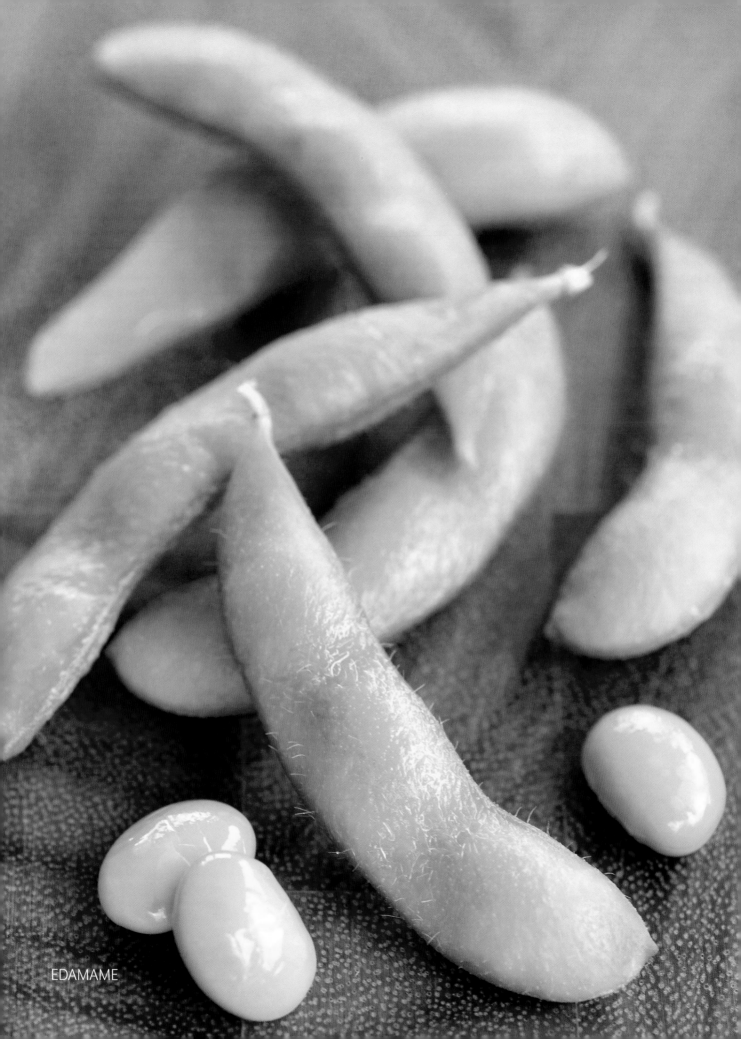

EDAMAME

Weight Watchers

In a study of 466 women, researchers found that excess weight was as damaging to the eyes as UV exposure, diabetes and aging. Those who were 30 to 40 pounds overweight were far more likely to develop cataracts at a younger age than their thinner peers.

SOYBEANS FOR ZINC

The eyes have one of the body's highest concentrations of zinc—particularly in the iris and retina. Preliminary research suggests a link between low zinc intake and eye maladies such as color blindness, cataract formation and optic neuritis, the inflammation of the optic nerve. While the most traditionally cited sources of zinc include oysters, Dungeness crab and red meat, most vegetarians enjoy adequate levels of zinc, despite the absence of such animal proteins in their diet. Soybean products such as tofu, soy milk and soy cheese might well be the reason, as soy not only contains zinc but also has other compounds that aid the mineral's absorption as well.

It should also be noted that findings from the Centre for Eye Research Australia in Melbourne indicate that despite the zinc content in red meat, carnivorous habits may significantly increase the risk of AMD. Researchers examined the diets and eye health of 5,604 men and women over the course of a decade and found that those who reported eating red meat more than 10 times a week had a 50 percent higher risk of AMD than those who ate meat fewer than five times a week. Those in the study who ate a lot of processed meats (e.g., salami and sausage) were the most strongly predisposed to AMD. But chicken intake showed no association with early AMD—and, in fact, actually appeared to be protective in a late form of the condition.

Other zinc sources include peanuts, peas, lima beans, summer squash, potatoes, corn, Napa cabbage and bok choy

EATING ANTIOXIDANT-RICH FOODS IS KEY TO PROTECTING THE EYES FROM THE DAMAGE CAUSED BY AGING.

Conclusion

The ability to see the wondrous world around you is often taken for granted. Aging affects your eyes—just like it affects your joints and bones—stiffening the lenses so that it can be harder to focus your gaze. But by taking measures to protect your eyes today, you can maintain your vision along with the joy and independence it affords. Eating more antioxidant-rich fruits and vegetables—like those highlighted in this chapter—is the most important thing you can do to preserve your eyesight over the course of a lifetime.

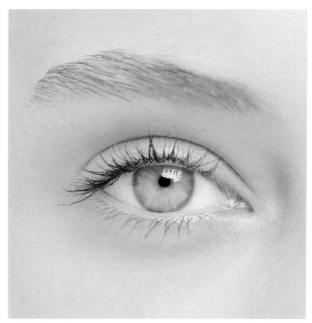

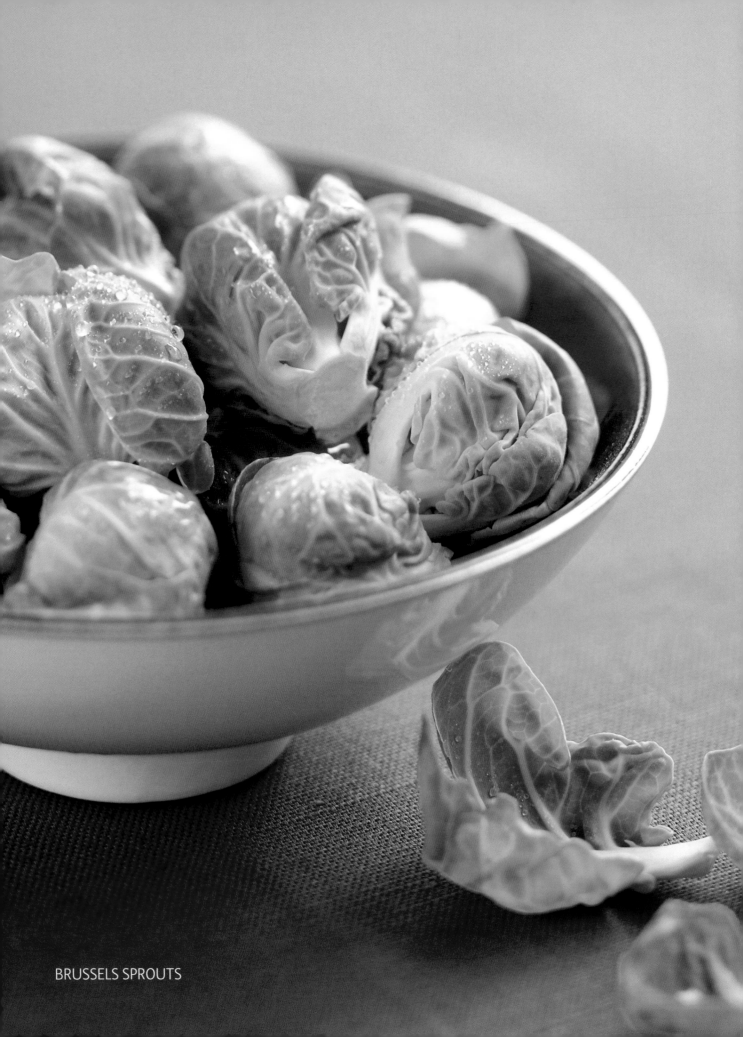

BRUSSELS SPROUTS

CHAPTER 7

Pregnancy Health

You Need: FOLATE, CHOLINE, BETAINE, VITAMIN D, CALCIUM, IRON, ANTIOXIDANTS

Eat These:

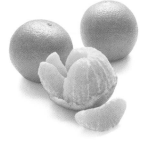

ORANGES

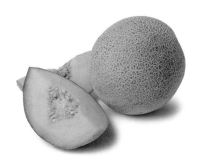

CANTALOUPE

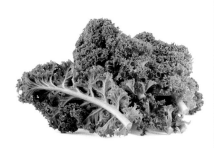

KALE

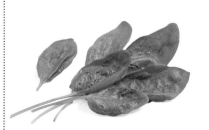

SPINACH

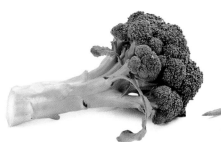

BROCCOLI

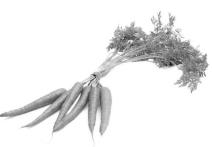

CARROTS

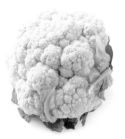

CAULIFLOWER

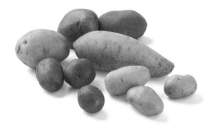

POTATOES

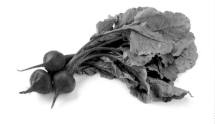

BEETS

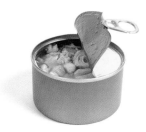

CANNED SALMON

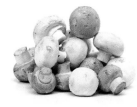

BUTTON MUSHROOMS

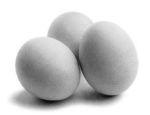

EGGS

▶ Steven Zeisel

Steven Zeisel, MD, PhD; Kenan Distinguished Professor, Department of Nutrition; professor, Department of Pediatrics; and Associate Dean for Research, School of Public Health at the University of North Carolina at Chapel Hill, is director of the University of North Carolina's School of Public Health's Nutrition Research Institute at the newly formed North Carolina Research Campus.

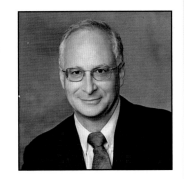

Q: How did you come to focus on the role of nutrients like choline in fetal brain development?

SZ: We found that the placenta has been designed to deliver choline to babies in large amounts, and then we discovered that breast-feeding does the same thing—drawing choline out of the mother and delivering it to the baby in high concentrations. That led us to ask: Why would this happen? Why did evolution develop this mechanism that delivers a lot of choline to babies? It must be important.

Q: What did you do next?

SZ: We looked at animal tests to see what happens to the offspring of mothers fed either high-choline or low-choline diets. We found that there is a critical period when a little extra choline in the diet results in a 30 percent improvement in memory that lasts for the offspring's entire life.

Q: Are you saying that an old rat, originally born to a choline-fed mother, would be smarter than a young rat whose mother had been deprived of choline?

SZ: Yes, certainly they would appear to be younger in terms of their memory than their age would have predicted, because they wouldn't have become senile as they grew older. Another thing that happened when we took choline away: The animals had much more trouble doing the complicated maze running. They were okay on simple stuff; but as soon as you added any complications, they just fell apart and had trouble running.

Q: What's the equivalent for humans?

SZ: Timewise, the equivalent in humans would begin 25 weeks into the pregnancy, when the memory center starts developing, and continue through the first year after birth. So there's a longer period with humans, because it's not only the placenta that gives choline to the human baby, but also the mother's breast milk.

The take-home message is that pregnancy is a time when nutrition is exceedingly important. And the old idea that you can make up for deficiencies during pregnancy by providing the child with better nutrition later in life isn't accurate. Folic acid, choline and betaine are three of the nutrients that mothers have to make sure they get in their diet during pregnancy.

Q: What are some good sources of choline? What about choline supplements?

SZ: Top choline sources include eggs, cauliflower, peanuts, potatoes and oranges. I wouldn't take supplements. There's something called phosphatidylcholine that people sprinkle on their food. It may be okay, but it breaks down in your gut into something that smells fishy, and you'll smell fishy after taking it, so I don't recommend that. I feel that getting choline in foods is always a better approach than taking it as a supplement—you not only get the nutrients, but you also get all the other good things that come along with the food.

> The old idea that nutrient deficiencies during pregnancy can be made up for later in the child's life isn't accurate.

During pregnancy, the old adage "You are what you eat" takes on heightened significance. An expectant mother's food and beverage choices have the potential to impact the health of the growing baby both positively and negatively. Cravings can sometimes be signals that point to foods with the nutrients your body and your baby need during a particular phase of fetal development.

But it's important to use discretion in honoring those signals, so cravings don't become an excuse to overindulge. Why? Because obesity poses a serious health threat during pregnancy. A gain of more than 40 pounds raises the risk for a number of complications, including gestational diabetes and preeclampsia, also known as pregnancy-induced hypertension, which is the leading cause of premature delivery as well as maternal and fetal death. Other risks of excess pregnancy weight gain include congenital malformations and an increased likelihood of the child becoming overweight later in life.

According to the March of Dimes, normal-weight women should gain only 25 to 35 pounds during pregnancy, and overweight women just 15 to 25 pounds. So, it's important for moms-to-be to find a healthy balance between indulging their cravings and resisting them—and to make sure that, regardless of the foods they're drawn to, they get plenty of the nutrients that are vital for their health and their baby's healthy development. Awareness is key; so with that in mind, some of the essentials follow.

Folate (or Folic Acid)

This B vitamin helps prevent malformation of the fetal neural tube, the precursor to the brain and spine. Since 1998, when the FDA mandated folate fortification in breads, cereal and pasta, neural tube defects have plummeted 30 percent in the United States, sparing thousands of babies from spina bifida (abnormal spinal cord development) and anencephaly (impeded brain development). A daily dose of folic acid during the first trimester of pregnancy has been found to reduce neural tube defects by at least 50 percent. Adequate intake prior to pregnancy and during the second trimester can also significantly lower the risk of preterm delivery as well. Doctors recommend increasing folic acid before pregnancy, because brain and spinal cord defects typically develop during the first weeks of gestation, often before a woman knows that she's pregnant. In fact, a 1991 study published in the *Lancet* found that supplementation with folic acid beginning around the time of conception reduced the likelihood of having a baby with a neural tube defect in women who were at high risk for this abnormality (due to a previous affected pregnancy). The importance of folic acid underscores the dangers of low-carb diets, given that such regimens eliminate foods that are fortified with folic acid. Scientists worry that the declining consumption of folate-rich foods could have grave consequences for the next generation.

Top whole food folate sources include spinach, asparagus, collard greens, broccoli, turnip greens, Brussels sprouts and beets

Choline and Betaine

Like folate, choline and betaine have a protective effect, and researchers suspect that the three may work synergistically. In fact, the *American Journal of Epidemiology* reported that babies born to women whose diets were highest in choline and betaine were 75 percent less likely to have neural tube defects than babies born to women with the lowest levels of these nutrients. In addition, choline has been receiving increasing recognition as a nutrient necessary for the proper formation of the developing brain's memory center.

Top betaine sources include wheat bran, cereals and fresh veggies, such as beets and spinach

Top choline sources include beef liver, wheat germ, cod, eggs and wild salmon

NUTRITION TIP

Harvard researchers found that fish-eating moms had brainier kids—but they warn that the benefits must be balanced against the mercury risk. Pregnant women, those who may become pregnant and nursing moms should eat two servings of fish per week, opting for low-mercury varieties (like salmon and sardines) over fish high in mercury (like swordfish, shark, king mackerel and tuna).

GINGER

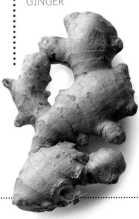

A Spicy Solution

An Australian study found that ginger can relieve morning sickness. While the root has long figured in folk remedies, these findings are among the first to confirm ginger's ability to reduce nausea and vomiting among pregnant women. Researchers caution that further study is needed to address concerns regarding ginger's safety for fetuses.

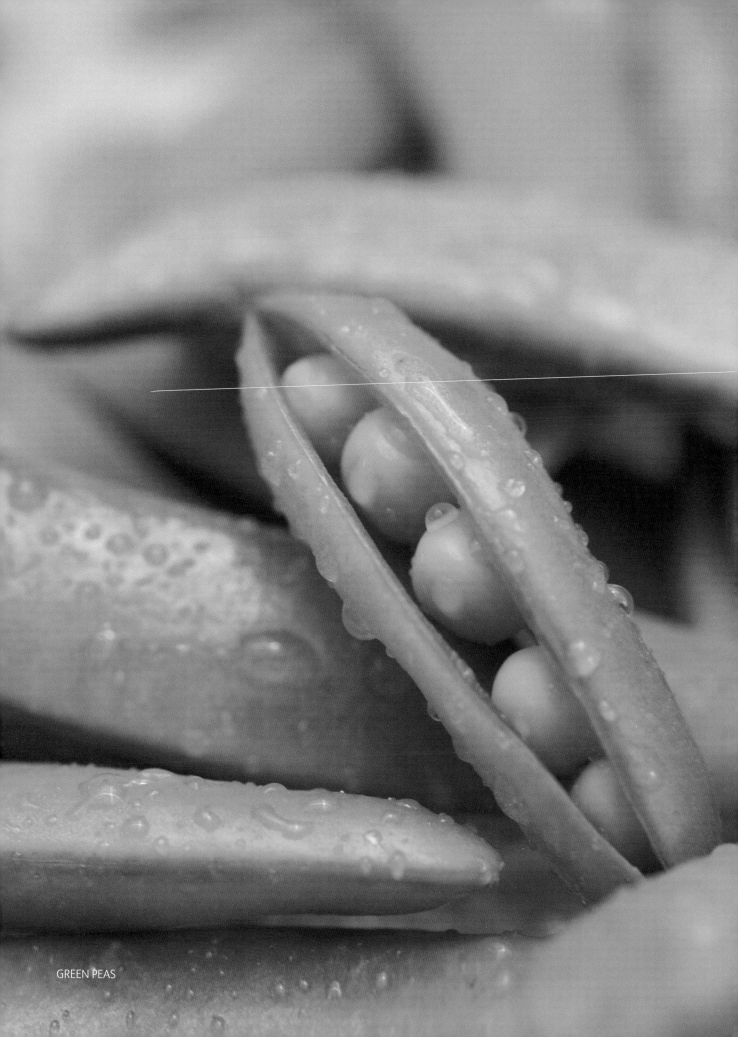

GREEN PEAS

Bananas and Baby Boys

BANANAS

Dietary research on potassium intake during pregnancy may bolster the old wives' tale linking eating bananas with having boys. Compared with those who gave birth to girls, mothers of boys consumed an average of 300 milligrams more potassium per day. (One banana contains 450 milligrams of potassium.)

Vitamin D

In one study, children whose mothers had the lowest levels of vitamin D during pregnancy were found to have thinner, weaker bones by the age of 9. Although your body can produce vitamin D if exposed to adequate sunlight, you may want to consider adding dietary sources of it as well.

Top vitamin D sources include canned sardines, cooked oysters and DOLE Portobello mushrooms (which naturally contain 100 percent of your vitamin D requirements)

Calcium

Calcium is another bone-healthy nutrient that's beneficial for mothers as well as babies. Your calcium needs double during pregnancy, and low intake is associated with increased risk of preeclampsia and preterm delivery. In one study, 1,500 milligrams of calcium per day was enough to reduce the most serious consequences of preeclampsia by approximately 25 percent. Preterm births were also reduced and survival rates increased for mothers and babies.

Top plant-based calcium sources include collard greens, kale, peas, navy beans and sardines

Copper

Chinese researchers found that many mothers of premature babies were low on copper. It's possible that deficient copper could undermine collagen production, contributing to a more precarious pregnancy. In addition, animal research suggests that copper deficiency during pregnancy may lead to lower levels of certain enzymes needed for infants' brain development.

Top copper sources include oysters, shiitake mushrooms, cashews and sunflower seeds

CASHEWS ARE HIGH IN COPPER, WHICH RESEARCH SUGGESTS PROTECTS AGAINST PRETERM DELIVERY.

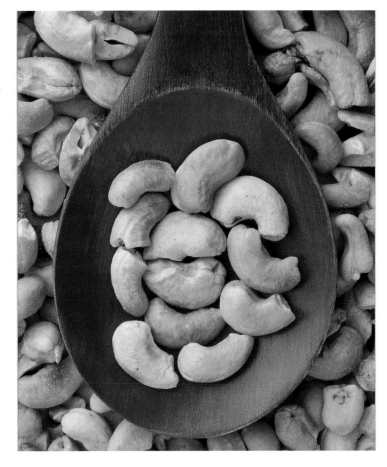

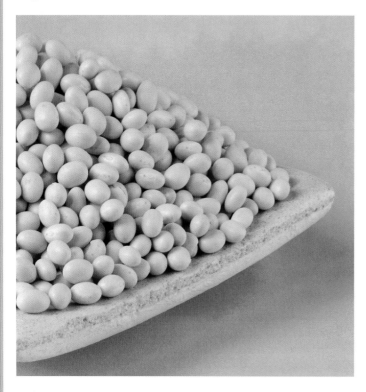

FITNESS TIP
Is having a baby in your future? Then start exercising today. According to a study in *Clinical Obstetrics* and *Gynecology*, women who exercised regularly before they conceived had half the risk of gestational diabetes than their non-exercising peers did.

Zinc

Zinc is essential for the normal development of the fetus and placenta during pregnancy. Zinc deficiency has been linked to neural tube defects and certain kinds of retardation and learning impairments. (Note: Although sufficient iron is important during pregnancy, supplementation with large amounts of iron can interfere with the absorption of zinc.)

Top zinc sources include Alaskan king crab, white beans and lentils

Iodine

Iodine is essential for the normal development of the fetus and newborn, and it helps prevent neonatal hypothyroidism (a condition marked by decreased production of thyroid hormones, possibly leading to mental retardation and heart problems).

Top iodine sources include cod, shrimp and potatoes (with skin)

Antioxidants

About 2,200 children are diagnosed with acute lymphocytic leukemia in the United States each year, making it the most common cancer in children and adolescents. Advances in treatment have greatly improved survival rates, but research into the prevention of this disease through proper diet is opening up a promising new frontier. A study funded by the National Institute of Environmental Health Sciences (NIEHS) found that the higher a woman's intake of carotenoid-rich foods—carrots, cantaloupes, sweet potatoes and spinach—in the 12-month period prior to conception, the lower her chances of giving birth to a child with leukemia. "This is the first time researchers have conducted a systematic survey of a woman's diet and linked it to the risk of childhood leukemia," Kenneth Olden, PhD, director of NIEHS, announced upon the study's completion.

Obesity and Reproductive Health

Even before conception, excess weight interferes with reproductive health. For example, unwanted pounds may increase your risk of unwanted pregnancy. Researchers at the Fred Hutchinson Cancer Research Center compared the body mass index (BMI) of 248 women who became pregnant while taking birth control pills and found that overweight women are 60 percent more likely, and obese women 70 percent more likely, to conceive than slimmer women. While oral contraceptives have never provided fail-safe protection against pregnancy, previous studies had identified a failure rate of less than 1 percent for the general population. These findings suggest that up to 7 percent of heavier women may get pregnant, even when conscientiously taking their contraceptive pills.

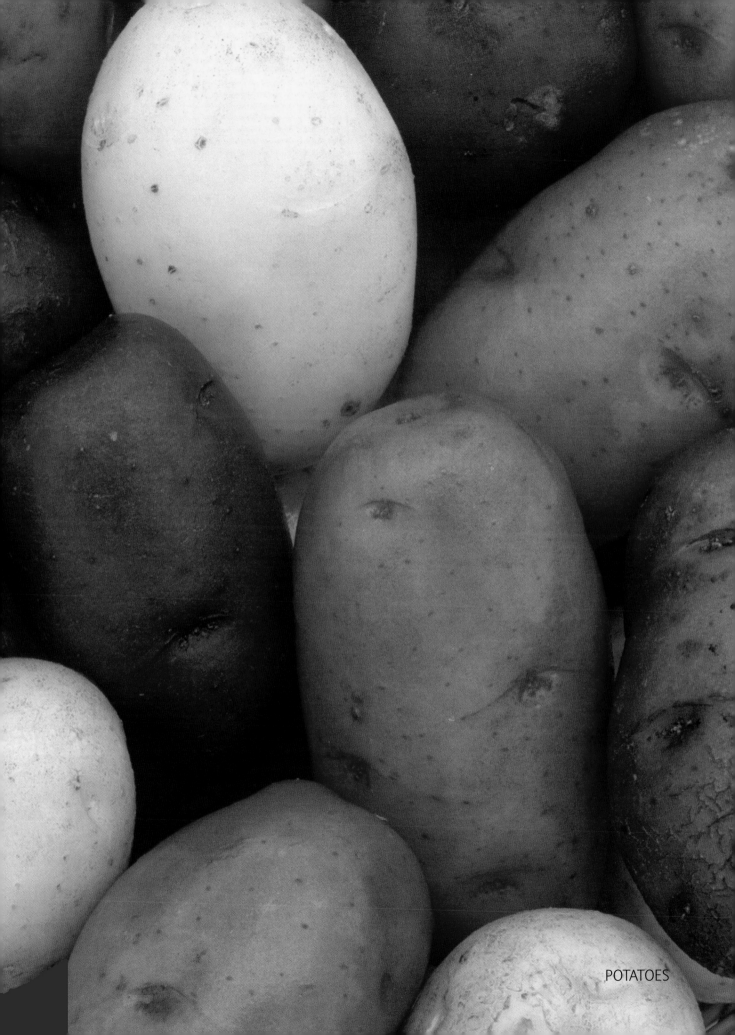

POTATOES

FITNESS TIP

Although research shows that morning exercise can rev up your metabolism and even improve your sleep, experts at the American Council on Exercise say that an afternoon workout may be even more effective. That's when the body is at peak performance— higher temperature, more flexibility and lower blood pressure and heart rate— priming you to burn more calories.

Scientists have yet to determine the exact biological mechanism at work, but they suspect several factors may contribute to the higher rate of failure. For one thing, the more you weigh, the higher your metabolism—which may shorten the duration of a medication's effectiveness. This may be unwelcome news for those who like to blame a sluggish metabolism—as opposed to overeating or inactivity—for excess pounds, but it's simple physics: It takes more muscle to lug around more fat, and more muscle means a higher metabolic rate. Another possible explanation is that fat-soluble birth control hormones (estrogen and progesterone) may get "trapped" in excess fat and not be properly processed in the body.

In addition, new research suggests that entering pregnancy with extra pounds increases your chances of miscarriage by 67 percent. British researchers analyzed 16 studies with a combined 16,000 female subjects and found that those with a BMI of 25 or higher were dramatically more likely to suffer miscarriage within the first five months of pregnancy. In real terms, that means a 5-foot-4-inch woman weighing 145 pounds (prior to pregnancy) would be two-thirds more likely to miscarry than a woman who weighed 15 pounds less. To calculate your risk, check out the BMI chart on page 247.

Overweight women, according to University of Pittsburgh researchers, also are twice as likely—and obese women three times as likely—to develop preeclampsia as their normal-weight peers. And the risk rises sharply even with small increases in prepregnancy body fat.

Other reproductive risks posed by excess prepregnancy weight include infertility, gestational diabetes, congenital malformations and an increased likelihood of the child becoming overweight later in life.

Alcohol Undermines Nursing

One of the weirdest old wives' tales holds that drinking beer can stimulate lactation in nursing mothers. It may sound incredible to modern ears, but faith in the brewer's contribution to breast-feeding was once so widespread that in 1895 Anheuser-Busch produced Malt-Nutrine, a beer that physicians would prescribe as a tonic for breast-feeding women.

New research, however, debunks the beer-benefits myth and demonstrates the detriments of alcohol consumption while nursing. Upon testing lactating women for prolactin and oxytocin levels, the two key hormones that influence lactation performance in breast-feeding mothers, University of Pennsylvania researchers discovered that using alcohol (of any kind) disrupted the hormonal balance required for the optimum yield of breast milk—thus reducing the quality and quantity available to the nursing infant. What's more, other studies have established that when a breast-feeding mother consumes alcohol, it shows up in her milk. Like blood levels of alcohol, milk levels of alcohol eventually dissipate. Still, infants who consume even small amounts of alcohol may suffer problems with motor development, including a weak suckling reflex, which, along with the reduced yield of breast milk, may prevent proper weight gain.

Breast-Feeding Benefits

Consider these statistics: Compared with babies who are not breast-fed, babies who are breast-fed for three to five months are a third less likely to be obese at age 6; those breast-fed for six months are 43 percent less likely to be obese at age 6; and those breast-fed for more than a year are 72 percent less likely to be obese at age 6. Some studies point to the presence of leptin, a satiety hormone, in breast milk, while certain researchers theorize that the modulations in a mother's milk—due to variety in her diet— helps babies develop an appetite that's more attuned to taste and satiety signals.

Babies also enjoy a range of health-protective benefits from breast milk, which make them less vulnerable to certain allergies, ear infections, pneumonia and meningitis. They may also be better protected from heart disease and diabetes down the road. Researchers in Scotland found that children who were fed formula as babies were more likely to develop higher cholesterol and glucose levels later in life, raising their risk of heart disease and diabetes, respectively.

Breast-feeding might also make your baby smarter, according to a study in the *Journal of the American Medical Association* which linked the duration of breast-feeding with significantly higher scores on various verbal and intelligence tests later in life.

In addition, according to the American Academy of Pediatrics, breast-feeding helps mothers return to their prepregnancy weight faster, because it burns more calories. Other benefits to the mom include a reduced risk of ovarian cancer, osteoporosis prevention and a lower incidence of premenopausal breast cancer.

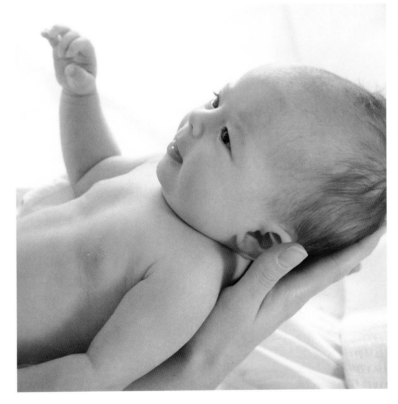

But breast-feeding mothers need to be sure to take precautions, such as drinking lots of fluids and avoiding imported or unpasteurized soft cheeses, cigarette smoke, alcohol, and large or longer-living fish (which tend to be high in mercury) like tuna, swordfish, shark and orange roughy. The Institute of Medicine's (IOM) discussion of energy requirements for lactating mothers estimates a 4 to 5 percent (80 to 100 calories for a 2,000 calorie diet) increase in a woman's metabolic rate during milk production, much lower than the 200 to 500 calories recommended in the early 1990s and the 700 to 1,000 before that. Currently, the U.S. Department of Health and Human Services (HHS) recommends lactating women stick with the same number of calories they were consuming before their pregnancy as a strategy for weight loss after giving birth.

BREAST-FED BABIES ENJOY A HOST OF HEALTH-PROTECTIVE BENEFITS THAT LAST WELL BEYOND INFANCY.

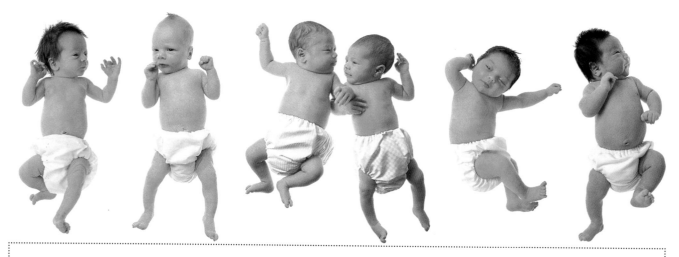

Dairy Double

The dairy industry's marketing mantra of "three-a-day" could take on a whole new meaning in light of a 2006 study in the *Journal of Reproductive Medicine*, which links milk consumption with multiple births. Study author Gary Steinman, MD, PhD, of the Long Island Jewish Medical Center, compared the twinning rates of vegan mothers with the general population of mothers and found the latter to be five times more likely to give birth to twins. Of 1,042 vegan women, only four had experienced multiple births—about 0.4 percent—compared with nearly 2 percent of the general population of mothers. And when Dr. Steinman had 66 women with a history of multiple births rate their dairy consumption on a scale of one to four (one being none, four being a lot of milk), the moms of multiples averaged about a three.

Dr. Steinman speculates that the increased tendency to twin among milk-drinking moms can be attributed to the growth hormones that commonly have been given to cows in the United States since the 1990s—when the rate of multiple births began to rise significantly. Does the data support his hypothesis? Perhaps, though additional factors, such as more women giving birth later in life, likely play a role as well.

FOOD TIP

Go baby crazy with baby veggies—baby carrots, baby turnips, baby squash, baby artichokes and baby cauliflower. In addition to their cute-appeal, baby veggies are often milder in taste. Plus, being more tender, they require less time to cook.

Make your calories count by choosing nutrient-rich fruits and vegetables, whole grains, monounsaturated fats and lean proteins. If your eating habits have been less than healthy in the past, let your new arrival be the inspiration you need to overhaul your diet. When it comes to preparing your child for a lifetime of proper nutrition, keep in mind that what and how you eat will continue to have a profound influence long after your baby is weaned.

Given the benefits of breast-feeding, in 2000—after a decade in which only 64 percent of American mothers were breast-feeding at hospital discharge and just 29 percent were still doing so six months later—the Surgeon General issued a call for action with the goal of raising those figures to 75 percent and 50 percent, respectively, by 2010. According to a 2008 Centers for Disease Control and Prevention report (based on the most current, available numbers from 2005), that goal is in sight, with about 74 percent of mothers breast-feeding their newborns and 43 percent still doing so six months after giving birth.

Programmed to Be Fat

Eating ice cream and other fatty foods during your pregnancy may raise the chances of your child becoming obese later in life. A Rockefeller University animal study demonstrated that even short-term exposure to a high-fat diet in utero could prompt genetic fetal changes that dictate an increased appetite, higher fat intake, earlier puberty and a higher body weight later in life. The offspring of rats fed a 50 percent fat diet for two weeks during pregnancy were up to 140 percent more likely to be fat than those whose moms ate a balanced diet during the intervention period.

But there are still discrepancies among socioeconomic, ethnic and age groups, which suggests that education is the key to bringing the benefits of breast-feeding to a wider population of mothers and children. More than 85 percent of college-educated mothers breast-feed, compared with 66 percent of those mothers who haven't completed high school. In terms of race, 76 percent of Caucasian mothers breast-feed, in contrast with 61 percent of their African-American peers. And, of mothers age 30 and older, 79 percent breast-feed, as opposed to 51 percent of mothers under the age of 20. But if past is prologue, recent rate gains among lagging groups promise continued progress in the years to come.

A HEALTHY DIET BEFORE AND DURING PREGNANCY, AND WHILE NURSING, GIVES YOUR BABY A HEALTHY HEAD START.

Conclusion

Good nutrition is perhaps more important during pregnancy than at any other time in a woman's life, not simply on account of the health of the child, but also because a child's gestation makes tremendous demands on the mother's body. Eating right can help ensure that essential nutrient levels aren't drained from the mother in response to the baby's needs. In addition, a diet rich in fruits and vegetables can help expectant mothers avoid unnecessary weight gain, and thus avoid risks to both their and their child's health. Plus, this kind of diet will make it easier for the mother to return to a healthy weight after delivery.

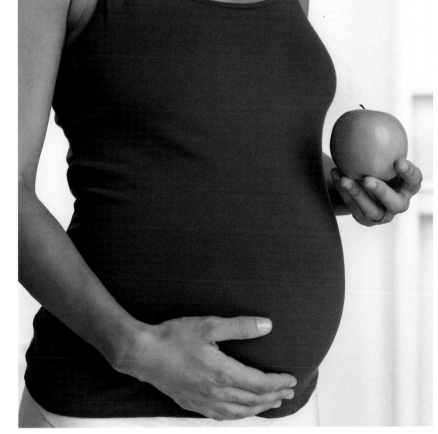

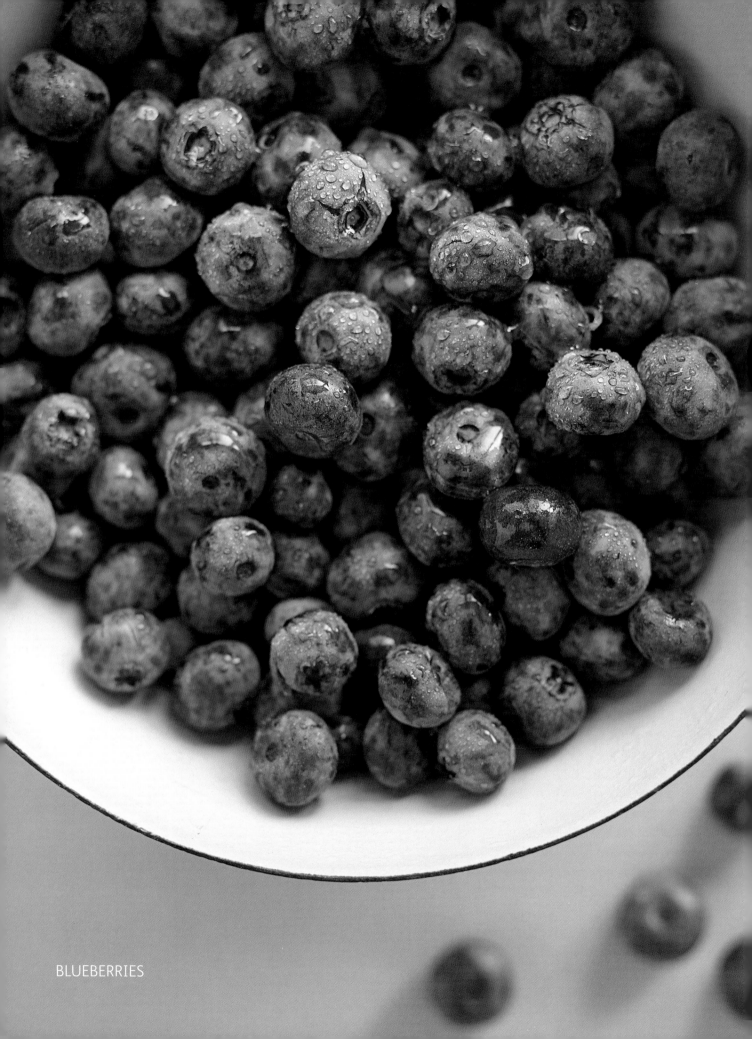

BLUEBERRIES

CHAPTER 8

Brain Health

You Need: ANTIOXIDANTS, ANTHOCYANINS, FOLATE, VITAMIN C, CHOLINE

Eat These:

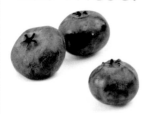

BLUEBERRIES

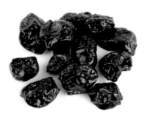

POMEGRANATES

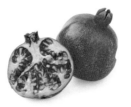

PRUNES

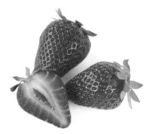

STRAWBERRIES

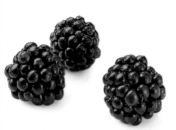

BLACKBERRIES

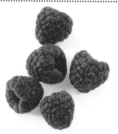

RASPBERRIES

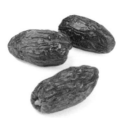

DATES

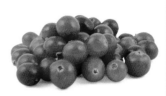

CRANBERRIES

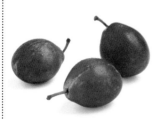

PLUMS

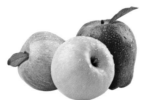

APPLES

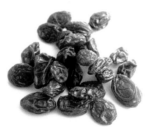

RAISINS

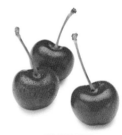

CHERRIES

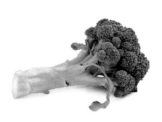

BROCCOLI

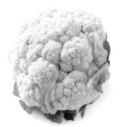

BROCCOLI SPROUTS

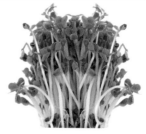

CAULIFLOWER

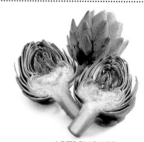

ARTICHOKES

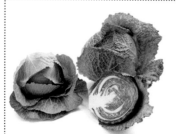

CABBAGE

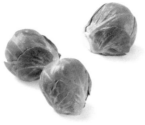

BRUSSELS SPROUTS

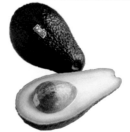

AVOCADOS

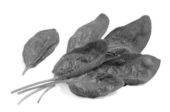

SPINACH

▶ James Joseph

James Joseph, PhD, is an expert on aging and has done extensive research on the role of diet in preserving brain health. He is currently director of the Neuroscience Laboratory at the USDA Human Nutrition Research Center on Aging at Tufts University.

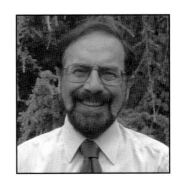

Q: What is the main cause of decline in brain function as we age?

JJ: One of the major theories of aging attributes physiological deterioration to the accumulated damage that free radicals cause our cells over time—and neurons, the interconnected networks of nerve cells that the brain relies on to function, are particularly vulnerable to free-radical damage.

Q: What are free radicals, and how do they work?

JJ: Free radicals are highly unstable molecules, due to the fact that they're missing an electron. They react with oxygen, bonding with other molecules and swiping electrons from them, which initiates a chain reaction as successive molecules lose and gain electrons. This disruption of normal cellular processes causes oxidative stress to cell membranes, DNA and other important tissue components (similar to the rusting of metal or the browning of a sliced apple exposed to the air). Over time, this oxidation can cause inflammation and other unhealthy cellular changes, which are characteristic of every major disease. In terms of the brain, free radicals interfere with neuron function, causing a reduction in the number of synapses. But studies indicate that eating fruits and vegetables that are high in antioxidant activity can help offset the free-radical damage that accelerates the aging process. Every major disease has an oxidative stress and inflammatory component.

WALNUTS SUPPLY A HEALTHY COMBINATION OF FIBER, FATTY ACIDS, B VITAMINS, VITAMIN E, MAGNESIUM, PLANT STEROLS AND MORE.

Q: Are there any particular foods you recommend?

JJ: The fruits with the highest antioxidant activity are the berry fruits—such as blueberries, raspberries, strawberries, boysenberries, blackberries and cranberries. The high-antioxidant vegetables include spinach and artichokes. Nuts also contain beneficial fatty acids, polyphenols and vitamin E. With walnuts, one not only gets vitamin E but also combinations of fiber, B vitamins, magnesium, plant sterols and omega-3 fatty acids—the "good" fats—as well as the beneficial polyphenols. The same is true for avocados.

Q: Are supplements as good a source of antioxidants as food?

JJ: The problem with supplements is that they don't overcome the negative effects of a bad diet. Additionally, when we obtain our antioxidants from foods, we are not getting just one or two antioxidants but a whole array of compounds that have beneficial properties. There's increasing evidence that when you take these nutrients out of the food matrix, they may be ineffective or even harmful.

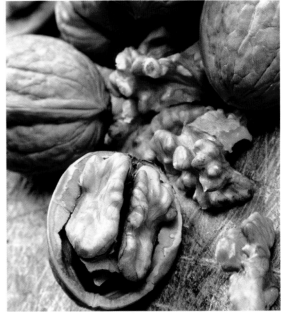

Whether you simply want to remember where you left your keys or you're looking to ward off debilitating and life-threatening cognitive disease, it's important to know what habits and lifestyle factors can impact brain function and accelerate—or decelerate—age-related mental decline.

Conveniently, the same actions you can take to preserve brain health over time are beneficial to day-to-day performance as well. So, whether the advice in this chapter arises from a study on Alzheimer's disease, depression or cognitive function, it can be applied across the board to improve brain development; mood; focus; mental clarity; concentration; visual, verbal, and spatial acuity; and more.

Obesity

Increasingly, clinical studies are indicating that excess weight is bad for the brain. An international group of researchers found that among more than 400 healthy adult men and women, those with an elevated body mass index (BMI) performed consistently worse on cognitive tests than those with a normal BMI. The results, reported in a 2007 issue of *Comprehensive Psychiatry*, echo previous findings linking obesity to impaired executive skills, verbal fluency and short- and long-term memory. Moreover, a five-year French study of 2,223 participants connected higher BMIs with lower cognitive test scores, also finding that the heavier test subjects were at the beginning of the study, the greater their cognitive decline by its conclusion.

And it's not only *adult* brains that are affected. A 2008 study in the journal *Obesity* reported that among 2,519 children, ages 8 to 16, increased body weight was associated with decreased visuospatial organization and general mental ability.

Researchers have also found that obese or even overweight women are more susceptible to losing brain tissue as they age, which makes sense in light of the many studies showing an elevated incidence of Alzheimer's disease among obese and overweight adults. In 2004, after following 1,500 subjects for 21 years, Swedish researchers concluded that obesity doubles the risk of developing dementia.

Fortunately, taking action to reduce the risk factors now—losing excess weight, improving your diet and exercising—gives you a far better chance of avoiding these minute neural injuries and maintaining your mental edge through the years.

HEALTH TIP
Night Eating Syndrome (NES), a condition characterized by waking several times during the night to eat, is 10 times more prevalent among the obese than the adult population at large. Research suggests that night eating contributes to obesity over time.

Brain Calisthenics

Exercising your mind is just as important to brain health as exercising your body. A study published in the *New England Journal of Medicine* monitoring 470 older Americans for five years found that those who played board games several times a week with others enjoyed a 74 percent lower risk of developing dementia. Other protective activities include playing a musical instrument (which yielded a 69 percent lower risk) and doing crosswords regularly (which conferred a 47 percent lower risk). Scientists believe such activities help maintain mental fitness by stimulating connections between brain cells—and building up new brain cells which replace those that die.

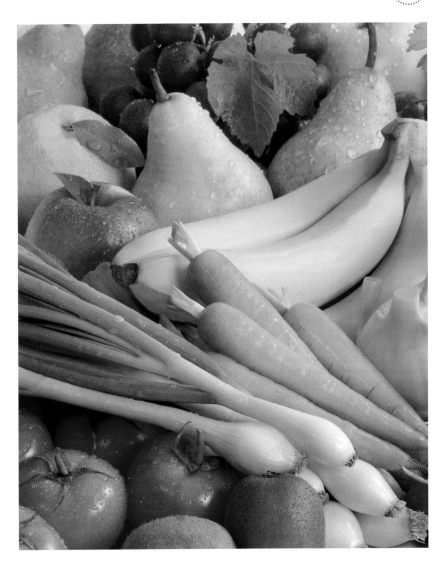

What to Choose

EATING FOR BRAIN HEALTH

Fruits and vegetables provide a two-in-one weapon against brain decline. First, they help with weight control: Low in calories and rich in nutrients, they fill you up and fight deficiency-fueled cravings. Second: They provide antioxidants and other key compounds that help protect the brain.

Other elements of a brain-healthy diet include nuts, seeds, fatty fish and foods high in omega-3 fatty acids

FRUITS AND VEGETABLES ARE FULL OF BRAIN-PROTECTING ANTIOXIDANTS AND COMPOUNDS.

Alzheimer's Epidemic

One in 45 Americans will ultimately suffer from dementia, the most common form of which is Alzheimer's disease. There are more than 5 million cases of Alzheimer's in the United States today, and that number is expected to more than triple by 2050—due not only to an increase in the aging population but also to expanding waistlines.

DIET TIP
Brainiacs eat breakfast! Researchers at the University of Health Sciences/ Chicago Medical School found superior cognitive performance and memory recall among breakfast eaters compared with those who skipped the morning meal.

ONE SMART VEGGIE

Research confirms that seniors who eat more vegetables experience significantly less age-related cognitive decline. Researchers at Rush University collected dietary data from 3,718 adults, ages 65 and older, and administered memory tests over the course of six years. It turned out that those adults who ate more than four servings (that's 2 cups) of vegetables daily had a 38 percent lower rate of mental deterioration than those who ate less than one serving (half a cup) of vegetables per day.

These findings constitute yet more evidence of the protective power of produce, following on the heels of Harvard research which found that middle-aged women who ate the most leafy greens, cruciferous veggies or a combination of both boosted their odds of maintaining mental sharpness in later years. Specifically, the women who ate eight or more servings of vegetables per week, like spinach and broccoli, scored higher on cognitive tests than those who consumed just three servings.

DON'T FORGET FRUIT

Blueberries might help you outsmart Alzheimer's. In the first major study on the effect of fruits and vegetables in reversing neural cell damage, researchers at the Neuroscience Laboratory at Tufts University found that blueberry-supplemented animal subjects exhibited improved brain- and motor-function coordination.

Fresh apples—the peel in particular—have some of the highest levels of quercetin (which is also found in onions, broccoli, kale, blueberries, cranberries and red grapes). Some of the most exciting studies of this flavonol suggest it may help fight Alzheimer's disease by protecting brain cells against oxidative stress. In an animal study at Cornell University, quercetin proved more powerful than the antioxidant vitamin C in neutralizing the kind of neural damage done by free radicals. "Fresh apples have some of the highest levels of quercetin … and may be among the best food choices for fighting Alzheimer's," says study author and professor of Food Science and Technology, C.Y. Lee.

Eating and IQ

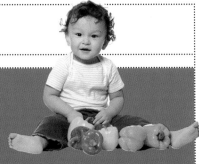

Eating certain foods may help boost brainpower, but what about the obverse: Are geniuses predisposed to eat certain foods? Quite possibly, according to one British study that found children with higher IQs were more likely to grow up to be vegetarians.

Researchers tested 8,000 10-year-olds for mental ability back in 1970 and then followed up with the subjects 20 years later to ask about their diet. It turned out that the adults who had become vegetarians were more intelligent as kids—about 6 percent smarter, at least as measured by IQ points. The study authors speculate that smarter folks are more likely to think through the consequences of what they eat—both in terms of health *and* ideology.

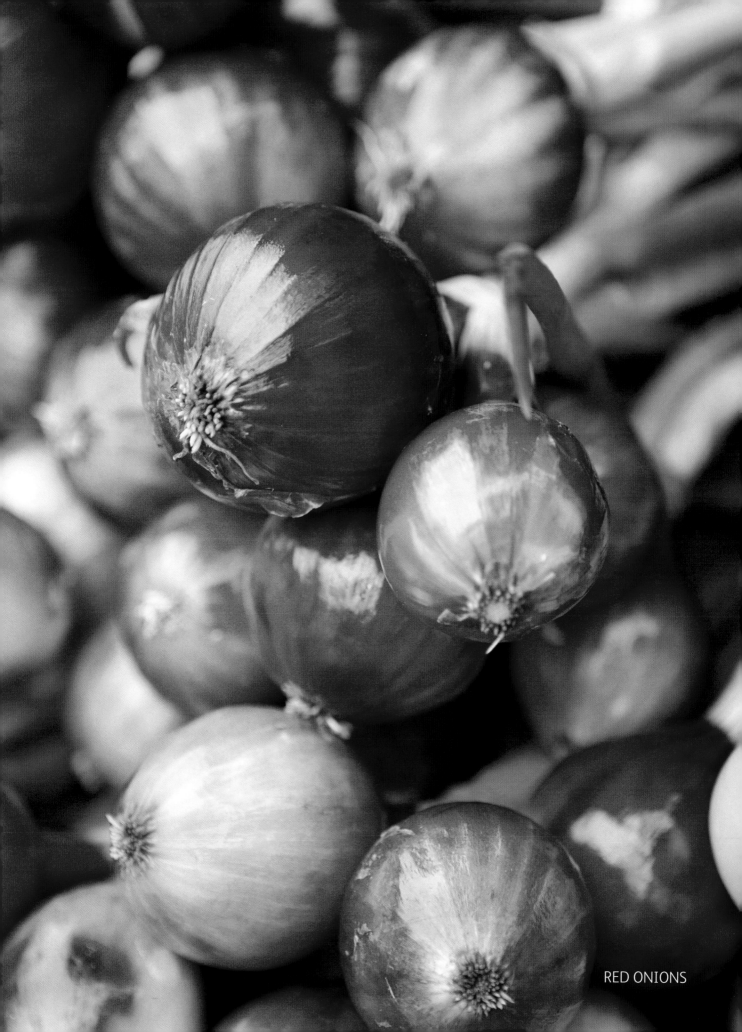

RED ONIONS

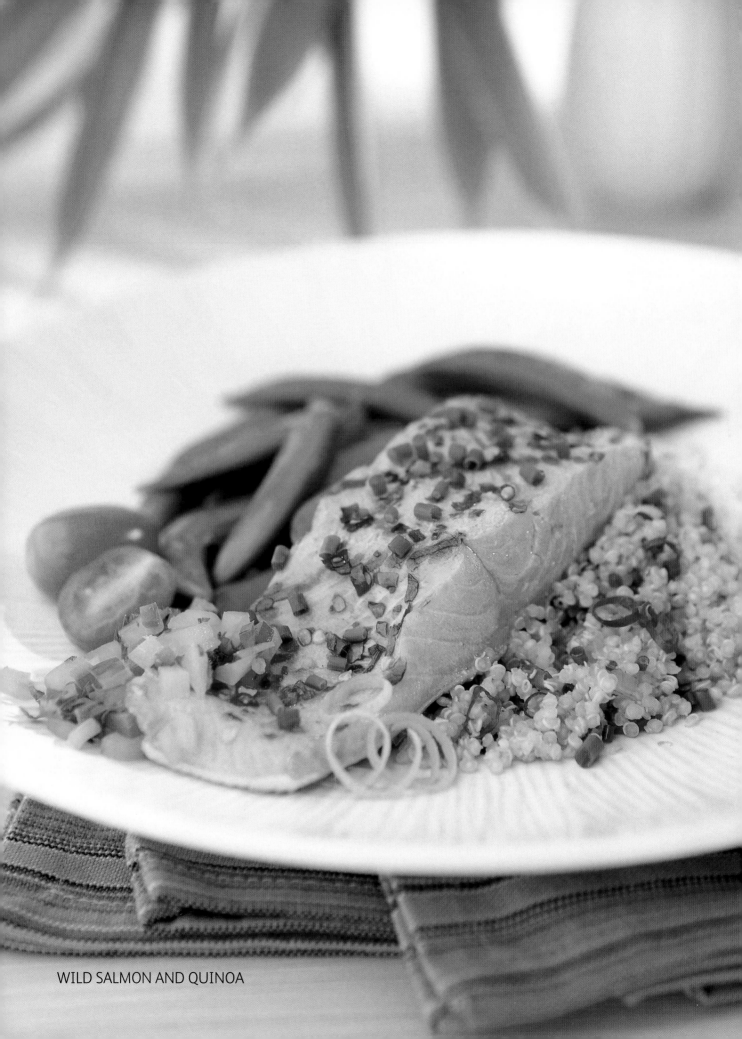

WILD SALMON AND QUINOA

JUICE IT UP

Research suggests that fruit and vegetable juice may offer powerful protection against Alzheimer's. A Vanderbilt University study found that those who drank fruit or vegetable juice more than three times per week were an astounding 75 percent less likely to develop Alzheimer's than once-a-week or non-juice drinkers. Researchers believe that the antioxidant polyphenols contained in juice guard against the oxidation (or rust, if you will) of brain tissues.

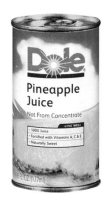

FISH FOR PROTEIN

According to researchers at Rush University Medical Center, seniors who eat as little as one serving of fish per week slow age-related mental decline by an equivalent of three to four years and reduce their risk of Alzheimer's by half. And a study at Harvard that retested blood samples taken 20 years earlier found that people with higher blood levels of a type of omega-3 found in fish oil were least likely to have developed Alzheimer's two decades later.

The omega-3 fatty acids found in fish (especially fatty fish, such as salmon, sardines, flounder and cod), nuts, seeds and some oils (such as canola and olive oil) have also been shown to help with depression and other mental states. In a study of 3,600 adults conducted by Kaiser Permanente, those who ate a serving of fatty fish were 20 percent less likely to register aggravation, resentment, mistrust or cynicism. Fish is also a great source for lean protein and B vitamins—crucial for brain health.

THE NUTRIENTS IN BROCCOLI HELP PRESERVE MENTAL FUNCTION AND PROTECT THE BRAIN AFTER TRAUMA.

VITAMIN E FOR EXTRA ACUITY

"Vitamin E is one of the most potent antioxidants in animal and lab studies," says Martha Clare Morris, ScD, an epidemiologist at Rush-Presbyterian-St. Luke's Medical Center in Chicago. In her three-year study of more than 3,000 people over age 65, those who had the highest vitamin E intake (from food, not supplements) showed 37 percent less decline on tests of memory, attention and abstract thinking, and they also had a 70 percent lower risk of developing Alzheimer's.

Top vitamin E sources include sunflower seeds, almonds, hazelnuts, spinach and broccoli

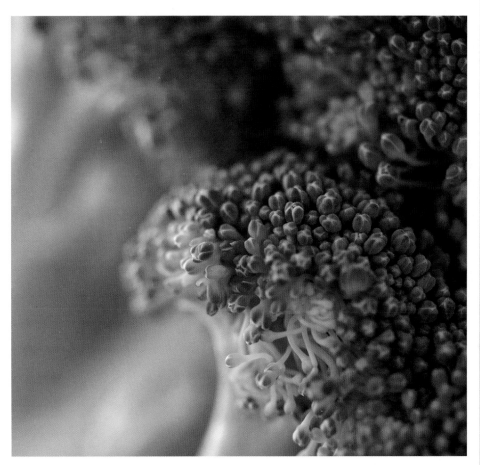

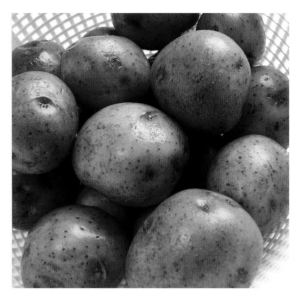

RED POTATOES ARE A TOP SOURCE FOR NIACIN, WHICH RESEARCHERS SAY MAY HELP WARD OFF ALZHEIMER'S.

NIACIN FOR YOUR NOGGIN

In a four-year study of 800 seniors, those with the highest intake of niacin—also known as vitamin B3—had an 80 percent lower risk of developing Alzheimer's disease.

Top niacin sources include portobello and button mushrooms, red potatoes and salmon (an all-around superfood for seniors)

What to Avoid
EXCESSIVE ALCOHOL CONSUMPTION

While there's ample research documenting the heart-health benefits of moderate alcohol consumption, heavy drinking has been shown to do lasting damage to the brain. A Saint Louis University animal study suggests that several years of heavy drinking not only slows down learning ability, but can also permanently impair memory as well. Researchers fed two groups of rodents an alcoholic solution for either four or eight weeks—the human equivalent of a daily bottle of wine or a six-pack of beer for either three or six years. Both groups were tested for long-term memory and learning ability after being "off the bottle" for three weeks. Significant long-term memory impairment occurred in the eight-week rats but not the four-week rats. What's more, the impairment hadn't improved when the rats were retested nine weeks later.

German researchers who used computerized tomography scans to examine the brains of 158 human subjects—which included both alcoholics and a control group—found that women drinkers develop brain atrophy faster than their male counterparts. Lead researcher Karl Mann, MD, observed, "Women developed equal brain-volume reductions as the men after a significantly shorter period of alcohol dependence than the men." In other words, although women typically start drinking at an older age, consume less and are less likely to develop alcohol dependence than men, their brains are more vulnerable to neurochemical damage from excess drinking.

Broccoli and the Blood-Brain Barrier

Can diet help protect you from the effects of a head injury? Quite possibly. If the injury breaches a network of capillaries called the blood-brain barrier, toxins that would otherwise be kept out can seep into the brain and cause further damage well after the initial event. In a Texas A&M University study, researchers used a rodent model to show that sulforaphane—an indirect antioxidant formed when broccoli is chewed—helps rally certain proteins that strengthen the impaired blood-brain barrier after physical trauma.

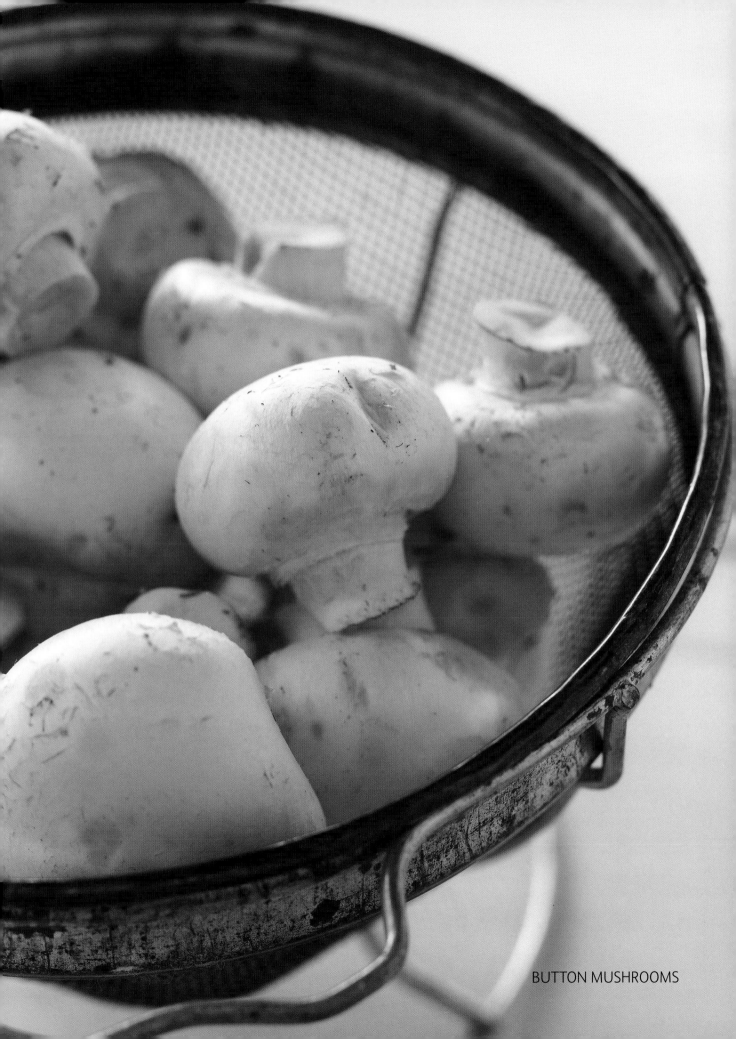

BUTTON MUSHROOMS

Exercise Your Faculties

Diet is one key to maintaining a brain-healthy weight; exercise is another. But the latest research indicates that the benefits of physical activity extend well beyond body mass. Exercise promotes blood flow to the brain and supplies the cells with oxygen and nutrients; in addition, it seems to boost brain hormones that help keep you focused, lowers memory-damaging amino acids and prevents—or possibly reverses—the natural brain shrinkage that begins in middle age.

Taiwanese researchers found that middle-aged mice trained to work out on a treadmill every day for five weeks grew 2.5 times more new brain cells than mice that didn't work out. Not only was the quantity of brain cells superior in the mice that worked out, but the quality of these cells was as well. Also, mice that began exercising in early middle age fared even better than mice that took to the treadmill in later middle age.

Researchers at the University of Edinburgh in Scotland studied physical fitness and cognitive function in 460 human subjects, all surviving participants of the 1932 Scottish Mental Health Survey. They reviewed IQ data from the earlier study and administered the same cognitive test that participants had taken at age 11 to the 79-year-olds, looking at verbal reasoning, numerical and spatial skills. Then they tested their physical prowess, including grip strength, 6-meter walk time and lung function. What the researchers found was that higher fitness levels at age 79 were a significant predictor of higher cognitive test scores, indicating that physical fitness has a direct correlation to successful cognitive aging.

KEEP YOUR WITS BY WALKING

A University of Illinois study used magnetic resonance imaging (MRI) to measure brain volume in nearly 60 seniors. Half of the group was then put on a brisk walking regimen—one hour per day, three times a week—while the rest were assigned stretch-and-tone exercises. "After only three months, the people who [walked] had the brain volumes of people three years younger," observed study coauthor Arthur Kramer, PhD. MRIs revealed no such improvements for the stretch-and-tone group, leading researchers to believe that walking pumps more blood to the brain, which in turn fuels the growth of new neurons.

EXERCISE TO THE BEAT FOR AN EXTRA BOOST

A study in the *New England Journal of Medicine* found that among 450 seniors, all age 75, those who danced several times per week had the best defenses against mental deterioration. And researchers at Ohio State University report that adults participating in a cardiac rehabilitation program who exercised to music not only reported feeling better emotionally postworkout, but they also *doubled* their verbal fluency test scores, while the control group's scores remained flat.

"The combination of music and exercise may stimulate and increase cognitive arousal while helping to organize cognitive output," said study author Charles Emery, PhD, who used

HEALTH TIP
Factors that help protect the heart may also help protect the brain, suggests results from the large-scale Framingham Heart Study. A series of cognitive tests revealed that those with the highest risk factors for stroke scored far behind their peers in reasoning, attention span and the ability to plan ahead. The good news is that by losing excess weight, improving diet and exercising, you have a far better chance of maintaining your mental edge as the years go by.

Meditation, Mind Modification

Cutting-edge research indicates that regular meditation may thwart age-related deterioration of the prefrontal cortex. In a Harvard University–led study, magnetic resonance imaging revealed superior brain structure in 25- to 50-year-olds who meditated for 40 minutes per day compared with a nonmeditating control group. The thinner cortices of control-group participants reflect the kind of brain shrinkage that occurs with age. Researchers hypothesize that regular meditation may help preserve the integrity of those areas of the brain involved with sensory perception, rational thinking and emotional processing.

Vivaldi's *The Four Seasons* for the experiment and cited the symphony's moderate tempo and positive effects in previous research.

VARY YOUR WORKOUT TO MAXIMIZE BENEFITS
Variety of exercise—opposed to intensity, in terms of total calorie burn—may reduce the risk of developing dementia later in life, according to researchers at Johns Hopkins. They conducted the Cardiovascular Health Cognition Study, which asked 3,375 seniors to list the frequency and duration of their participation in 15 physical activities—including walking, biking, hiking, dancing, bowling and golfing—that are common among older adults. While 450 new cases of dementia were reported during the course of the eight-year study, only 84 occurred in those seniors who took part in four or more activities, and 130 struck those who participated in no activities or only one. "It could well be that maintaining a variety of activities keeps more parts of the brain active," says Constantine Lyketsos, PhD, senior study author.

DANCING IS NOT ONLY A GREAT WAY TO GET SOME EXERCISE AND BOOST YOUR MOOD—IT'S BEEN FOUND TO HELP WARD OFF MENTAL DECLINE.

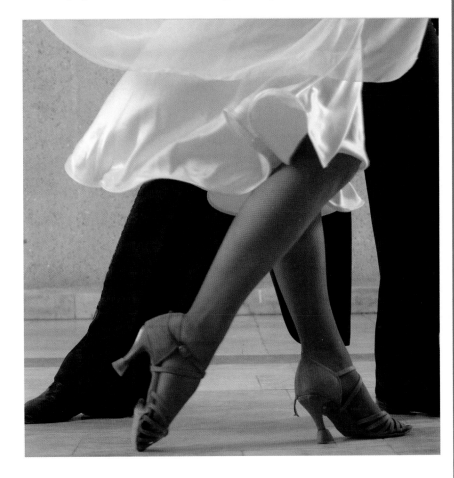

Conclusion
Maintaining a healthy weight throughout life is one of the most important factors in preserving cognitive function into a ripe old age—particularly if it's achieved by maintaining a diet rich in fruits and vegetables and getting plenty of vigorous, varied exercise.

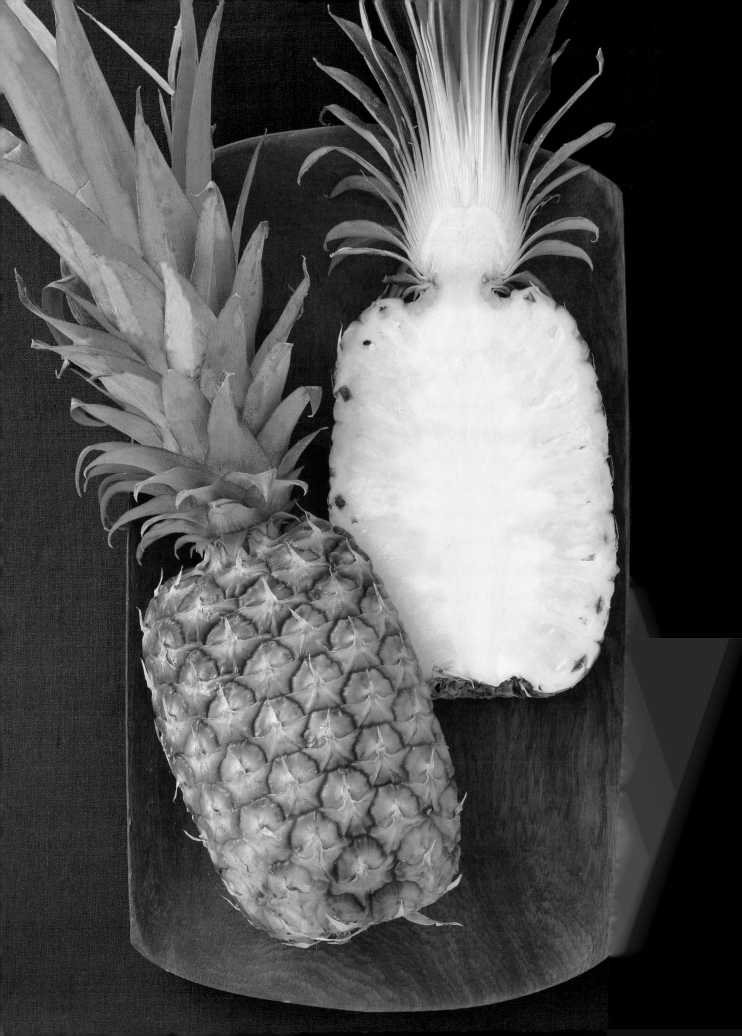

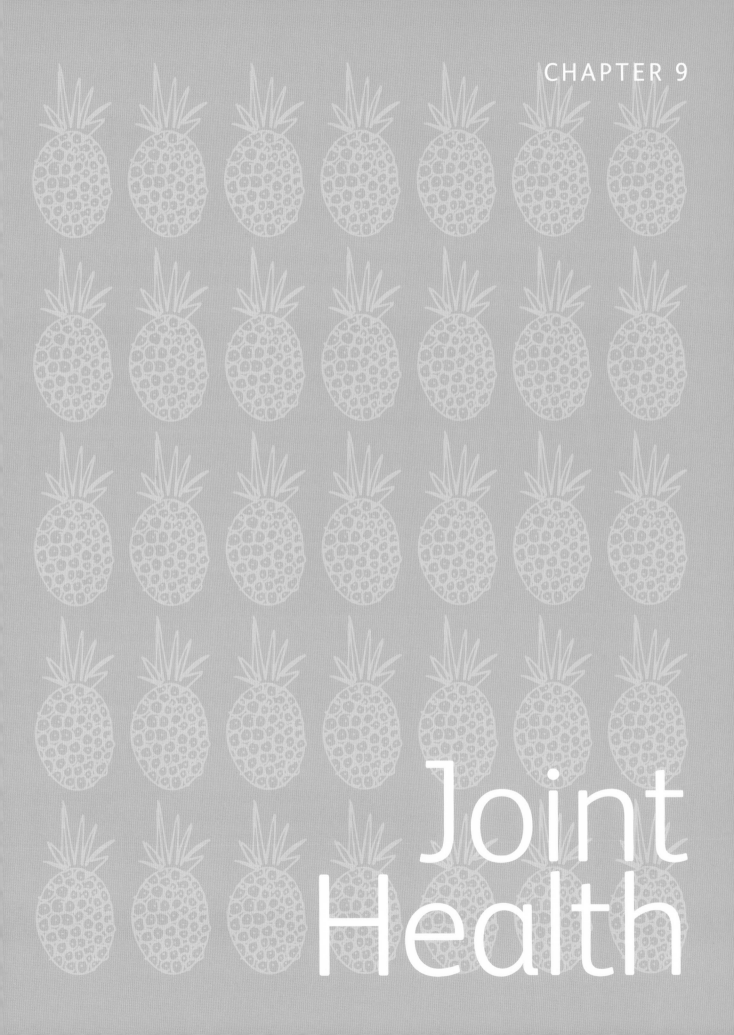

CHAPTER 9

Joint
Health

You Need: BROMELAIN, ANTHOCYANINS, BETA-CRYPTOXANTHIN, SULFORAPHANE, VITAMIN C, CALCIUM, VITAMIN D, SELENIUM

Eat These:

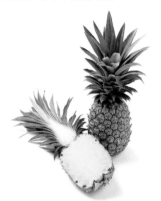

PINEAPPLE

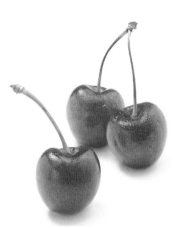

CHERRIES

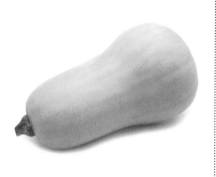

BUTTERNUT SQUASH

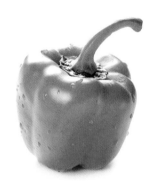

RED BELL PEPPER

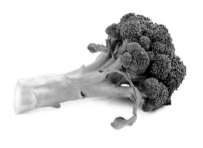

BROCCOLI

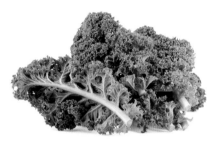

KALE

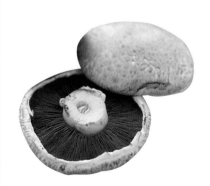

PORTOBELLO MUSHROOMS

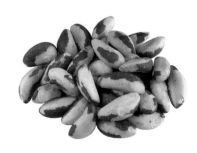

BRAZIL NUTS

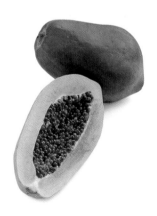

PAPAYAS

The two most common forms of arthritis, osteoarthritis (OA) and rheumatoid arthritis (RA), afflict one in three American adults. Osteoarthritis, the more prevalent joint condition, often occurs as cartilage wears down over time, causing swelling and pain as bone rubs against bone. Rheumatoid arthritis is an autoimmune disease in which the immune system mistakenly attacks healthy joint tissue, causing inflammation and joint damage.

Diet and lifestyle habits have the potential to either aggravate or alleviate the symptoms of both conditions. In studies where severe rheumatoid arthritis sufferers switched to a low-fat diet and adopted regular exercise, symptoms decreased dramatically—so much so that patients required less medication. Apparently, dietary changes provide the biggest benefits; symptoms reappeared as soon as patients returned to bad eating habits. This chapter walks you though the latest scientific findings on nutrients and lifestyle choices that can help reduce the inflammation and pain associated with arthritis.

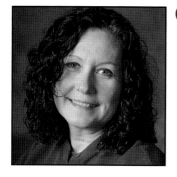

▶ Deborah E. Kipp

Deborah E. Kipp, PhD, RD, is professor and chair of the Department of Nutrition at the University of North Carolina at Greensboro. She received her PhD from Cornell University and her RD from Miami Valley Hospital in Dayton, Ohio. Her current research focuses on how nutrient deficiencies (vitamin C and iron) and hormone activity affect the skeleton.

Q: What's the scope of osteoarthritis as it afflicts the American population?

DK: According to the National Osteoporosis Foundation, osteoarthritis is the most common type of arthritis, affecting nearly 27 million Americans. It's caused by a breakdown of cartilage in joints, resulting in reduced cushioning and, consequently, pain, stiffness and loss of movement in the affected joint. Major risk factors for the development of osteoarthritis include heredity, joint trauma, aging and obesity.

Q: How significant is obesity to this problem?

Obesity increases pressure on the joints and is a common risk factor for osteoarthritis.

DK: It's one of the most common risk factors for osteoarthritis. Obesity causes an increase in mechanical stress and pressure on joints, which wears away the cartilage that normally protects the joints and causes pain and inflammation. Weight loss reduces the stress and the load on the hips, knees and lower back, thereby preventing or slowing the development of osteoarthritis in those joints.

Q: How does exercise impact joint health?

DK: Exercise helps protect joints by building strong muscles around them. Stretching exercises improve their range of motion. And activities like swimming, walking and weight lifting increase flexibility and endurance—and also help with weight control, boost energy and improve overall health and fitness.

Q: What role does diet play?

DK: A well-balanced diet with a variety of foods—including plenty of fruits, vegetables, grains, non-fat dairy and other calcium-rich foods, and lean proteins like fish, turkey and beans—is important for promoting health and preventing disease. The food we eat provides essential nutrients, such as vitamins, minerals, fatty acids and protein. We also must balance energy sources (calories consumed) with energy expenditure in order to maintain appropriate body weight (or lose weight if needed). There are other components, called phytochemicals, in some of the food we eat; they aren't essential nutrients, but they have health-protective effects (for instance, working as antioxidants or to enhance immunity) and help reduce our risk of diseases. Phytochemicals are found in plant-based foods such as fruits and vegetables. A well-balanced diet includes a variety of colorful fruits and vegetables that provide essential nutrients as well as phytochemicals.

Q: How important are antioxidants to joint health?

DK: Antioxidants help prevent free-radical formation, which can cause cartilage damage and inflammation. So a diet containing a variety of fruits and vegetables rich in antioxidants, such as vitamin C, alpha-tocopherol (vitamin E), beta-carotene and other carotenoids and phytochemicals, will help prevent joint damage and pain. Vitamin C is also essential for the formation of cross-linked collagen, which is a protein found in cartilage.

Q: How do enzymes, such as bromelain in pineapples or papain in papayas, impact the joints?

DK: In general, these enzymes have anti-inflammatory properties and may help reduce the joint pain of osteoarthritis. These foods also contain essential vitamins and minerals, including those with antioxidant properties, which would be important to include in a well-balanced diet to promote joint health.

Q: What's the importance of good fats in maintaining joint health?

DK: Fish oils, which are excellent sources of omega-3 fatty acids, may help in reducing pain and inflammation of stiff joints in some people with arthritis. Fish oils are obtained in the diet by eating fish like mackerel, salmon, herring and tuna.

Q: What's your opinion of all these joint-health supplements that we see on the shelves these days?

DK: Scientific research on the possible benefit of over-the-counter supplements containing glucosamine and chondroitin in reducing joint pain and improving function with osteoarthritis is very limited and inconclusive. Some physicians suggest that their patients try a supplement for a period of several weeks to a couple of months, and if they don't feel any relief in that time, to discontinue using it. Supplements should not be taken without close medical supervision due to potential side effects and interactions with medicines, so anyone trying these or any other over-the-counter supplements should consult their physician first.

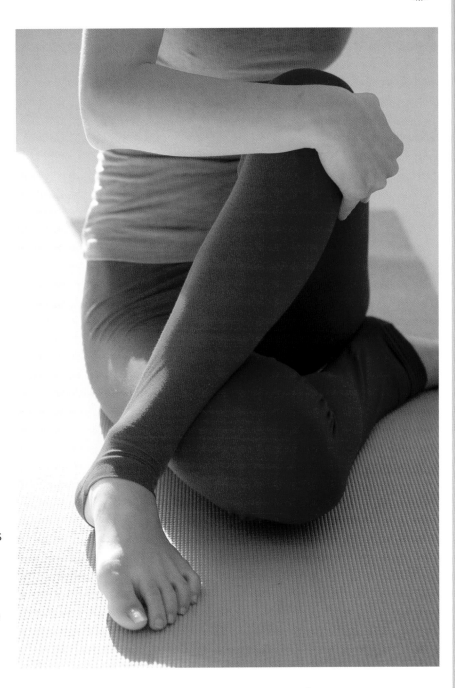

STRECHING CAN HELP IMPROVE RANGE OF MOTION AND PROTECT JOINT HEALTH.

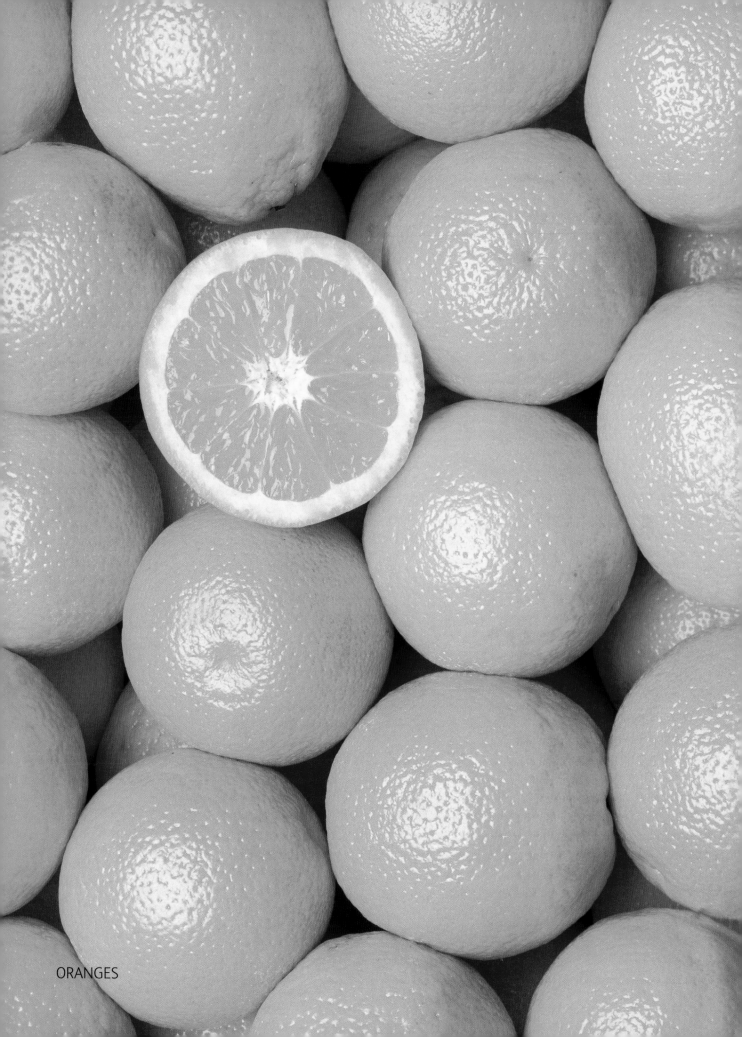

ORANGES

What to Choose

A diet high in fruits and vegetables helps protect the joints in a variety of ways, supplying nutrients like vitamin C, which is needed for calcium and iron absorption, collagen formation and protection against free-radical damage. The high fiber, water and other nutrient content in plant-based foods also help with weight management, making it easier to avoid obesity, which places unhealthy stress on vulnerable joints. And Harvard researchers have found a link between low fruit and vegetable consumption and the higher risk of rheumatoid arthritis.

Certain fruits and vegetables also supply particular nutrients with more targeted joint benefits. For example:

PINEAPPLE

This tropical fruit is the only natural source of bromelain, an enzyme that acts as a cleanup crew, digesting dead protein cells in the case of injury or run-of-the-mill microtears that are part of the muscle-building process. Research suggests that the bromelain in pineapples can also help reduce inflammation and relieve muscle soreness. Scientists at the Dole Nutrition Institute found that both fresh and frozen pineapples have as much, if not more, bromelain activity than supplements. Pineapples are also an excellent source of vitamin C—which helps improve iron and calcium absorption and promotes collagen formation—and manganese, which supports metabolism and bone density.

NUTRITION TIP
In addition to its joint benefits, vitamin C is good for the heart. It combats the oxidation of LDL (bad) cholesterol and is thought to help lower blood levels of C-reactive protein (a marker of inflammatory heart disease).

The Healing Touch

After two months of regular Swedish massages, osteoarthritis sufferers reported better knee function as well as less stiffness and pain, according to a study in the *Archives of Internal Medicine*. Researchers believe that massage helped improve joint flexibility and blood circulation, leading to this positive outcome.

CHERRIES

Cherries are a top source of anthocyanins, thought to reduce inflammation and lower blood levels of uric acid, which can crystallize and accumulate in the joints, causing the type of pain along the lines of that associated with gout attacks. A U.S. Agricultural Research Service study found that five hours after consuming about 45 Bing cherries, women's plasma-urate levels decreased by approximately 15 percent.

BUTTERNUT SQUASH

Butternut squash is rich in beta-cryptoxanthin, a provitamin A carotenoid. In a study in the *American Journal of Clinical Nutrition,* subjects with the highest intake of fruit and vegetables containing beta-cryptoxanthin reduced their risk of developing polyarthritis by 50 percent. **Other beta-cryptoxanthin sources include** oranges, pumpkins, tangerines and papayas

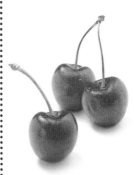

CHERRIES

RED BELL PEPPERS ARE LOADED WITH VITAMIN C, WHICH STUDIES SUGGEST HELPS LOWER OSTEOARTHRITIS RISK.

DIET TIP

It seems no part of the body is immune to the damaging effects of excess weight. Even the hands can bear the consequences in the form of unsightly, oversize knuckles caused by a joint-deforming condition called osteoarthritis. French researchers have linked the joint distortion to leptin, a hormone released by fat cells. To keep your hands svelte, stay active and avoid calorie overload that leads to weight gain.

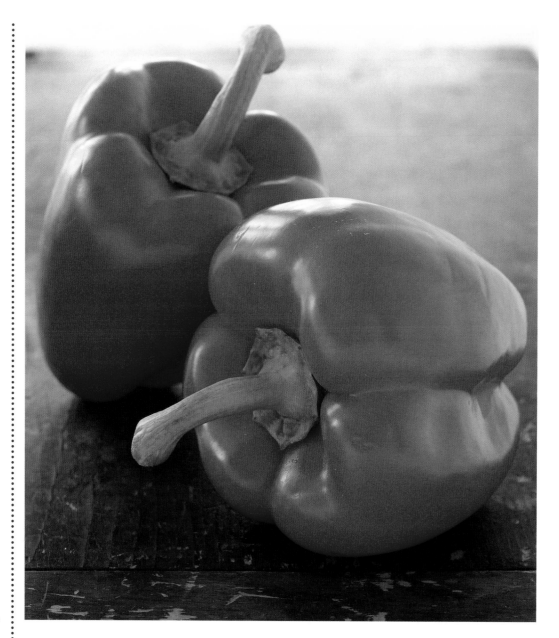

RED BELL PEPPERS

One large red bell pepper can supply 340 percent of your daily vitamin C—and high vitamin C intakes have shown promise in reducing later risk of osteoarthritis of the knee. For 10 years, Australian researchers tracked the diets of 293 healthy adults and then used MRIs to test for osteoarthritic markers. The results showed that those adults with the highest fruit and vitamin C intakes were least likely to develop the kind of bone abnormalities that indicate incipient arthritis of the knees. Additionally, in a Boston University study, people who got less than 150 milligrams daily of vitamin C had faster cartilage breakdown.

Other vitamin C sources include citrus fruits, pineapples, kiwis, broccoli, cauliflower, cantaloupes, papayas, strawberries, tomatoes, sweet and hot peppers, kale, collard greens and sweet potatoes

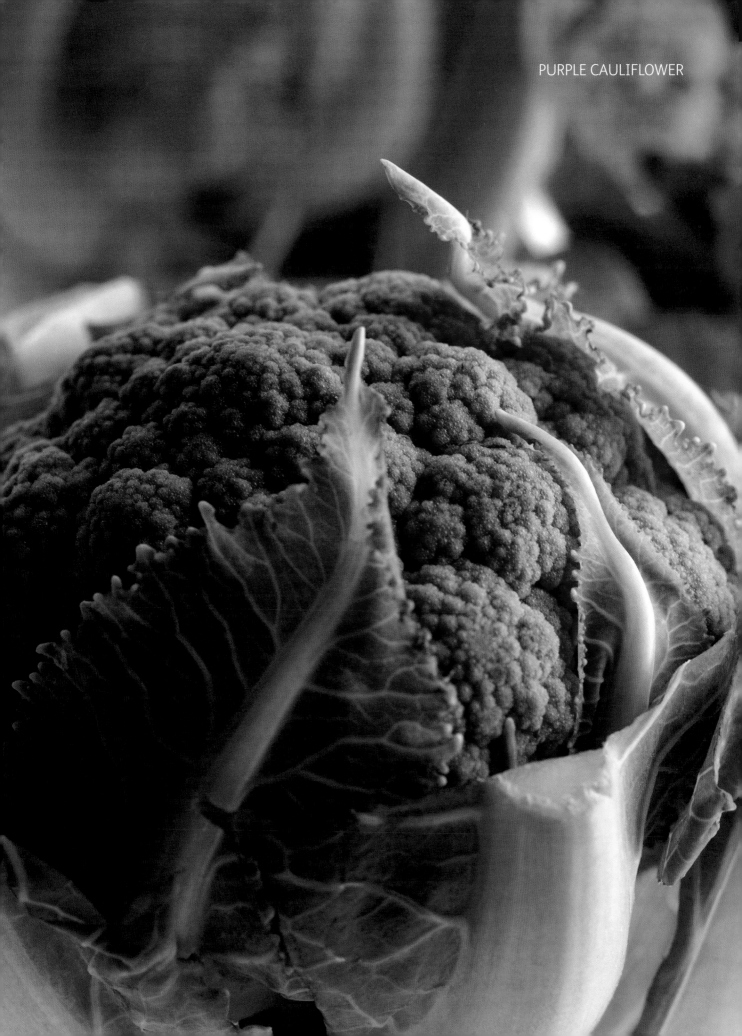

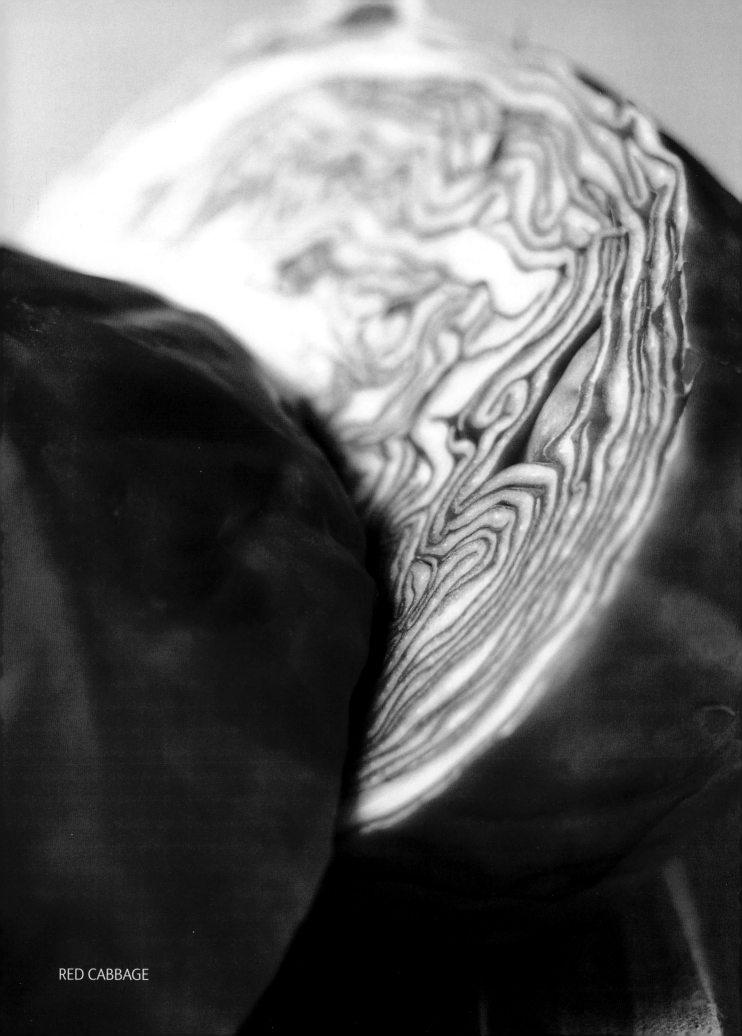

RED CABBAGE

BROCCOLI

When broccoli and other cruciferous veggies are eaten, they release a compound called sulforaphane that triggers the body's own antioxidant defenses. Research suggests that this process may block the COX-2 enzymes which cause inflammation. Broccoli sprouts are one of the most potent sources of these compounds.
Other sources include cabbage, cauliflower and Brussels sprouts

KALE

Kale holds the line against osteoarthritis due to its high-calcium content, which helps slow bone loss.
Other sources include nonfat dairy products, collard greens, soybeans and arugula

FOOD TIP

Nuts are a great source of heart healthy omega-3 oils and vitamin E antioxidants. But if you buy them crusted with blood-pressure-boosting salt, fattening sugar or artery-clogging trans fats, you'll cancel out any potential benefits. So eat your nuts au naturel!

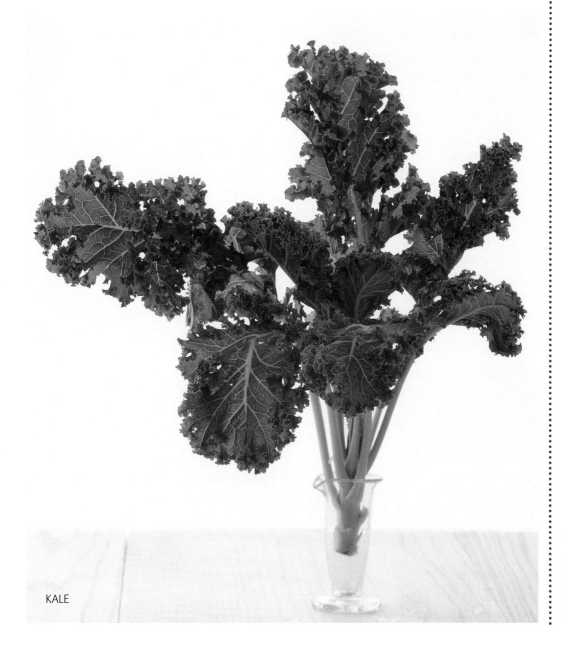

KALE

EATING KALE IS A SIMPLE WAY TO ADD CALCIUM AND HELP SLOW DOWN BONE LOSS.

A high dietary selenium intake is associated with a 40 percent reduction in risk for developing osteo- arthritis in the knees.

YOU CAN GET A FULL DAY'S SUPPLY OF SELENIUM FROM JUST ONE BRAZIL NUT.

DOLE PORTOBELLO MUSHROOMS

Research suggests that those who meet their daily vitamin D requirements are less vulnerable to arthritis pain. This may be due to vitamin D's anti-inflammatory benefits and its promotion of calcium absorption. Your body makes vitamin D in response to sun exposure, and it's difficult to get 100 percent of your daily requirement from food—at least it was until recently. Dole researchers have pioneered a process using an ordinary flashbulb to boost the vitamin D content in mushrooms (which produce the nutrient upon exposure to light, just as humans do). Now, DOLE Portobello Mushrooms are a top vitamin D source, supplying 100 percent of daily requirements in just 3 ounces (85 grams).

Other vitamin D sources include oysters, sardines and fortified nonfat milk

FISH

Omega-3 fatty acids help reduce the inflammation associated with rheumatoid arthritis. Many studies have found that regular consumption of fatty fish, which are high in omega-3s, helps alleviate joint pain, swelling and morning stiffness—sometimes making drugs unnecessary.

Other omega-3 sources include salmon, halibut, sardines and black cod

BRAZIL NUTS

Brazil nuts are a potent source of selenium, which is thought to fight inflammation and help counter the free radicals that attack the joints. In a Belgian study, women with rheumatoid arthritis who increased their selenium intake for four months experienced significant improvement in joint movement and strength compared with a control group.

Additionally, in a study from The Thurston Arthritis Research Center at the University of North Carolina, those with higher levels of selenium in their toenails were 40 percent less likely to have osteoarthritis in their knees. Study author Joanne M. Jordan, MD, MPH, comments: "Our preliminary results suggest that we might be able to prevent or delay osteoarthritis of the knees and possibly other joints in some people if they are not getting enough selenium. That's important because the condition, which makes walking painful, is the leading cause of activity limitation among adults in developed countries."

Keep in mind, selenium can be toxic in large amounts, so doctors advise against consuming more than 100 micrograms per day The amount found in just one Brazil nut provides about 96 micrograms—137 percent of your daily value for selenium.

Other selenium sources include cod, shrimp, tuna, shiitake mushrooms and whole grains

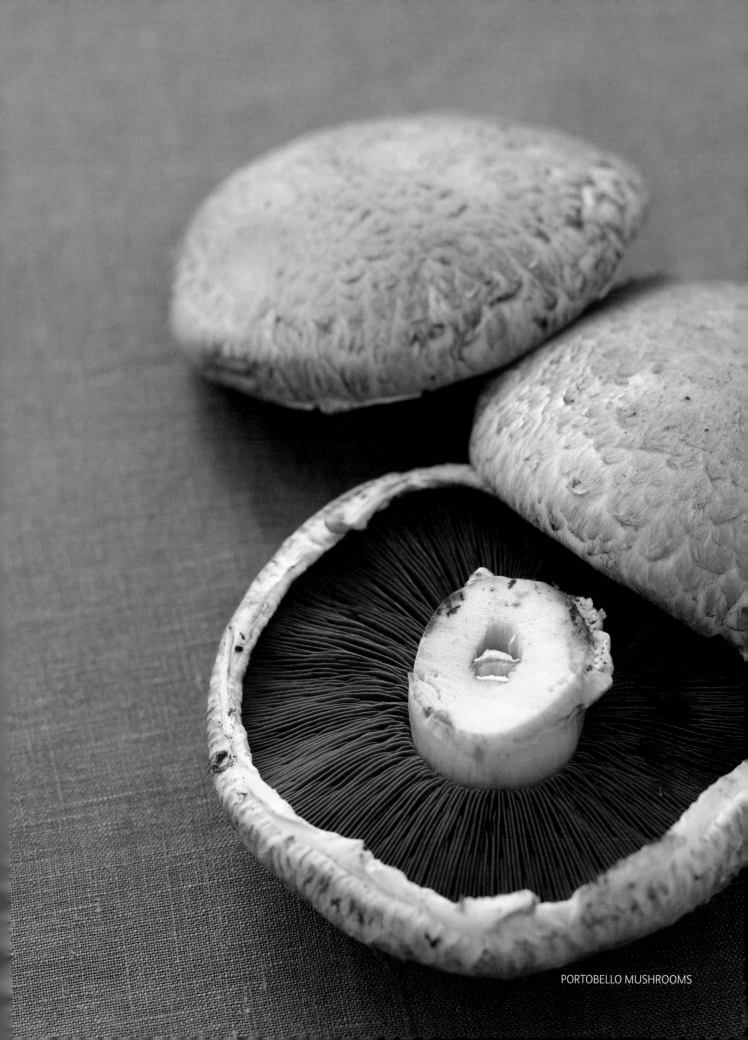

PORTOBELLO MUSHROOMS

Turmeric Tea Treatment

TURMERIC POWDER

Green and black teas contain flavonoids, antioxidant compounds thought to block the production of a type of prostaglandin that exacerbates inflammation and pain.

Try adding turmeric to your tea for an extra dose of relief. For centuries, this deep-yellow spice (common in Indian dishes) has been used to treat wounds, infections and other health problems. In recent years, researchers have attributed antioxidant, anticancer, antibiotic and antiviral properties to curcumin, the compound responsible for turmeric's yellow pigment, as well.

Turmeric tea is thought to lubricate the joints and help relieve pain in arthritis, bursitis and tendonitis sufferers—or in anyone with chronic joint pain.

¼ cup spring or distilled water
⅛ tsp turmeric powder
3 cardamom pods
1 cup soy milk
2 Tbsp cold-pressed almond oil
Honey or maple syrup to taste

Bring water to a boil; then add the turmeric powder and cardamom pods. Reduce heat to low, and allow the mixture to simmer for 5–10 minutes.

Add soy milk and almond oil to the liquid. Heat just to the boiling point, but do not allow the mixture to come to a boil.

Remove from heat and strain the tea into a clean coffee mug. Add honey or maple syrup to sweeten, if desired, and drink immediately.

What to Avoid

EXCESS WEIGHT

If you're among the majority of Americans who are overweight or obese, slimming down can significantly slow the progression and ease the pain of joint degeneration. In fact, according to the *Arthritis Advisor,* you can reduce knee stress by 40 to 80 pounds with a mere 10-pound weight loss. That may sound like a lot, but it's estimated that the knee actually supports four times the body weight when you're walking, so a 10-pound loss can reduce the load at least fourfold. In addition, French researchers have linked the joint distortion caused by osteoarthritis to a hormone called leptin that's released by fat cells, and they have discovered that the higher the body mass index, the higher the concentration of leptin in the joints.

Exercise Rx

It might seem counterintuitive, but one of the best ways to relieve achy joints may be by increasing your activity. While weight lifting and aerobic exercise have proven pain-relieving benefits, so have some gentler options, like tai chi and aquatic exercise. And the latter two may be better alternatives for those who have been inactive for a while.

In an Australian study, reported in a 2007 issue of *Arthritis & Rheumatism*, researchers divided 152 sedentary adults with painful hip or knee osteoarthritis into three groups. One group attended tai chi classes, another took hydrotherapy classes and the third remained inactive. After 12 weeks, those in the exercising groups showed increased mobility and significant decreases in pain—and the pain-relieving benefits continued for three months after the classes ended. According to the study authors, the gentle, continuous movements of aquatic exercise and tai chi can help improve strength, balance and posture without putting too much pressure on the joints.

EXCESS SATURATED FAT

Most saturated fats trigger an inflammatory reaction in the body, which exacerbates arthritis symptoms. Many doctors recommend that arthritis patients limit their consumption of whole-dairy products (such as whole milk, cheese and ice cream) and animal products (such as red meat and poultry), and replace them with healthier choices, like cold-water fish rich in omega-3 fatty acids. Doctors who recommend fish to alleviate joint pain and stiffness say the benefits are maximized when other animal fats are minimized. In addition, in a 2004 study published in *Arthritis & Rheumatism*, British researchers identified a high level of red meat consumption as an independent risk factor for rheumatoid arthritis after finding that the subjects who ate the most red meat were twice as likely to develop the disease as those who limited their intake to less than an ounce per day.

OVER TIME, THE GENTLE, CONTINUOUS MOVEMENTS OF TAI CHI CAN PROVIDE RELIEF FOR ACHY JOINTS.

Conclusion

For a long time, dietary approaches to preventing and managing arthritis were ignored—or worse, ridiculed—by the medical establishment. But with the rise of the joint-crushing obesity epidemic and the emergence of a new frontier in nutrition research, the connection between food and joint health can no longer be denied. An arthritis diagnosis no longer has to mean a life of pain, limitation or dependence on medication. A healthy diet and regular exercise can keep you mobile, comfortable and independent over the long haul.

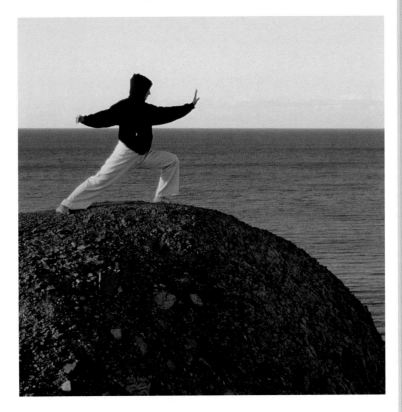

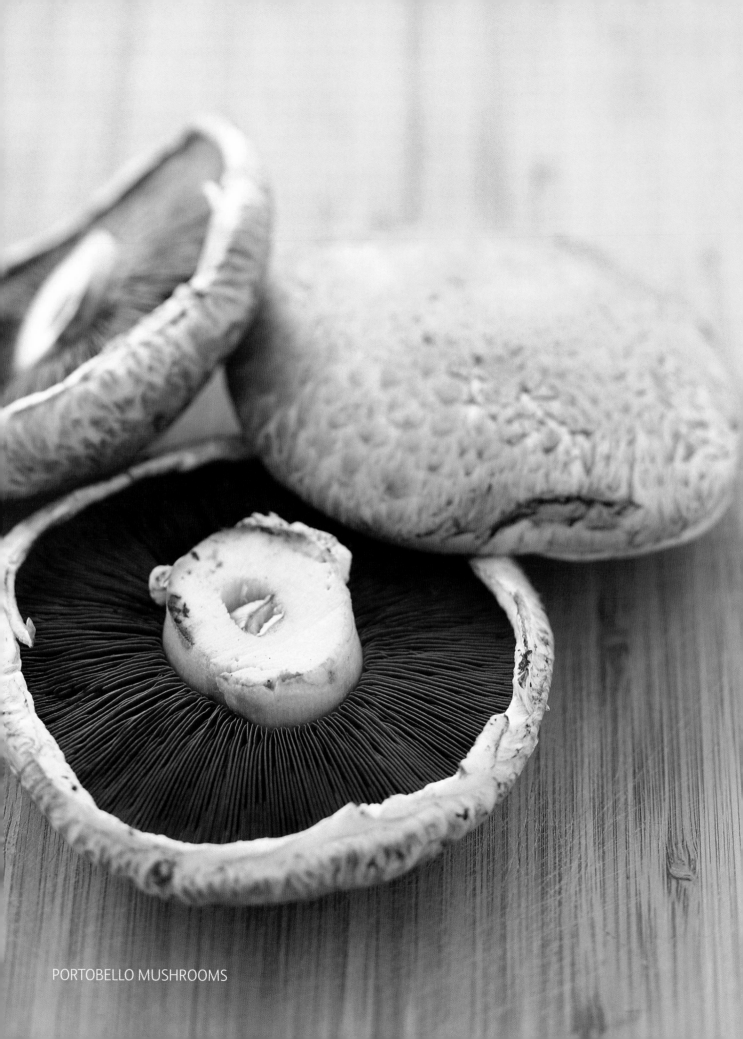

PORTOBELLO MUSHROOMS

CHAPTER 10

Bone Health

You Need: CALCIUM, VITAMIN D, VITAMIN K, FOLATE, MANGANESE, MAGNESIUM, VITAMIN C, POTASSIUM

Eat These:

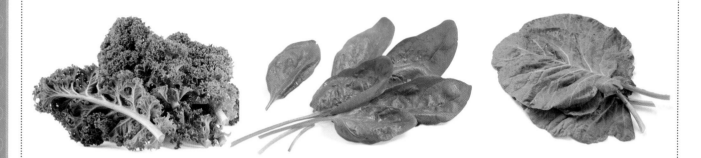

KALE   SPINACH   COLLARD GREENS

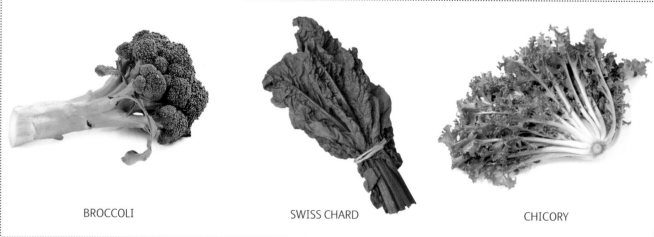

BROCCOLI   SWISS CHARD   CHICORY

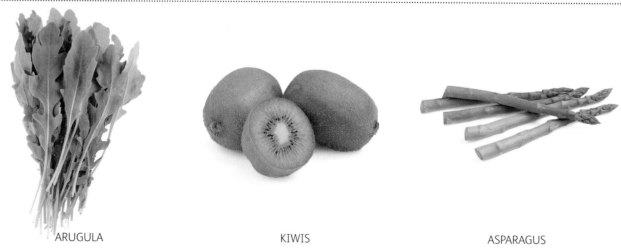

ARUGULA   KIWIS   ASPARAGUS

▶ John Anderson

John Anderson, PhD, is a professor in the Department of Nutrition at the University of North Carolina at Chapel Hill and a member of the American Society for Nutritional Sciences, the American College of Nutrition, the American Society for Nutrition, the American Society for Bone and Mineral Research and the International Bone and Mineral Society.

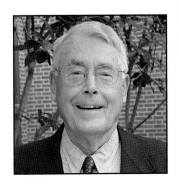

Q: Why is calcium so important to bone health?

JA: If insufficient calcium is ingested, the amount of calcium in the skeleton declines until the skeleton itself—or vulnerable locations such as the vertebrae and hips—becomes increasingly at risk for fractures. This typically happens at a slow rate, so we tend to see the effects later in life, rather than right away.

Q: What other nutrients are important to bone health?

JA: Phosphorus and a number of other minerals, such as magnesium, potassium and zinc, have critical roles in bone tissue. Vitamins—particularly vitamin D and other fat-soluble vitamins, the B vitamins and vitamin C—and macronutrients, including omega-3 polyunsaturated fatty acids, are utilized by bone cells or tissues in support of the skeleton as well. Almost all of these nutrients are available in substantial amounts in each serving of plant-based foods, including vegetables, fruits, whole grains, nuts and seeds. In addition, nonfat dairy foods—milk, cheese and yogurt—are good sources for calcium; ocean fish are good sources for vitamin D and omega-3 fatty acids; and fish is also a good source for protein.

Q: Are there foods we should avoid?

JA: Processed foods and beverages tend to be too high in phosphorus (as phosphates), sodium and sugar (or high-fructose corn syrup)—all of which are considered adverse risk factors for bone health. Too much phosphorus stimulates an increase in the parathyroid hormone, which in turn increases bone breakdown or resorption. If this breakdown is not balanced by new bone formation or an increase in bone mineralization, bone mass and density decline. Too much sodium, in combination with too little dietary potassium, directly interferes with the normal function of bone cells and may also alter their acid-base balance. Too much sugar yields too much fructose, which may increase renal losses of calcium in the process of renal-stone formation. And too much animal protein may contribute to a greater metabolic generation of acid that must be excreted, which results in acidic urine. Yet acidic urine can be readily neutralized by increasing daily consumption of base-generating fruits and vegetables.

Q: Can alcohol intake impact one's bone health?

JA: Alcohol (ethanol), when consumed in excess, may generate so much acid that neutralization of the extra acid load becomes too slow. Consequently, the acid begins to degrade bone tissue, reduce bone density and place the chronic drinker at risk of osteoporosis and fractures.

Calcium, phosphorus and a number of other minerals have critical roles in bone-tissue health.

> **Q: Your recent research discusses the role of antioxidants in bone health. Which antioxidants help us maintain healthy bones?**
> **JA:** Plant foods contain both nutrient and phytochemical-nonnutrient antioxidants. In fact, probably more than 10,000 phytochemical antioxidants exist among the myriad of plant foods. For example, onions, garlic, soy, tomatoes and many other plant foods contain these protective molecules, but typically in small amounts. When sufficient servings of fruits and vegetables are consumed each day, plenty of the antioxidants are absorbed and penetrate the various tissues and cells of the body. We have examined several types of plant antioxidants, such as those from soy, tea and ginkgo biloba, in the tissue cultures of bone cells and have found them to be as potent, if not more so, than vitamin C as an antioxidant. Other published reports of human studies support our in vitro work.

According to the Human Nutrition Research Center on Aging at Tufts University, 10 million Americans over the age of 50 have osteoporosis and more than 33 million have low bone mass, a problem responsible for 1.5 million fractures of the spine, hip and wrist every year in the United States.

We naturally experience some amount of bone loss as we age, but there are lifestyle factors that can slow the process—and others that can speed it up. The latter include smoking, excessive alcohol intake, lack of exercise, some nutrient deficiencies and excess body fat. It used to be thought that being overweight—despite all the associated risks, from diabetes to cancer and cardiovascular disease—had, at least, the advantage of generating stronger bones. But alas, emerging research shows that fat—far from being a bone bolsterer—actually undermines them. A study presented at the 2008 annual meeting of the American Dietetic Association found that among postmenopausal women, higher fat mass also meant lower bone-mineral density.

But hold on … isn't weight-bearing exercise supposed to increase bone density? Then why wouldn't carrying around an extra 50 pounds of fat have the same effect? As it turns out, adipose tissue is an active organ, and it produces toxic substances that impair the body's ability to maintain strong bones. In addition, excess fat induces an inflammatory response that inhibits bone building and multiplies *osteoclasts* (cells that break down bones). In contrast, packing extra muscle—as opposed to fat—actually does strengthen bones.

And fortunately, a proper diet and lifestyle can go a long way toward protecting your skeleton. It's well-known that calcium is important for strong bones. But researchers increasingly believe that other nutrients found in fruit and vegetables play a big role in boosting bone strength as well. A 2006 study published in the *American Journal of Clinical Nutrition* found that female seniors and adolescents of both sexes bolstered their bone strength by doubling their produce intake. And an earlier study at the University of Tennessee found that girls, ages 8 to 12, who consume more than three servings of fruit per day have greater bone mass (and less calcium excretion) than those who consume fewer than three servings.

Here's a list of further dietary recommendations for achieving and maintaining optimum bone health.

NUTRITION TIP
Osteoporosis isn't confined to the elderly. In one study, 67 percent of children, ages 6 to 13, who experienced frequent fractures already had the disease. To make sure kids' growing bones stay strong, add healthy calcium sources and plenty of fruits and vegetables to their diet.

Benefit the Bones with Exercise

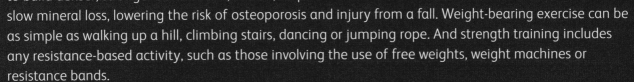

Bone mass and strength naturally diminish with age. But exercise can halt and even reverse this process. The most bone-beneficial exercises are those that involve weight bearing and strength training, because when muscles pull on bones, the skeletal system is prompted to build denser, stronger bones. That, in turn, helps slow mineral loss, lowering the risk of osteoporosis and injury from a fall. Weight-bearing exercise can be as simple as walking up a hill, climbing stairs, dancing or jumping rope. And strength training includes any resistance-based activity, such as those involving the use of free weights, weight machines or resistance bands.

Several studies indicate that high-intensity training is even more beneficial than basic strength training. In a 2004 *Journal of Applied Physiology* report, researchers compared the effect of strength training (slow resistance exercises) and power training (fast resistance exercises) on bone-mineral density in two groups of postmenopausal women. The latter group showed markedly better results.

Note: If you have osteoporosis, high-impact activities that increase compression in the spine and lower extremities (such as jumping, running or jogging) are not recommended, because they can lead to fractures in weakened bones. Instead, opt for exercises with slow, controlled movements, such as tai chi or aqua therapy.

COLLARD GREENS

Calcium from Food, Not Pills

Here's a trick question: If person A consumes 200 milligrams more calcium than person B, who would have stronger bones? Though it would seem that the person with higher calcium intake would naturally have stronger bones, well, *naturally* is the operative phrase. Because studies indicate that people who get their calcium from natural—i.e., whole food—sources may actually have stronger bones than those who rely on supplements. In fact, a study from the Washington University School of Medicine found that women who relied on their diet for calcium had higher bone-mineral density than women who got calcium from supplements, even though their total intakes were 20 percent lower!

Why would more calcium from supplements translate into less of the mineral in the bones? For one thing, only about 35 percent of the calcium in supplements makes it into the bones, due primarily to the lower absorbability of this type of calcium in these often-untested, over-the-counter formulations. For another, fruits and vegetables supply many of the other oft-neglected nutrients needed for bone health, such as potassium, folate and vitamin C. And produce consumption has been linked to higher bone-mineral content—so it's possible that the group that relied on food sources for nutrients also had a higher produce intake.

FITNESS TIP
Researchers at the University of Wolverhampton in England found that walking was effective in warding off osteoporosis in the lower limbs—but not in the upper body. So, add some free weights and push-ups to your routine to protect your upper body as well.

What to Choose

CALCIUM

Calcium is essential for strong, healthy bones. If there's not sufficient calcium in the blood (to maintain normal heartbeat, blood coagulation and nerve-muscle function), it will be leached from the bones. Although we tend to think of milk as a top calcium source, there's evidence that protein from animal products increases calcium loss, weakening the bones. So, it's preferable to get your calcium from plant-based sources.

Top plant calcium sources include broccoli, kale, collard greens, beans and butternut squash

MAGNESIUM

Magnesium is also essential for bone health, helping to convert vitamin D into its active form in the body and get calcium into the bones. It has also shown promise in treating osteoporosis. Researchers in Israel had 31 women with osteoporosis increase daily magnesium intake for two years. At the end of that period, 22 of the women had increased their bone density up to 8 percent (five women experienced decreases in their rate of bone loss). A control group of 23 women experienced significant decreases in bone density.

Top magnesium sources include wheat germ, sunflower seeds, seafood, nuts and green, leafy vegetables

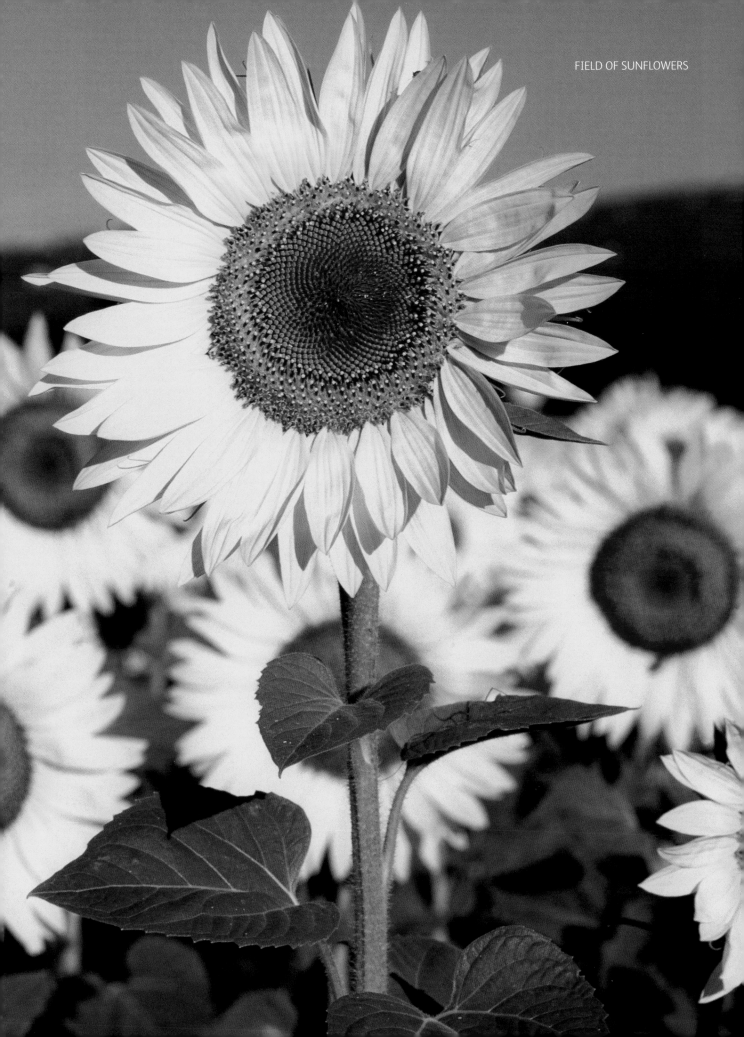

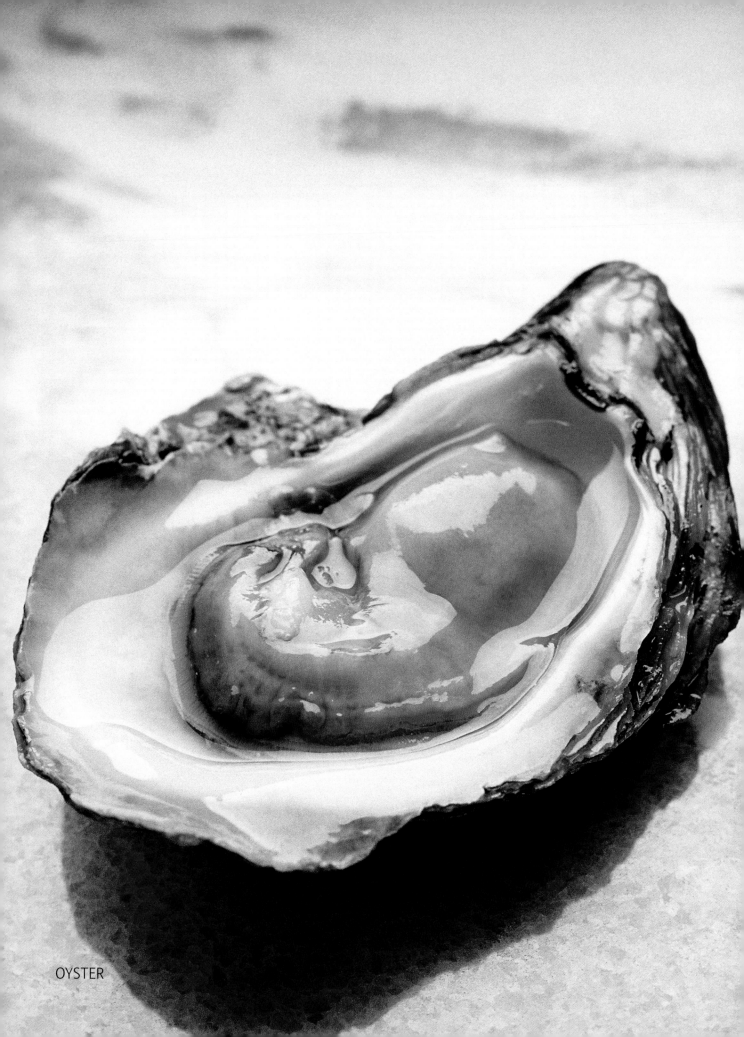

OYSTER

VITAMIN D

Vitamin D helps the body maintain healthy blood levels of calcium by allowing the bones to absorb calcium more efficiently, and thus it's linked to stronger bones (as well as to stronger muscles). A vitamin D deficiency is associated with the increased risk of fractures, particularly hip fractures, in the elderly. And, while there are no conclusive studies pointing to vitamin D deficiency as a direct cause of osteoporosis, it's a well-documented cause of osteomalacia, or soft bones, which also can lead to fractures.

Until recently it's been difficult to get sufficient vitamin D from diet alone, because sun exposure is needed for the body to synthesize it. But Dole scientists have discovered that mushrooms produce vitamin D upon exposure to light (just as you do), which allowed them to develop a process that uses an ordinary flashbulb to increase the vitamin D content in mushrooms. So, now it's possible to get 100 percent of your daily vitamin D requirement from DOLE Portobello Mushrooms.

Top vitamin D sources include DOLE Portobello Mushrooms, sunshine, canned sardines, canned pink salmon, fortified orange juice and oysters

VITAMIN B12

Vitamin B12 has an important role in bone-cell formation and function, and it helps keep homocysteine levels from rising and weakening bones. Deficiencies are linked with lower bone density. In fact, when Tufts University scientists measured the bone-mineral density and blood levels of vitamin B12 in nearly 2,600 men and women, they found that among those with low B12 levels, women had less-dense bones in the spine and men had less-solid hip bones, putting both groups at risk for osteoporosis.

Top vitamin B12 sources include poultry, seafood, eggs and nonfat dairy products like yogurt and milk

POTASSIUM

This mineral helps maintain a healthy acid-alkaline balance in the body, leading to reduced calcium excretion. In a 2005 study in the *American Journal of Clinical Nutrition,* British researchers found that perimenopausal women (those in the several years preceding menopause) with the highest potassium intake had 8 percent greater bone-mineral density than those with the lowest intake. The researchers projected that if the women maintained their high intake into old age, they could lower their fracture risk by 30 percent.

Top potassium sources include bananas, spinach, broccoli, potatoes, kiwifruits and plantains

NUTRITION TIP
Is drinking cola bad for your bones? Diet, regular and decaffeinated colas contain phosphoric acid, which studies indicate inhibits calcium absorption. While these findings are preliminary, you can play it safe by switching to noncola alternatives, such as sparkling flavored waters, or make your own by adding juice to a glass of club soda.

KIWIFRUIT IS HIGH IN POTASSIUM AND OTHER NUTRIENTS.

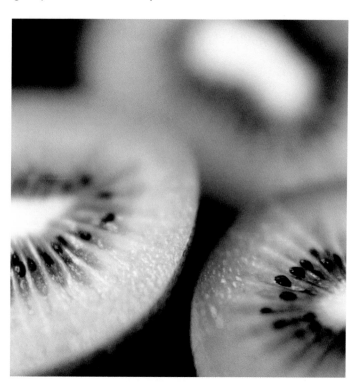

NUTRITION TIP
Japanese researchers studying the effects of vitamin K in protecting bones found that this vitamin may also help protect against liver cancer. Female subjects with viral liver cirrhosis who increased vitamin K intake were 90 percent less likely to develop liver cancer than those in a control group. Just 1 cup of spinach provides nearly 1,000 percent of a woman's daily vitamin K needs.

FOLATE

Folate helps lower levels of homocysteine, an amino acid linked to increased risk of fractures (as well as cardiovascular and Alzheimer's disease). In the Danish Osteoporosis Prevention Study, which tracked nearly 2,000 perimenopausal women over 10 years, a high dietary intake of folate was shown to have a positive impact on bone-mass density.

Top folate sources include spinach, asparagus, broccoli, romaine lettuce and oranges

VITAMIN K

Vitamin K helps strengthen the bones and is thought to lower the risk of fractures. Research shows that people with osteoporosis have low blood levels of vitamin K. In a Dutch study, 70 postmenopausal women who were given 1 milligram (1,000 micrograms) of vitamin K daily for three months experienced significant decreases in urinary calcium loss.

Top vitamin K sources include broccoli, arugula, collard greens, cabbage, grapes, blueberries and leafy green vegetables like kale, spinach and romaine lettuce

VITAMIN C

Vitamin C, a powerful antioxidant, has been linked to greater bone-mineral content, particularly in children and postmenopausal women. Vitamin C also supports collagen production, which is thought to be related to calcium absorption.

Top vitamin C sources include citrus fruits like grapefruit and oranges, as well as strawberries, broccoli and red bell peppers

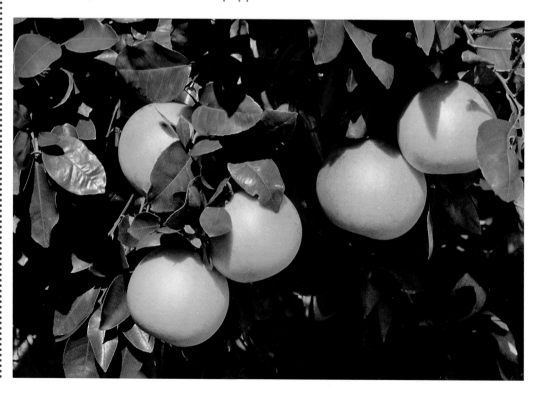

GRAPEFRUIT IS CHOCK-FULL OF VITAMIN C, THOUGHT TO HELP IMPROVE CALCIUM ABSORPTION AND BONE-MINERAL DENSITY.

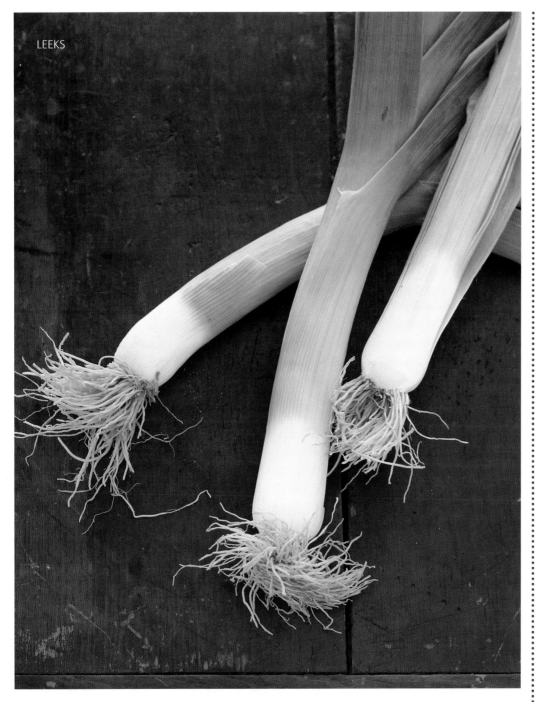

LEEKS

PREBIOTIC FIBER, FOUND IN LEEKS AND ONIONS, IS THOUGHT TO HELP BOOST BONE-MINERAL DENSITY.

FOOD TIP

In addition to prebiotic fiber, onions contain the peptide GPCS, another compound that bolsters the bones. In a 2005 *Journal of Agricultural and Food Chemistry* study, Swiss researchers reported that GPCS "significantly inhibited the loss of bone minerals, including calcium," in isolated bone cells from newborn rats. These findings indicate that regular onion consumption may help prevent osteoporosis.

PREBIOTIC FIBER

Prebiotic fiber is thought to improve bone-mineral density. In a Baylor College of Medicine study, researchers examined the cumulative effects of prebiotic-fiber intake in a test group of 100 children, ages 9 to 13. After one year, those children who had been on a regimen of 8 grams of supplemental prebiotic fiber per day had increased calcium retention and bone density compared with those who had been given a placebo.

Top prebiotic fiber sources include bananas, leeks, onions, garlic, artichokes and asparagus

Calcium Pore

While vigorous exercise can bolster bone health, profuse perspiration leads to some calcium loss. Drafting college basketball players as his test subjects, a University of Tennessee professor analyzed the amount of calcium they lost during training sessions. By literally squeezing sweat from the athletes' jerseys, Robert Klesges, PhD, found an average calcium loss of nearly 250 milligrams per athlete per practice (a significant drain on the recommended intake of 1,000 to 1,200 milligrams per day). The consequence of such excessive calcium exudation was an average loss of more than 6 percent of bone-mineral density over the course of just one basketball season!

NUTRITION TIP

You know cholesterol clogs the arteries, but did you know it can compromise bone health too? Italian researchers found that high LDL (bad) cholesterol levels were linked to osteopenia, a bone-thinning precursor to osteoporosis in postmenopausal women. Their theory is that excessive LDL levels cause bone to break down faster than it can be rebuilt. So, keep "bad" cholesterol in check with fiber-rich fruits and veggies, which have antioxidants that prevent the oxidation of LDL.

What to Avoid

SUGAR

Excessive sugar intake can increase kidney stone formation, a process which in turn leaches calcium from the bones. Too much sugar can also block absorption of magnesium and calcium, making them unavailable for the formation of bone cells.

TOO MUCH MEAT

Research has linked excess retinol, the fat-soluble form of vitamin A found in animal foods, to increased risk of fracture. Instead of getting vitamin A—which is essential to the absorption of calcium—from animal sources, opt for beta-carotene (a precursor to vitamin A) from fresh fruits and veggies like carrots, sweet potatoes and cantaloupes; there's no link between beta-carotene and fracture risk.

EXCESS DIETARY FAT

There's mounting evidence indicating that both the amount and type of fat in the diet have an impact on bone health. In a 2006 review of data from the National Health and Nutrition Examination Survey, researchers looked at the relationship between dietary fat and bone-mineral density in the hip and found that higher saturated-fat intake was associated with lower bone-mineral density, particularly in men under the age of 50.

Other studies have shown that fish oil, flaxseeds and flaxseed oil significantly reduce cytokine production and increase calcium absorption, bone calcium and bone density, but scientists say that further research is necessary to gather more evidence and determine the mechanism for this benefit.

TOO MUCH ALCOHOL

Excessive alcohol intake can inhibit calcium absorption as well as bone formation. It can also generate so much acid that the body degrades bone tissue to neutralize the imbalance. Researchers have found osteoporotic fractures and reduced bone mass in a significant percentage of men with chronic alcoholism.

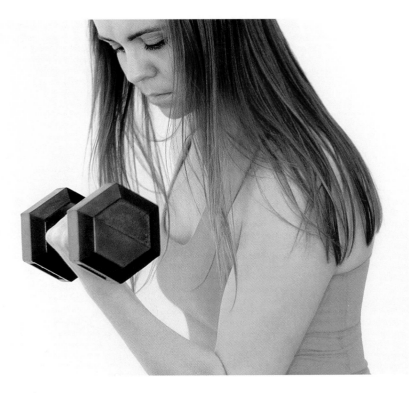

WEIGHT-BEARING
EXERCISE SIGNALS
BONE CELLS TO
INCREASE IN MASS.

Conclusion

Building stronger bones begins in the mind: Instead of thinking of the skeleton as only the hard, static scaffolding of the body, we need to recognize that our bones are in a constant state of flux. The skeleton is a porous, flexible structure—made up of living tissue formed by collagen, calcium and other minerals—which is incessantly being torn down and built up. Once the dynamic nature of our bones is understood, it becomes clear that a variety of important nutrients are required to feed this vital process. You need enough calcium, in conjunction with the other vitamins and minerals listed in this chapter, to optimize bone mass and reduce fracture risk later in life. Exercise—especially the kind that offers bone-building impact—is also crucial to this equation.

Bikers' Bones

For all its benefits, cycling as your sole exercise may leave your bones vulnerable to osteopenia, according to a study from the University of Missouri. Researchers tested the bone-mineral density of 27 cyclists and 19 runners, ranging in age from 20 to 59. While one might expect both groups of athletes to have hardy bones, it turned out that 63 percent of the cyclists had osteopenia (lower-than-normal bone density) compared with 19 percent of the runners. Osteopenia was not confined to the older study subjects—several cyclists in their 20s and 30s were already experiencing significant bone-density loss. Unlike cycling, activities like jumping rope, lifting weights and playing contact sports (e.g., soccer or volleyball) provide bone-building impact, which signals bone cells to increase in mass.

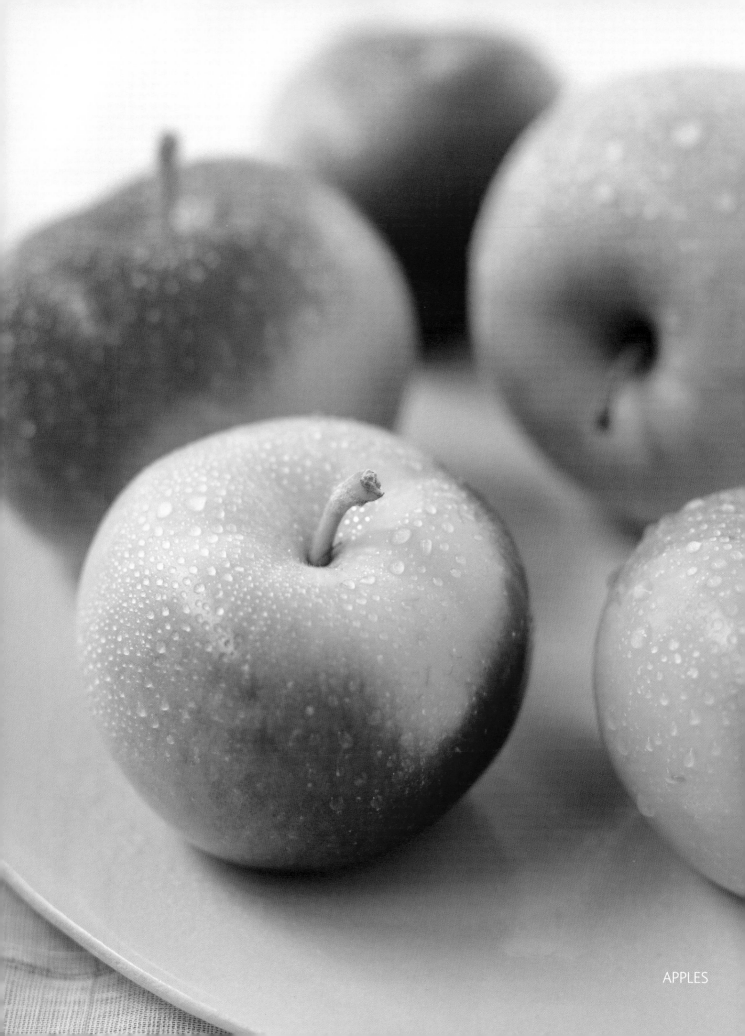

APPLES

CHAPTER 11

Immunity

You Need: VITAMIN A, VITAMIN C, SELENIUM, ZINC, ANTIOXIDANT FLAVONOIDS

Eat These:

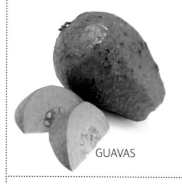

GUAVAS

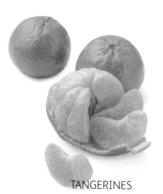

TANGERINES

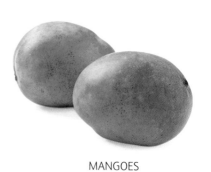

MANGOES

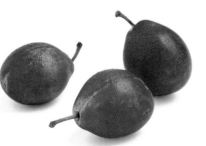

PLUMS

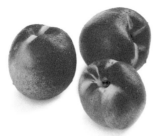

NECTARINES

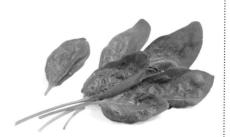

SPINACH

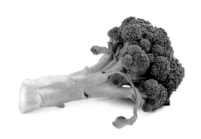

BROCCOLI

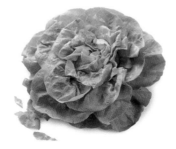

GREEN LETTUCE

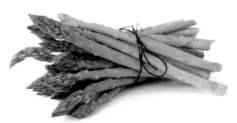

ASPARAGUS

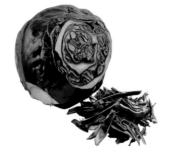

RED CABBAGE

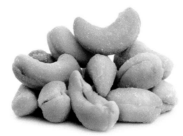

CASHEWS

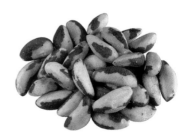

BRAZIL NUTS

▶ Dr. David C. Nieman

David Nieman, DrPH, FACSM, is a professor of health and exercise science, and director of the Human Performance Labs at Appalachian State University in Boone, North Carolina, and the North Carolina Research Campus in Kannapolis. His current research is focused on how nutrition can affect exercise-induced immune dysfunction. Dr. Nieman has published more than 230 peer-reviewed publications and is the author of nine books on health, exercise physiology and nutrition.

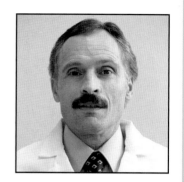

Q: What kind of impact does diet have on the health of the immune system?

DN: If you have a deficiency of any nutrient, the immune cells will function less well. The immune system needs nutrients to do their work, and a regular diet should provide enough nutrients for the immune system to get along.

Q: Tell us about your own diet.

DN: I live on a dairy farm, and I grow blueberries and raspberries, so I eat huge quantities of berries. I'm also a vegetarian.

Q: Are there dietary practices that can wear out the immune system?

DN: Studies show that children who are going through protein-calorie malnutrition in Africa suffer more infections of just about every variety, from gastrointestinal to lung and eye infections. People with anorexia nervosa show suppressed immunity and a higher rate of infections, pneumonia and other such ailments. They often die from lung infections.

As you know, our problem in America is not a lack of food, but rather too much of it. We have compared immunity in obese, overweight and normal-weight individuals and found that obesity causes slight impairments in some aspects of immunity. But I have been more impressed with how very *few* differences there are.

BERRIES CONTAIN ESPECIALLY HIGH CONCENTRATIONS OF IMMUNITY-BOOSTING QUERCETIN.

Q: What can be done to support immunity as we get older?

DN: Aging has a huge effect on the immune system, especially on T cells—a type of white blood cell that selectively searches out and destroys infectious agents like germs and viruses. The thymus gland is like the university for T cells—it's where they go to mature—but age-related thymus decline begins when we're around 30 years of age. By the time we're between ages 60 and 65, the T cells suffer, and by our 70s and 80s, they don't function well at all—and that's when infection and cancer rates start to go up.

In a study I was involved in, we compared the immune function in a group of normal elderly women, with an average age of 73, with that in a group of highly fit older women. The T cells in the thin, active women functioned significantly better—67 percent better, at a rate equal to that in 40-year-old women—

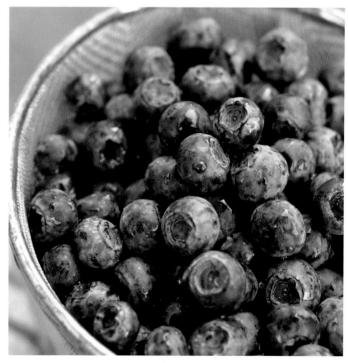

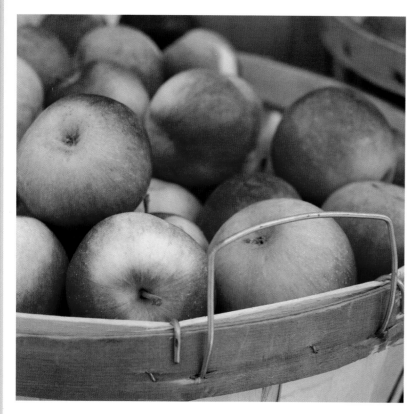

APPLES ARE A GOOD SOURCE OF QUERCETIN, WHICH RESIDES PRIMARILY IN THE SKIN OF THE FRUIT.

FITNESS TIP

Can't walk to work? Try parking a mile away and walking to and from your car. You'll burn up to 1,000 calories per week, which translates into losing a pound in under a month. Plus, a recent study found that brisk walking every day can cut your chance of getting a cold in half.

than in those of the less active women. And, their natural killer cells functioned at a 56 percent higher level. Our study showed that if you stay fit and lean, those T cells function really well compared with those of people who are sedentary and overweight.

Q: What about quercetin? Can it help support immunity?

DN: If you mix quercetin with just about any virus or bacteria, it stops their replication early on. The most common quercetin food source in the United States is apples, where it's found in the peel. The U.S. Department of Defense conducted some in vitro and animal studies, and then wanted me to do some of the first human studies to see if quercetin could help buoy soldiers' immunity. We simulated the fatigue soldiers' experience during a three-day war mission by having cyclists train to exhaustion for three hours per day for three days. After they'd gone through nine hours of heavy exertion, we followed up with a series of muscle biopsies and blood analyses over the following two weeks and found infections in only 5 percent of the quercetin group compared with 45 percent of the placebo group. We have since found that, in the general community, quercetin knocks infection rates down by about a third.

Q: Are berries a top quercetin source?

DN: Yes, the highest concentrations of quercetin are found in berries and onions. Elderberries, of all the berries, are very rich in quercetin, but blueberries—and all other berries—also contain substantial amounts of quercetin. So, while the average American consumes only 20 milligrams of quercetin per day, vegetarians who eat a lot of apples, onions, berries and that sort of thing have been found to get 100 to 200 milligrams daily.

As you know, the average American is quite deficient in fruits and vegetables. Through our studies, in both animals and humans, we've found that 1,000 milligrams per day—500 milligrams in the morning and 500 milligrams in the afternoon—is the optimal amount of supplementation for quercetin to exert its antiviral effects. Although I'm not a supplement guy—because I think your diet can give you just about everything you need for day-to-day activity—we're talking about something different here. The average apple has 10 milligrams of quercetin; so in our study, we were essentially giving them 100 apples worth per day, and that's a lot. But there are a few gems out there in Mother Nature that, when they're isolated and given in doses that exceed what we can get through food, can be really helpful. So far, in this case the research is supporting that high quantities of quercetin from supplements works for the athlete, and we just have to determine whether or not the general population will benefit from taking extra amounts of these flavonoids.

Q: Do you think that the everyday, normal person who isn't an athlete and doesn't endure that kind of stress benefits from the quercetin in apples, strawberries and other sources?

DN: There are very well-conducted studies showing that people who eat lots of apples, onions and berries have higher-than-normal quercetin levels in their blood because of their diets. People with high quercetin intake have a 60 percent reduction in lung-cancer death rates. They have a third less incidence of heart disease, and research shows that they have less pancreatic and colon cancer as well.

What I hope every reader will get from this interview, at the very least, is that if they up their intake of apples, onions and berries, over the long term they should experience lower rates for various types of cancer and heart disease.

Q: What about the effect of physical activity on immunity?

DN: There's nothing more powerful than regular activity (even if it's just moderate) for getting the immune system to do a better job in detecting and fighting pathogens. Research has found that people who put in 45 minutes of brisk walking, five days a week, cut their number of sick days in half, mainly because walking enhances the circulation of neutrophils and natural killer cells. The effect lasts for about three hours, and then you're back to normal; but if you keep up the walking on a daily basis, you'll improve your body's overall immune surveillance against pathogens in a lasting way.

DIET TIP

Tufts research suggests an increased intake of white button mushrooms could enhance your body's natural killer cells, improving your immunity to tumors and disease-causing viruses.

The average American gets two to three upper respiratory infections each year, and one in five Americans comes down with the flu. While most people recover within a week or two, about 36,000 die from influenza-related complications and about 50,000 from respiratory infections (including pneumonia). On top of that, roughly 76 million cases of foodborne illnesses are reported each year, resulting in about 5,000 deaths. The bottom line: Human beings are greatly outnumbered when it comes to the bugs, viruses and bacteria that cause infections.

But fortunately, if you take some basic precautions—in terms of nutrition, exercise, sleep and hygiene—your robust immune system can protect you from the majority of these viral challenges.

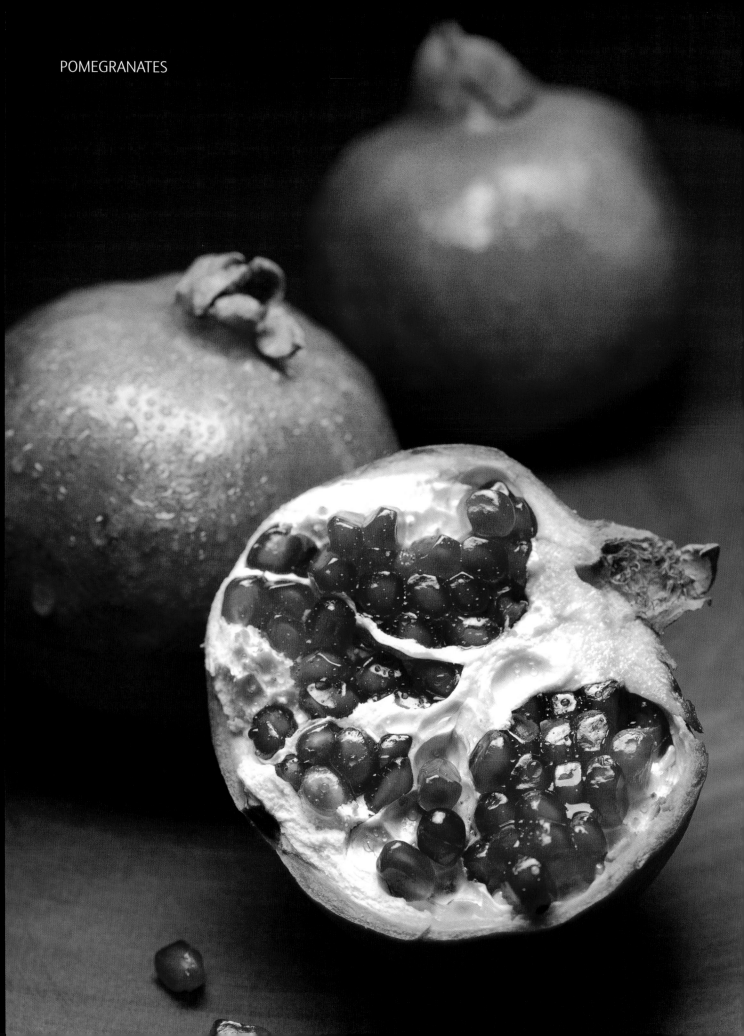

POMEGRANATES

Make Merry to Cut Cold Risks

Feeling down can make you more susceptible to sickness. Researchers at Carnegie Mellon University evaluated the temperaments of 300 healthy test subjects and then exposed them to an infectious virus. Those with the lowest happiness quotients were three times more likely to come down with a cold than their more buoyant peers.

While getting your flu shot and washing your hands frequently are the most important measures for avoiding the flu, you can also strengthen your immune system by eating powerhouse fruits and vegetables. The science of eating for immunity has come a long way since the days of relying on grandma's chicken-noodle soup remedy. Scientists have found vitamins A, C and E, antioxidants like quercetin, prebiotic fiber and zinc, to be potent defenders against germs, viruses and infections. So, adding the following fruits and vegetables to your diet is a good way to give your immune-health regimen a boost.

What to Choose

SPINACH FOR ANTIOXIDANTS
Along with kale, this leafy green packs a powerful punch; both are loaded with antioxidants that shield immune cells from environmental damage and encourage the production of bacteria-busting white blood cells. In addition, the antioxidants in spinach protect the enzymes that repair DNA damage, thereby enhancing your body's ability to rejuvenate itself.

Other antioxidant sources include pomegranates, Concord grape juice, blueberries, blackberries, raisins, red cabbage, prunes, raspberries, strawberries, oranges and carrots

BERRIES FOR QUERCETIN
In addition to quercetin's many other health benefits—ranging from detoxification to protection against Alzheimer's and lung cancer—this potent antioxidant found in berries also stops viruses in their tracks.

Other quercetin sources include red apples, onions, broccoli, kale and red grapes

ALMONDS FOR VITAMIN E
Well-known for its healthy-skin benefits, vitamin E, found in almonds, is another antioxidant that has been shown to support the immune system in addition to helping slow down the aging process. It acts as a "big brother" to other vitamins, protecting them from oxidation and, thus, allowing them to do their work.

Other vitamin E sources include sunflower seeds, avocados, vegetable juices, whole grains, and green, leafy vegetables

HEALTH TIP
Resistance training not only pumps up your muscles, but may also pump up your immunity. A Canadian study found that individuals who exercised with resistance bands three times per week boosted blood levels of natural killer cells. These cells are part of our body's defense system against infection.

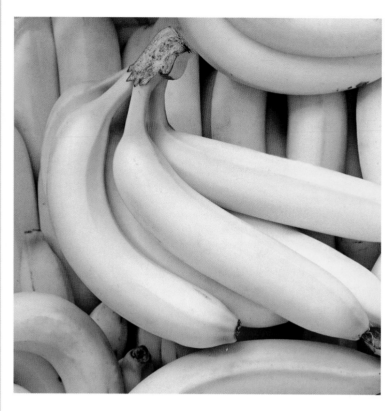

RED BELL PEPPERS FOR VITAMIN C

Evidence suggests that vitamin C can stave off the sniffles, particularly in people involved in extreme activities, such as marathon runners and soldiers. Research shows that the incidence of colds in these populations is reduced by 50 percent when subjects consume 250 to 1,000 milligrams of vitamin C per day. A single medium red bell pepper contains 152 milligrams, which fulfills 170 to 200 percent of your daily needs.

Other vitamin C sources include citrus fruits and juices, kiwifruits, pineapples, broccoli, cantaloupes, strawberries and tomatoes

BANANAS FOR PREBIOTIC FIBER

This wonder-fiber found in bananas, also known as resistant starch, selectively feeds the protective bacteria in your gut. In addition to guarding the intestinal tract against harmful pathogens, these "good" bacteria are thought to help stimulate immune-cell production.

Other prebiotic fiber sources include plantains, leeks, onions, garlic, artichokes and asparagus

BANANAS HELP FIGHT FOODBORNE ILLNESSES BY FORTIFYING THE PROTECTIVE BACTERIA IN YOUR GUT.

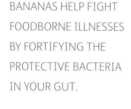

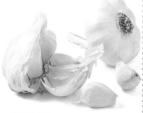

GARLIC

GARLIC FOR SULFUR

Referred to by some as Russian penicillin, garlic and its protective properties were once regarded as the domain of folk remedies. But research indicates that garlic has sulfur-containing antibacterial compounds, which fight infection by clearing away toxins and germs. In addition, garlic consumption seems to enhance the activity of white blood cells and T-helper cells, which are integral to a robust immune response.

Other sulfur sources include egg yolks, broccoli, cauliflower, kale, Brussels sprouts, watercress, radishes, leeks and onions

Meditation and Immunity

One study found that meditators produce more antibodies—an indicator of robust immune function—in response to a flu vaccine than nonmeditators. Other studies have linked meditation to reduced stress, better sleep, pain management, heart protection and even brain preservation—all of which are beneficial when it comes to warding off infection.

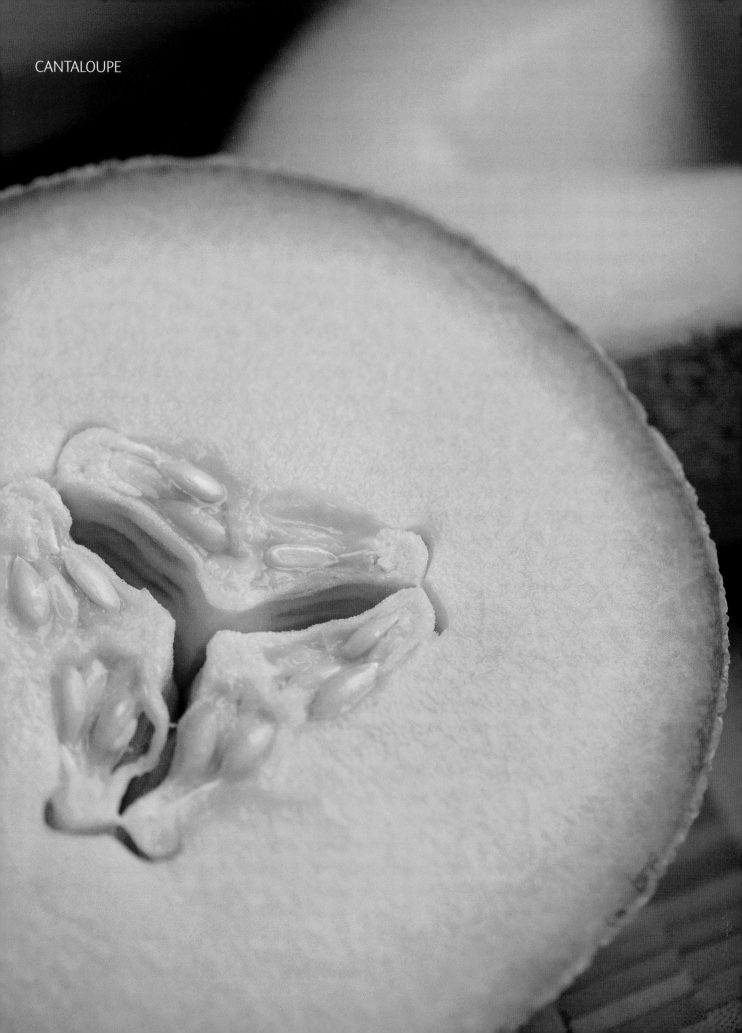

CANTALOUPE

One side effect of a power outage you may not have considered is food safety. If your refrigerator and freezer are without power for too long, you may need to toss some items. With doors closed, the fridge may maintain its temperature for about four hours. But err on the side of caution when it comes to perishables like poultry, dairy and leftovers. Better safe than sick!

NUTS FOR ZINC

This mighty mineral supports the immune system by enabling the synthesis of nucleic acids that are essential for cellular repair. Some studies have shown that zinc may reduce the duration of cold symptoms as well. While the most traditionally cited sources of zinc include oysters, Dungeness crab and red meat, other often-overlooked, healthy sources of zinc are soybeans, nuts and seeds. Researchers speculate that soy and nut consumption protects many vegetarians from zinc deficiency, given that they aren't able to derive it from animal sources.

Other zinc sources include peas, lima beans, summer squash, potatoes, corn, Napa cabbage, bok choy, pumpkin seeds, sunflower seeds and almonds

BUTTERNUT SQUASH FOR VITAMIN A

One cup of cooked butternut squash provides roughly 300 percent of your daily vitamin A needs. The same serving provides more than 50 percent of your daily vitamin C requirements as well, plus a substantial amount of vitamin E—which shields immune cells from free radicals and may boost production of bacteria-busting white blood cells.

Other vitamin A sources include sweet potatoes, carrots, spinach, kale, collard greens and pumpkins

Other Immune-Healthy Habits

WASH YOUR HANDS

Soap and water can remove bacteria from your hands and keep it from reaching your eyes, nose and mouth—and from infecting you. A University of Colorado study showed that students who washed their hands more often experienced fewer incidences of the common cold and flu.

Benefits of "Boo"

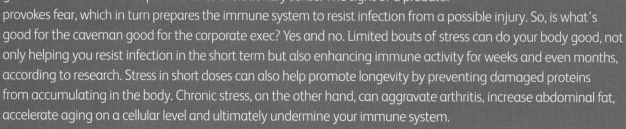

Could a Halloween fright help you fight winter colds? A study from Ohio State University suggests that exposure to acute stress triggers an increase in the number and activity of T cells—a type of white blood cell that seeks and destroys infectious germs and viruses. This response makes evolutionary sense: The sight of a predator provokes fear, which in turn prepares the immune system to resist infection from a possible injury. So, is what's good for the caveman good for the corporate exec? Yes and no. Limited bouts of stress can do your body good, not only helping you resist infection in the short term but also enhancing immune activity for weeks and even months, according to research. Stress in short doses can also help promote longevity by preventing damaged proteins from accumulating in the body. Chronic stress, on the other hand, can aggravate arthritis, increase abdominal fat, accelerate aging on a cellular level and ultimately undermine your immune system.

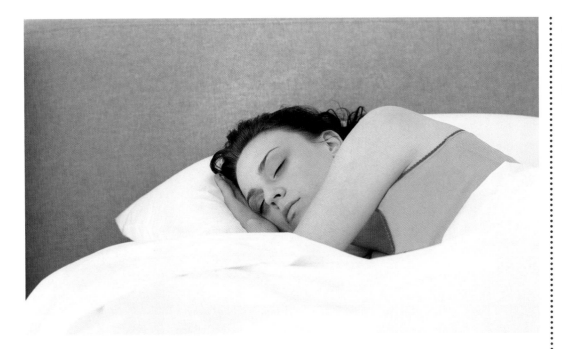

A GOOD NIGHT'S REST BOOSTS YOUR BODY'S ABILITY TO FIGHT INFECTION.

HIT THE HAY

Sleep deprivation dampens the production of the antibodies needed to fight infection; whereas allowing yourself to get adequate sleep will buoy your mood and give you more energy to exercise—both of which can help heighten your immune activity. A study in *Psychosomatic Medicine* found that even minor sleep disturbances cause a significant drop in the number of natural killer cells whose job is to destroy invaders.

TAKE TIME FOR TEA

Harvard researchers found that those subjects who drank five cups of black tea daily for two weeks had 10 times more interferons—a type of protein produced by the immune system in response to viral challenges—than those in a control group did. Interferons help fight infection by circulating in your system and blocking replication of the virus.

EXERCISE

While extreme overexertion (e.g., running a marathon or soldiering) can temporarily depress immune function, regular and moderate-to-vigorous activity has been found to help ward off infections. Research shows that seniors who practice tai chi have hardier immune responses than their inactive peers. Also, a number of studies demonstrate that aerobic activity among the elderly improves their antibody response to viruses.

Conclusion

While your immune system has evolved to function under even the worst kinds of dietary deprivation, there's no doubt that eating plenty of fruits and vegetables—particularly berries, leafy greens and nuts—will help enhance your overall health, including your ability to fight off infection and bounce back after illness. Being active, managing stress and having fun also play a role in maintaining a healthy immune system.

DIET TIP
Reduce fat intake to rev up your immunity. Tufts University researchers found that test subjects on a lower-fat diet (28 percent of calories from fat versus 38 percent in the test group) not only lowered their cholesterol but also boosted the activity of their T cells. These white blood cells selectively search out and destroy infectious agents like germs and viruses.

PART III

Slim Down, Shape Up with the Dole Diet and Fitness Plan

BLUEBERRY PLANT

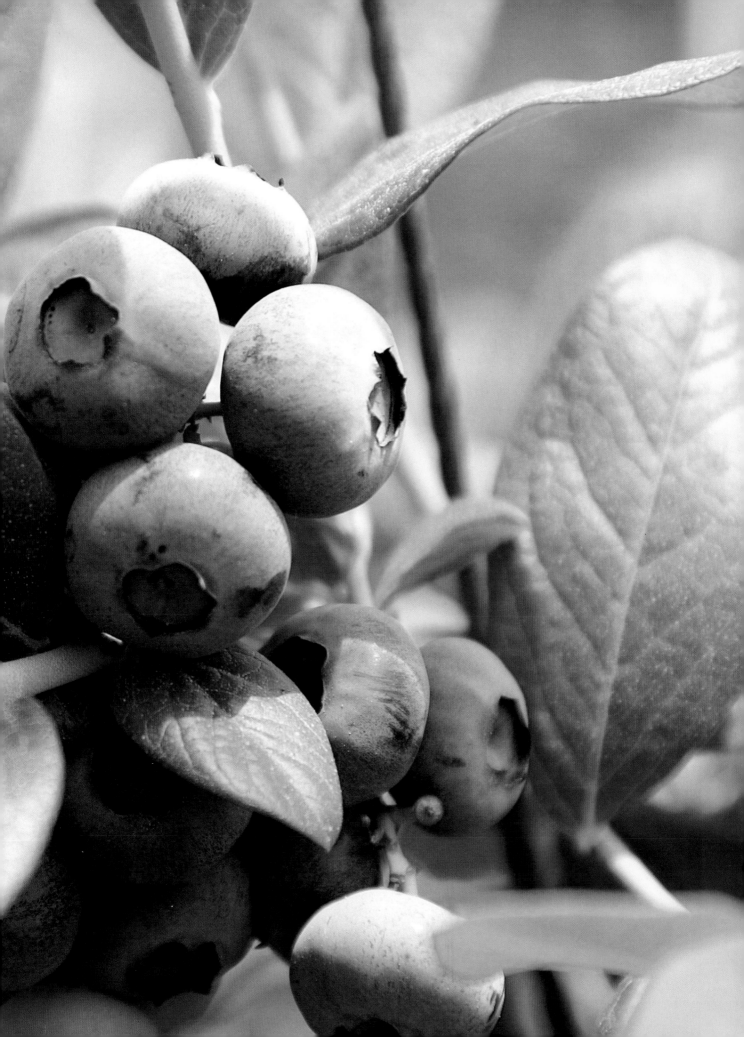

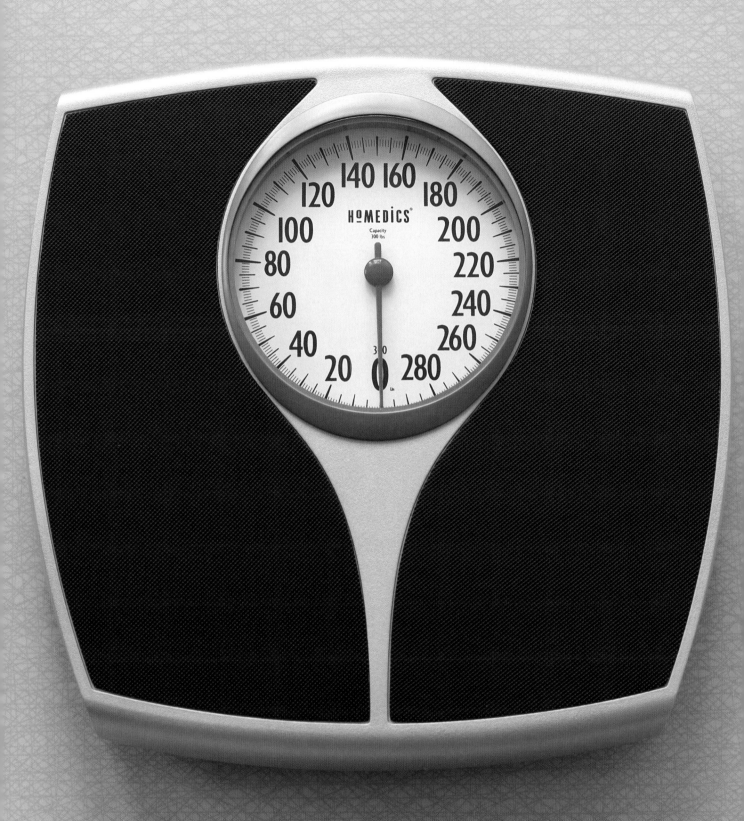

CHAPTER 12

Health Risks of Excess Weight

As a nation, Americans continue to get fatter and fatter. About two-thirds of adults in the country are either overweight or obese, according to the National Health and Nutrition Examination Survey. The fattest category is growing the fastest. A study published in *Public Health* found that between 2000 and 2005, the U.S. obese population (with a body mass index, or BMI, of 30 or more) increased by 24 percent. The morbidly obese population (with a BMI of 40 or more) increased twice as fast, while the supermorbidly obese population (with a BMI of 50 or more) increased three times as fast. If current trends continue, 30 years from now one-third of the U.S. population could be morbidly obese.

Why is this so alarming? Because obesity is the second-leading cause of preventable death in the United States and costs $117 billion in health care costs each year. But the cost to individuals' health is even more. Obese people are more likely to have high blood pressure and high cholesterol levels, major risk factors for heart disease and stroke. Several types of cancer are associated with being overweight, including cancer of the uterus, gallbladder, kidney, breast and colon. Other conditions linked with obesity include diabetes, sleep apnea, osteoarthritis, gout, gallbladder disease and infertility.

With that host of maladies, it's probably no surprise that those who are the most successful with losing weight—and more importantly, keeping it off—tend to be motivated more by a desire to improve their health rather than to simply improve their looks. If more people truly grasped just how harmful excess weight is to their health, they would have a lot more motivation both to start and to stick with a diet and exercise plan. Toward that end, this chapter shares some of the most compelling reasons to regain control of your weight.

What Is Fat, Anyway?

When a person is obese, he or she has a much higher amount of body fat than lean muscle mass. An excess of body fat results when the amount of calories you take in is greater than the amount you expend. Correspondingly, the formula for weight gain is pretty simple: You gain weight when you consume more calories than your body uses. Factors that promote obesity include genetic predisposition, family history, age and lifestyle—such as a high-calorie, high-fat diet or inactivity.

While body fat may be the extra baggage that makes your jeans tighter, scientific research is revealing that fat, technically known as adipose tissue, is far more than a lifeless layer of energy storage. Scientists have referred to fat as an endocrine organ, much like other glands that pump hormones into the bloodstream.

This new understanding of fat came with the discovery of leptin, a hormone released by the adipocyte (or fat cell) to signal satiety to the brain. Fat tissue also teams with macrophages (which are white blood cells in tissues) to trigger the body's inflammatory response, which in excess and over time can increase the risk of heart disease, arthritis, Alzheimer's, cancer and lots of other diseases.

Health professionals have long known that abdominal fat poses a greater health threat than lower-body largesse (the old apple versus pear comparison), but they didn't know why. These breakthroughs in understanding the nature of fat may finally provide the explanation. Fat deposited around the organs in the midsection, called visceral fat, might even be more metabolically active than the layer of fat under your skin.

That means that your internal organs essentially marinate in that sea of abdominal

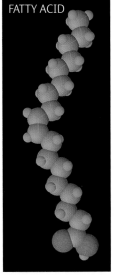

FATTY ACID

DIET TIP
Staying healthy doesn't mean eliminating all fats from your diet. Go for the *good* fats, monounsaturated and polyunsaturated, found in olive oil, canola oil, fish, nuts and avocados. These healthier fats boost heart health and may help lower the risk of Alzheimer's.

Heft Harder on Him

Obesity harms the health of both men and women, but it seems the excess heft weighs heavier on him than on her. Men were shown to have higher carbohydrate intolerance—the inability to process sugar found in carbs—and diminished exercise endurance, according to a Dutch study of 56 severely obese patients.

Fifty-nine percent of the men suffered from impaired carbohydrate intolerance compared with 35 percent of the women. Then, when these same subjects rode stationary bikes to test respiratory capacity, muscle strength and endurance, the women outperformed the men. One possible explanation: Women tend to store fat on the lower body, as opposed to around the midsection, where men do, and abdominal fat increases pressure on the lungs, making it harder to breathe when exercising.

fat, vulnerable to the toxic secretions from it that can wreak havoc with your metabolism. Even if a large percentage of body fat is removed through liposuction, the fat around organs still has a potentially toxic effect. The fat tucked around organs can't be removed through surgery; this is why liposuction won't address many health problems related to obesity.

Obesity can drive you to an early grave. Researchers from Brigham and Women's Hospital in Boston tracked 2,357 male doctors, monitoring five factors—inactivity, blood pressure, obesity, smoking and diabetes—until subjects either died or reached 90 years of age. Out of the original study group, 970 (or 41 percent) lived to the age of 90 or beyond. Those with all the risk factors (e.g., overweight, inactive, smoker, diabetic and having high blood pressure) had only a 4 percent chance of surviving the study period. Those with none of the risk factors had a 54 percent chance of making it.

Obesity itself reduces your survival rate to one in four—which might be optimistic, given that previous research found obesity to accelerate cellular aging even more than smoking, according to a study from St. Thomas' Hospital in England. Researchers looked at blood samples from more than 1,100 women (ages 18 to 76) and found that obese subjects were the equivalent of nine years older than their leaner peers, versus a 7.4 age increase for long-term smokers when compared with those who have never smoked. The researchers believe that fat itself actually accelerates the aging process. This may be why obese people are more susceptible to age-related diseases such as heart disease, osteoarthritis and diabetes.

Hearts Under Attack from Fat

Heart disease is America's No. 1 killer, and obesity is the leading cause of heart disease. Even if you have normal blood pressure and healthy cholesterol, being obese can increase your risk of dying of heart disease by 43 percent.

Trans Fat–Obesity Connection

When food manufacturers introduced an inexpensive hybrid sweetener called high-fructose corn syrup in the late 1960s, researchers began to notice a rise in obesity and diabetes rates. Now, trans fat is viewed as a major contributor to obesity, diabetes and heart disease.

Trans fats and high-fructose corn syrup are in 40 percent of the foods Americans eat every day. Trans fats turn up naturally in milk and meat—in tiny amounts. But the man-made version of trans fats causes most of the trouble. When vegetable oil and hydrogen are put together under tremendous pressure, the resulting fat is shelf-stable and inexpensive. Manufacturers now use it in nearly everything, from margarine and shortening to cookies, granola bars, bean dip and frozen French fries.

Look for the words *hydrogenated* or *partially hydrogenated oil*—code for trans fats—on labels. If partially hydrogenated oil is among the top three or four ingredients listed, you'll want to choose something else (the higher up an ingredient is on the list, the more the product contains of it).

How to Find Your Body Mass Index

Health care professionals use a calculation called the body mass index (BMI) to determine body weight relative to height. In adults, the BMI calculation strongly correlates with total body-fat content. Being overweight is defined as having a BMI between 25 and 29.9. Obesity is defined as having a BMI of 30 or more. Match your height and weight on this chart to find your BMI.

	NORMAL				OVERWEIGHT					OBESE	
BMI	21	22	23	24	25	26	27	28	29	30	31
HEIGHT (inches)	**BODY WEIGHT (pounds)**										
60	107	112	118	123	128	133	138	143	148	153	158
61	111	116	122	127	132	137	143	148	153	158	164
62	115	120	126	131	136	142	147	153	158	164	169
63	118	124	130	135	141	146	152	158	163	169	175
64	122	128	134	140	145	151	157	163	169	174	180
65	126	132	138	144	150	156	162	168	174	180	186
66	130	136	142	148	155	161	167	173	179	186	192
67	134	140	146	153	159	166	172	178	185	191	198
68	138	144	151	158	164	171	177	184	190	197	203
69	142	149	155	162	169	176	182	189	196	203	209
70	146	153	160	167	174	181	188	195	202	209	216
71	150	157	165	172	179	186	193	200	208	215	222
72	154	162	169	177	184	191	199	206	213	221	228
73	159	166	174	182	189	197	204	212	219	227	235

DIET TIP

Breakfast eaters in a Harvard study had a 35 to 50 percent lower rate for obesity, insulin resistance syndrome and heart disease. Experts theorize that breakfast may keep people from overeating later on or may even help balance hormones to control appetite.

Fat is especially harmful to your cardiovascular system because it assaults your heart on many different deadly levels. For example, having excess weight means your heart has to work much harder to pump blood through your body. The result is often high blood pressure, which is another risk factor for heart attacks and strokes. And those extra pounds can also raise blood cholesterol and triglyceride levels while lowering HDL (good) cholesterol. HDL (high-density lipoprotein) helps remove cholesterol from the bloodstream, reducing the risk of heart disease.

Obesity can trigger diabetes, which compounds all the heart-damaging effects of being overweight. And those who are only overweight but not obese are still likely to develop heart-related problems, even with no other risk factors. Excess body weight is linked with coronary heart disease, stroke, congestive heart failure and death from heart-related causes.

Obesity Linked to Nine Types of Cancer

Excess weight may contribute to 20 percent of deaths by cancer. Being overweight also increases the risk of developing cancers of the colon, breast, uterus, kidney,

State of the States

In 2007 only Colorado had an obesity rate of less than 20 percent, according to the Centers for Disease Control and Prevention. In 30 states, 25 percent or more of the population was obese. Alabama, Mississippi and Tennessee had obesity rates of 30 percent or higher.

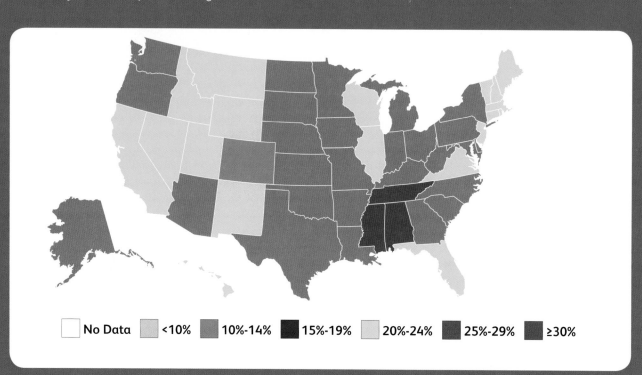

No Data   <10%   10%-14%   15%-19%   20%-24%   25%-29%   ≥30%

esophagus, pancreas, gallbladder and stomach, according to a study published in *Nature Reviews Cancer*. This examination of more than 200 epidemiological sources suggests overeating may be the biggest avoidable cause of cancer in nonsmokers.

Just how fat cells spur cancer growth is something scientists are only now beginning to figure out. The suspected mechanisms range from inflammation triggered by fat to overproduction of certain hormones and interference in insulin regulation. The good news is that unlike factors beyond our control—such as genetic predispositions to certain cancers—obesity is largely preventable.

Other research suggests that being as trim as possible is the best way to avoid cancer. The largest review of existing cancer research to date, jointly issued by the World Cancer Research Fund and the American Institute for Cancer Research, looked at 7,000 studies and found that those who maintained their BMI between 21 and 23 had the best odds of avoiding cancer. In fact, the accumulated findings suggested that the link between body fat and cancer risk was even stronger than previously believed.

How weight affects cancer varies by the type of cancer and gender. For example, being overweight means having up to two times the risk of developing colon cancer for men; for women, the risk is increased up to 50 percent. The largest obesity-related cancer affects only women: A heavy woman has twice the risk—and an obese woman up to five times the risk—of developing uterine cancer than a lean woman does.

Obesity also raises the risk of esophageal cancer. Researchers at the University of Melbourne in Australia followed 41,300 individuals, ages 27 to 75, for more than a decade. Obese subjects were nearly four times more likely to develop cancers of the upper stomach or esophagus than were those of normal weight. For example, a 5-foot-3-inch woman weighing 175 pounds or more has quadruple the esophageal cancer risk of a 5-foot-3-inch woman weighing 120 pounds. The results were similar for men.

DIET TIP
Diners consume 50 percent more calories, fat and sodium when they eat out compared with when they cook at home. Fifty years ago, Americans spent just a fourth of their food dollars outside the home; today a full half of the average food budget goes to meals and snacks eaten outside the home. So, be a homebody to have a healthy body as well.

STRAWBERRIES

Phytochemicals Fight Fat

Japanese researchers may have identified an antioxidant found in certain fruits and vegetables that could fight fat with double biological barrels. Spanish olives, strawberries, blackberries, blueberries, raspberries, red grapes, blood oranges, purple corn and açaí berries contain the phytochemical C3G, which was found to increase production of both adiponectin and leptin in animal trials at Doshisha University. Adiponectin is a protein that enhances fat burning. And leptin is a hormone that suppresses appetite and triggers thermogenesis—the conversion of calories to body heat. In fact, the word leptin derives from the Greek word *leptos*, which means thin.

A second study found that mice on a high-fat diet gained less weight when C3G was added to their food than a control group did. The data suggests that certain anthocyanins, long recognized for their free radical–scavenging prowess, could also have therapeutic potential in the prevention of obesity and diabetes. More research is merited to confirm the same benefits in humans.

Even if your weight falls in a normal range, studies warn against being too complacent: Every extra 22 pounds you put on doubles your risk for cancer, and as with heart disease risk, where you carry the weight matters. Additional inches around the waist raise your esophageal cancer risk. Every time you let your belt out four inches, your risk goes up 50 percent.

Fat Ages Children, Poses Health Risks

Kids seem to grow up too fast. Because of poor diets, they may be growing prematurely old on the inside, too. Alarming research from the University of Missouri-Kansas City suggests that the vascular systems (veins and arteries) of obese adolescents are three decades older than the rest of their bodies.

HANDY SNACKS LIKE CANTALOUPE SLICES HELP KIDS EAT HEALTHIER.

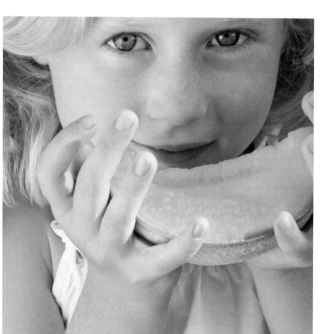

Ultrasound technology measuring the vascular age of 70 obese 10- to 16-year-olds revealed their arteries were more swollen with plaque and inflammation than their normal-weight peers. In fact, these obese adolescents had circulatory systems comparable to a normal 45-year-old.

Why? The same diet that leads to obesity also harms arteries. The saturated fat in fast-food meals ends up as cholesterol deposits, which obstruct and inflame arteries, inhibiting blood flow and restricting vascular flexibility. Junk food also tends to be coated in salt—contributing to rising rates of blood pressure among the young, which ages their arteries. And fatty buildup in heart valves has been seen in children as young as 3-years-old.

While high blood pressure is the leading cause of aging arteries, obesity by itself also raises blood pressure and cholesterol levels. Along with raising the risk of heart

Fresh Solutions for Kids' Diets

Fruits and vegetables are the best weapons against childhood obesity, filling kids up with healthy food while providing them vital nutrients, such as fiber and potassium, to keep their cholesterol and blood pressure levels normal.

The trick for most parents seems to be how to get their kids to eat more fruits and vegetables. A simple solution: Make them readily available. A study at the University of California, Los Angeles, found that when salad bars were introduced at three L.A. schools, the children increased their daily fruit and vegetable consumption by 40 percent.

The study also found an 11 percent drop in calories consumed, a 20 percent drop in cholesterol and a 27 percent decline in saturated-fat intake. With salad bars a potential secret weapon in the fight against childhood obesity, the Dole Nutrition Institute donated 50 salad carts to California public schools. Dole also provides healthy eating information to teachers and students at www.dole.com.

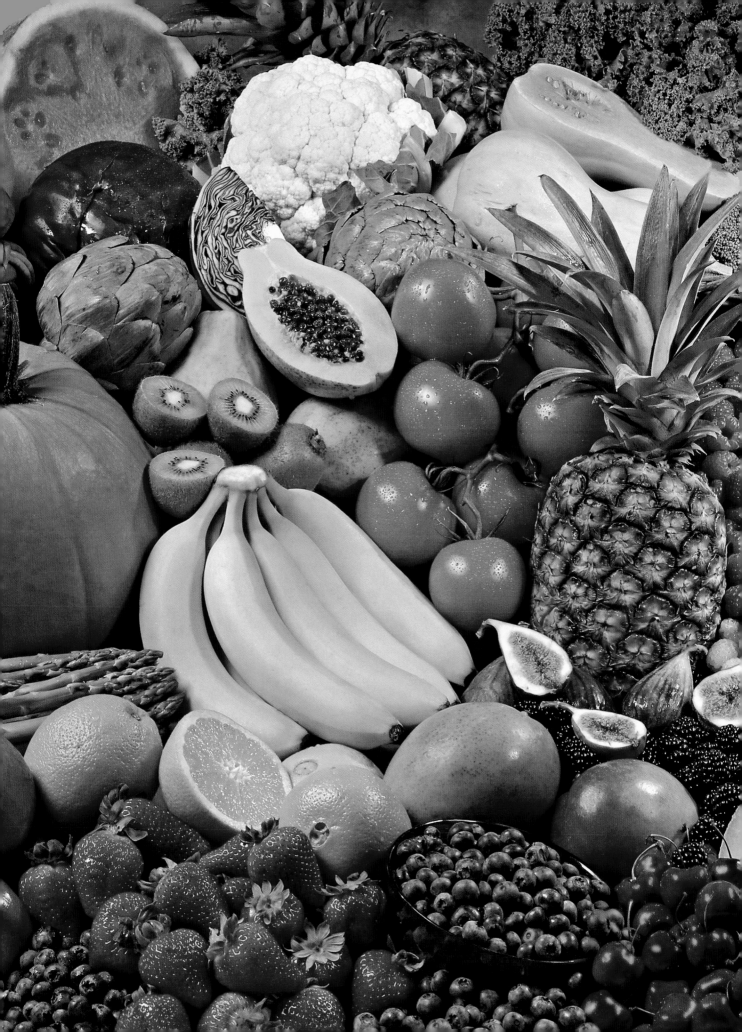

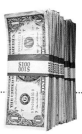

Being Big Costs, Skinny Saves

Along with adversely affecting your health, those extra pounds also impact your pocketbook.

Obese employees are paid $3.41 less per hour than their normal-weight counterparts, according to a Stanford University study. That pay difference isn't based on looks. The study found that the lower pay was a reflection of the higher medical and insurance costs for obese employees.

Beyond salary, there are tax implications for obesity as well. For example, there are potential tax breaks for certain weight-loss treatments, similar to how some medical expenses are deductible.

FITNESS TIP

Help your kids avoid summertime weight gain by limiting television and encouraging activity. Children's BMIs rise more than twice as fast during summer break versus during the school year. Increased summer tube time could add up to 1,000 extra calories per day.

attack and stroke for children, obesity may lead to an epidemic of type 2 diabetes among kids. The Centers for Disease Control and Prevention recently predicted that at least one in three American children born in the year 2000 will develop diabetes sometime in their lifetime.

As if the potential for manifesting heart disease and diabetes isn't bad enough, obese children also face an increased risk for a host of other ailments, including joint disorders, breathing constriction, emotional difficulties and frequent earaches. Plus, children who are overweight seem to do poorer on mental ability tests than their nonobese peers. Researchers at the University of South Carolina compared the body mass index of more than 2,500 kids, ages 8 to 16, with various measures of mental ability, including memorization and building block tests in which children use blocks to reproduce pictures of arrangements. Overweight children were nearly three times more likely to score poorly on tests measuring visuospatial organization.

Fatter Patients Mean Fuzzy Scans

Not only does excess weight raise the risk for disease, it can also make health problems harder to detect. During the past 15 years, the number of inconclusive radiology test results has doubled, despite increasingly sophisticated diagnostic equipment. It's no coincidence that America's obesity rate has also doubled. Increasingly, obesity hampers diagnostic accuracy by expanding the layer of fat tissue that scans must penetrate; in addition, sometimes patients are too big to fit into machines. A sign of the times: Manufacturers have begun modifying designs to accommodate patients who weigh up to 550 pounds.

Some doctors even predict that very soon one-third of patients will weigh 350 pounds or more—a serious consideration for doctors, medical equipment engineers and, most importantly, the patients themselves.

Bulge Bad for Bones

The common misconception is that being overweight strengthens bones, but alas, emerging research shows that fat actually undermines the skeletal system. For example, among postmenopausal women, higher fat mass also means lower bone-mineral densities, according to a study presented at the 2008 annual meeting of the American Dietetic Association.

You'd think that, since weight-bearing exercise increases bone density, then having, say, 25 pounds of extra body fat would have the same result, right? No. That's because adipose tissue produces toxic substances that impair the ability to maintain strong bones. Excess fat induces an inflammatory response that inhibits bone building and multiplies osteoclasts, which are cells that break down bones. By contrast, packing extra muscle instead of fat strengthens bones.

One way to tip that fat-muscle balance is to increase activity and eat more fruits and vegetables. Studies have linked eating fruits and vegetables with higher bone-mineral density. Such foods as leafy greens and broccoli supply a combination of bone-building nutrients while helping you get rid of that bone-harmful fat. Also incorporate more bananas and berries into your diet, both of which boost fat-burning potential.

Excess Pounds Double Infection Risk

Infections contracted in hospitals are the fourth-largest killer in the United States, according to the Committee to Reduce Infection Deaths. Research suggests that being obese can more than double your risk of wound infection.

If you are obese at the time of surgery, you are more than twice as likely to suffer an infection, states a study by the Washington University School of Medicine in St. Louis. The study, which looked at 2,316 cases of spinal surgery (46 of which resulted in infection), indicates that diabetes was another strong risk factor—making infection 3.5 times more likely. These results echo a Duke University study that found clinically obese patients to be 7.1 times more likely to experience a surgical-site infection.

These greater infection rates may help explain why gastric bypass surgery turns out to be far riskier than commonly believed. Obesity decreases the body's resistance to pathogens, which may in turn increase the risk of infection. Three studies appearing in the *Journal of the American Medical Association* call the safety—and supposed cost savings—of gastric bypass surgery into question.

HEALTH TIP
Boost bone health with resistant starch, found in bananas, leeks, onions, garlic and artichokes. In a study by the Baylor College of Medicine, increased resistant starch intake improved bone-mineral density by 15 percent among children.

More Pounds Equals Less Production

For companies, health care costs aren't the only place obesity takes a bite out of profits. A Center for Health Promotion study found that obese workers had more difficulty getting along with coworkers and also had more absentee days. These findings confirm similar correlations between obesity and absenteeism demonstrated in several other studies, including those done by the University of Nevada School of Medicine and Brigham Young University.

The data suggests that being active can increase productivity, improve workplace morale and drive return on investment that companies can give by providing opportunities and incentives for exercise, overhauling employee cafeterias and replacing vending machine junk food with healthier fare.

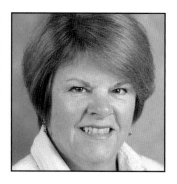

▶ Cheryl Lovelady

Cheryl Lovelady, PhD, MPH, RD, is a professor in the Department of Nutrition at the University of North Carolina at Greensboro (UNCG). Dr. Lovelady is also a consulting professor in the Department of Community and Family Medicine at Duke University. She is a member of the American College of Sports Medicine and a Fellow of the American Dietetic Association. She is a noted researcher in the area of women's health, with emphasis on energy needs and exercise in the postpartum period. Dr. Lovelady has received numerous awards for her research and teaching, including the Board of Governor's Outstanding Teaching Award and the Senior Research Excellence Award, School of Human Environmental Sciences at UNCG.

Q: What is causing the rise in obesity? What can reverse it?

CL: There are many factors affecting the rise in obesity. People are consuming more calories than they require. The rise in obesity corresponds to the increase in portion sizes over the years. Serving sizes of juice have increased from 4 ounces to 12 ounces. Children are bringing 20-ounce bottles of sports drinks in their school lunches or to their 45-minute soccer practices. One meal of a large cheeseburger with large fries and a large milk shake contains more calories than most adults require all day. We are eating less fruits and vegetables and more high-fat, energy-dense foods. In addition, there is easier access to low-cost foods high in fat and sugar. Fast-food restaurants are ubiquitous and often open 24 hours a day. Vending machines are in offices, schools and recreation centers.

WEIGHT-BEARING EXERCISE BURNS FAT AND BUILDS STRONG BONES.

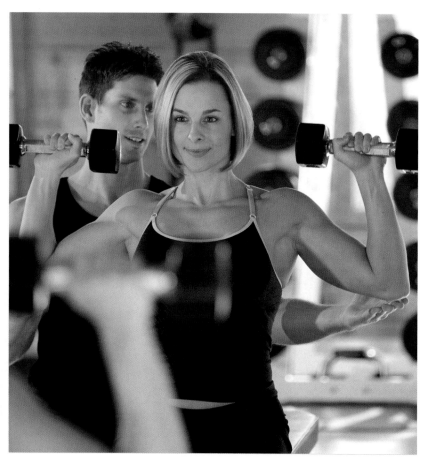

People are not burning as many calories as they were in the past. Less than half the adults in the United States meet the public health recommendations of accumulating 30 minutes or more of moderate-intensity physical activity on most, preferably all, days of the week. Twenty-five percent of Americans report no leisure-time physical activity. We are spending the majority of our time in sedentary activity. At the 2009 meeting of the American College of Sports Medicine, Dr. Neville Owen presented the President's Lecture on "The Science of Sedentary Behavior: Too Much Sitting and Too Little Exercise." He reported data showing that even performing the recommended minutes of physical activity cannot compensate for the harmful effects of sitting the rest of the day.

To reverse this rise, we must eat less, exercise more and be more active throughout the day.

Q: What determines if you are obese or merely overweight?

CL: The most common way to determine if you are overweight or obese is to calculate your body mass index (BMI). This is a ratio of your weight to your height. If your BMI is equal to or greater than 25, but less than 30, you are considered overweight. If your BMI is equal to or greater than 30, you are considered obese (see page 247 for a BMI chart).

Q: What is the difference between the athlete who may be heavy but strong and the TV-viewing couch potato, even though they may have the same BMI?

CL: BMI is calculated based on weight only. Body composition is not considered. So, the athlete who has a higher percent of muscle than the couch potato, who has a higher percent of body fat, can still have the same BMI. That is the problem with using BMI as an indicator of body fatness. But it is the simplest and least expensive way to estimate overweight and obesity.

Q: How does being obese affect longevity?

CL: Obesity increases the risk of many chronic diseases, which shorten our lives by a considerable number of years. Whether or not obesity by itself affects longevity remains controversial. When looking at the data, BMI is usually used as the surrogate for obesity. A report in 2006 found that obesity (a BMI greater than 30) and being underweight (a BMI less than 18.5), when compared with normal weight (a BMI greater than or equal to 18.5 and less than or equal to 25) were associated with excess deaths in the United States in 2000. However, it is very difficult to determine if it is obesity, or a poor diet and sedentary lifestyle, that is contributing to increased mortality.

Q: What other diseases does obesity increase the risk of?

CL: Obesity increases the risk of heart disease, type 2 diabetes, certain cancers, a fatty liver, high blood pressure and osteoarthritis.

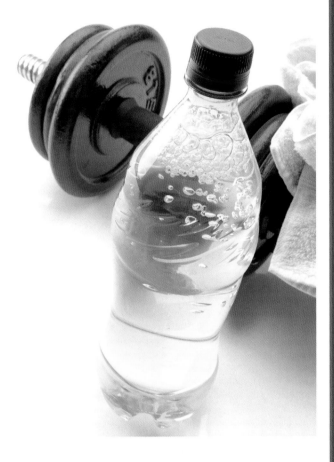

DRINKING WATER WHILE WORKING OUT MAY INCREASE CALORIE BURN.

Drink to the Benefits of Water

Not only is dehydration unhealthy—causing fatigue, constipation and toxicity—it may actually derail your diet. Thirst is often mistaken for hunger, which makes it harder to stick to limits and resist temptation. Moreover, water consumption may increase calorie burn. German researchers found that drinking about 17 ounces of water raised study subjects' metabolic rate by 30 percent.

APPLES

Filling Fruit Fiber Helps Fight Fat

You may know that pectin is the ingredient that helps make jams gel. But research suggests that this fruit-and-vegetable fiber may be a key ingredient to successful weight loss as well. A study from the State University of New York at Buffalo found that consuming more pectin—the connective fiber found in apples, oranges, plums, carrots and other produce—helps dieters feel more full. Researchers monitored the diets of 29 obese or overweight women to see whether their calorie intake would be affected by consuming 2.8 grams of pectin—roughly the amount found in a large apple—before breakfast and lunch. Those women who most benefited from the added pectin were those who historically had the hardest time dieting and controlling their weight. In fact, the extra pectin appeared to help these struggling dieters consume 12 percent fewer calories overall during the day—and 22 percent fewer calories during the evening.

Additional research confirms the body-weight benefits of fiber from fruit. Adding three apples or pears to their daily diet decreased calorie intake and spurred weight loss for women in a Brazilian fiber study. In contrast, women who added the same number of calories and fiber in the form of energy-dense oat cookies saw an increase in their calorie intake and no weight loss.

THE PECTIN IN PLUMS AND OTHER PRODUCE MAKES YOU FEEL FULLER LONGER.

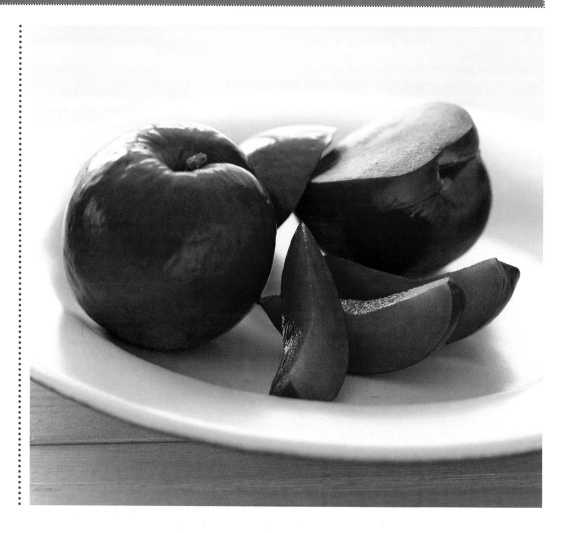

Q: What about the myth that carrying around this excess weight makes your bones stronger?

CL: Most epidemiological studies report a positive relationship between BMI and bone-mineral density. This is because weight-bearing exercise stimulates bone formation. However, when researchers look at excess body fat versus BMI, this relationship is not always consistent. A diet adequate in calcium, protein and vitamin D, as well as physical activity in the form of weight-bearing exercise, is a crucial determinant of strong bones.

Q: What's the difference between visceral and regular fat?

CL: Where your fat is located affects your metabolism and your risk of disease—in particular, for diabetes, high blood pressure, fatty liver and hyperlipidemia. Visceral fat is the fat surrounding your organs in your abdominal area. Fat deposition in this area is associated with the risk of these metabolic diseases, while fat located directly under the skin is not. However, this abdominal fat is very responsive to exercise and dietary changes. We conducted a study of overweight, sedentary women, 30- to 45-years-old. They began a resistance-training program, 25 minutes per day, three times per week. In addition, they decreased their calorie intake by only 250 calories per day. After 16 weeks on the program, each woman lost an average of 4 pounds. However, each lost approximately 6 pounds of fat, and 3.5 pounds of that loss was in the trunk area! Each also gained 2 pounds of lean body mass. These small changes in their diet and physical activity greatly decreased their risk of chronic disease.

Q: Fat has been described as behaving like an extra organ. Can you explain how and why?

CL: Fat is said to behave like an organ because the fat cells secrete hormones, which communicate with other parts of the body, as well as macrophages and cytokines, which can cause inflammation and lead to insulin resistance and osteoarthritis.

> Small changes in diet and physical activity have been found to reduce the risk of chronic disease.

Soup Is a Smart Snack

You probably know that having soup as an appetizer will help fill you up, making it easier to eat less. Now, according to researchers, a bowl between meals is better than other snacks in terms of controlling your hunger. When 24 women were served three different snacks that contained the same ingredients and calories—chicken rice casserole, the casserole with a glass of water, or a soup made with the casserole and water—the soup curbed their appetite the best. This group of women reported less hunger and ate 80 fewer calories at a meal two hours later.

Vegetable-based soups allow you to eat a large portion while still sparing calories. Your mouth likes the extra food, your brain is turned on by knowing you're having more, and now it seems that your stomach stays full longer than expected. All work together to keep you feeling satisfied.

So for fast and filling snacks, make soups using pureed vegetables to enjoy all week. When the weather is warmer, try chilled soup, such as gazpacho. Cold soups seem to have the same effect as the hot ones.

DIET TIP

Take the express lane to weight loss—literally—by choosing self-checkout. In a study of 500 consumers, grocery shoppers who scanned their own groceries were 43 percent less likely to make impulse buys. Self-checkout lanes generally have fewer snacks within arm's reach—limiting temptation, while saving time (on average lines are 66 percent shorter).

Q: Is it possible to be "fit but fat"—or does excess weight pose independent risks, regardless of fitness levels?

CL: This answer is dependent on how fitness is defined. Many studies use measures of blood pressure, blood glucose and blood lipids as indicators of fitness. You may have normal levels of these parameters and exceed the normal BMI of 25. However, we are now recognizing that "fitness" extends beyond these blood values. In addition to expanding the definition of fitness to include cardiovascular fitness, resistance to infection and other factors, researchers are also looking at body composition (body fat and where it's located) and finding that the fatter you are (in particular the more visceral fat you have), the less fit you are.

Q: What's the most effective way to maintain—or lose—weight?

CL: The only way to lose weight is to be in "negative energy balance." This means you consume fewer calories than you expend. And weight loss should only be 1 to 2 pounds per week. More than this usually results in loss of lean body mass. There are many diets that can achieve this; however, the most effective one varies among individuals. The key to successful weight loss is to achieve a way of eating that you can live with for the rest of your life. The diet should be well-balanced, containing moderate amounts of food from all food groups. It should contain adequate servings of fruits, vegetables and whole grains to supply you with required nutrients, fiber and other bioactive compounds. Protein and moderate amounts of healthy fats from olive and vegetable oils are also necessary.

Exercise must complement a decreased calorie intake. Exercise alone usually does not result in weight loss, because it takes a considerable amount of time and effort to burn an extra 500 calories a day. That is the amount of calories that will result in 1 pound of fat loss per week. A combination of decreasing calorie intake by 250 calories and increasing physical activity by 250 calories per day is the most effective way to lose weight. Guidelines from the American College of Sports Medicine state that moderate-intensity physical activity between 150 and 250 minutes per week will improve weight loss in studies that use moderate diet restriction.

In addition, the most effective way to maintain your weight loss is to do at least 250 minutes per week of moderate physical activity. Maintaining weight loss is difficult because you weigh less and, therefore, require fewer calories. That is why more physical exercise is required to maintain your weight at its new, lower level. Recording your food intake and weighing yourself weekly have also been shown to aid in weight maintenance.

Extra Pounds Aggravate Reflux Symptoms

What goes up must come down—but when it comes to overeating and acid reflux, what goes down may come up! If too many extra servings lead to even a few extra pounds, you could be setting yourself up for increased risk of gastroesophageal reflux disease.

This is a syndrome in which your stomach regurgitates acids into the esophageal area, causing painful symptoms ranging from heartburn to a persistent dry cough and a rise in your risk of esophageal cancer. Reflux symptoms doubled with only a 3.5-point increase in body mass index, according to one Boston University study that followed 10,000 women between 1984 and 1998.

These findings demonstrate that weight gain within "normal" range can cause the kind of gastrointestinal problems that are commonly associated with obesity. On the brighter side, the study also found that women who lost 3.5 BMI points experienced a 40 percent drop in gastroesophageal reflux disease symptoms.

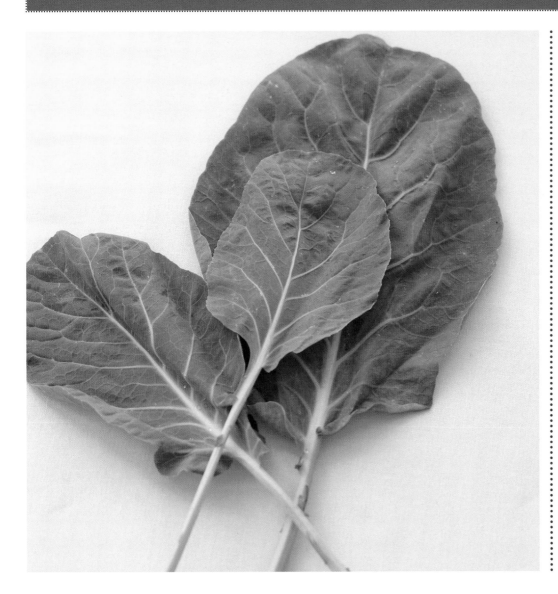

DIET TIP
Here are a few rules of thumb for your new dietary approach: Start meals with a big salad—lots of veggies, no croutons or creamy dressing; have double portions of fruit and vegetables at meals; and skip or cut back on calorie-dense starches, fats and fatty meats. Opt for a fruit dessert, with a dab of sorbet for flavor.

A DIET RICH IN FIBER FROM FOODS SUCH AS COLLARD GREENS CAN HELP LESSEN ACID REFLUX SYMPTOMS.

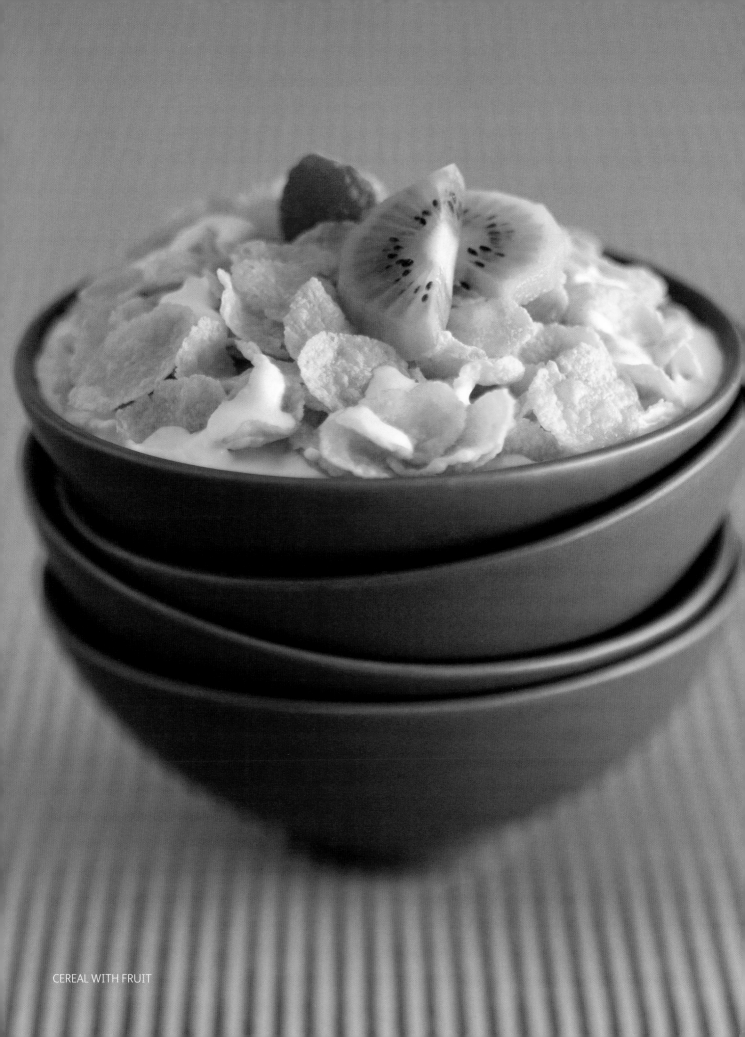

CEREAL WITH FRUIT

Simple Ways to Begin

Committing to a new diet plan may seem daunting, but you can easily incorporate a few simple changes into your current eating habits—beginning with breakfast. According to researchers at Queens College, the City University of New York, women who eat calorie-dense breakfasts report eating denser meals and more fat during the rest of the day, as well as having lower micronutrient intake and poorer diet quality. But it doesn't pay to skip breakfast entirely, because women who eat no breakfast are heavier than breakfast eaters.

Another way to shift your eating pattern is to go vegetarian, beginning with just a few days a week. The fact that fruits and vegetables tend to fill you up with fewer calories and more nutrition may explain why a study found that vegetarian women tend to weigh less. After evaluating the diet and health data of 56,000 Swedish women, Tufts University researchers found that the meat eaters were significantly more likely to be overweight than their vegetarian peers. According to the report, published in the *American Journal of Clinical Nutrition*, 40 percent of the carnivores were overweight, compared with 25 percent of the vegetarians and 29 percent of the flexitarians, pescatarians or semivegetarians—those who may avoid meat but eat fish and eggs. Though obesity is a bigger problem in the United States than in Sweden, the inverse relationship between weight and meat consumption would likely be comparable.

Inactivity Linked with Tummy Trouble

Want to lose weight with exercise, but worried that symptoms of gastrointestinal distress might hold you back? Research suggests that plugging away at your fitness resolution may be key to diminishing gastrointestinal symptoms over time.

While previous studies have found a much higher incidence of gastrointestinal distress (e.g., abdominal pain, diarrhea and bloating) among the obese, this investigation looked at a variety of weight-loss behaviors and found that physical activity stood out as the strongest protective factor. The study tracked the diets, activity levels and gastrointestinal symptoms of nearly 100 obese participants in a weight-loss program. While other healthy eating behaviors (i.e., fruit and vegetable consumption) and reduced fat intake were also linked to less discomfort, exercise appeared to confer the most significant benefit.

Conclusion

If current trends continue, 30 years from now one-third of the U.S. population could be morbidly obese! Hard to believe? Three decades ago, it would have been hard to imagine the present state of affairs: Two-thirds of the population is overweight or obese.

As if that wasn't enough cause for concern, the numbers of those who are morbidly obese and supermorbidly obese continue to skyrocket. The higher the BMI, the higher the growth rate of that group. But hopefully, armed with knowledge of some of these alarming health consequences, more Americans will take up the fight against fat—for their own sake, and for those they love.

DIET TIP

Overweight—and overwhelmed? Even modest weight loss can result in major health gains. In one large-scale study, participants who lost an average of 12 pounds and walked 20 minutes per day cut their risk of getting type 2 diabetes in half. So don't be defeated before you begin. Start taking small steps toward a healthy lifestyle today.

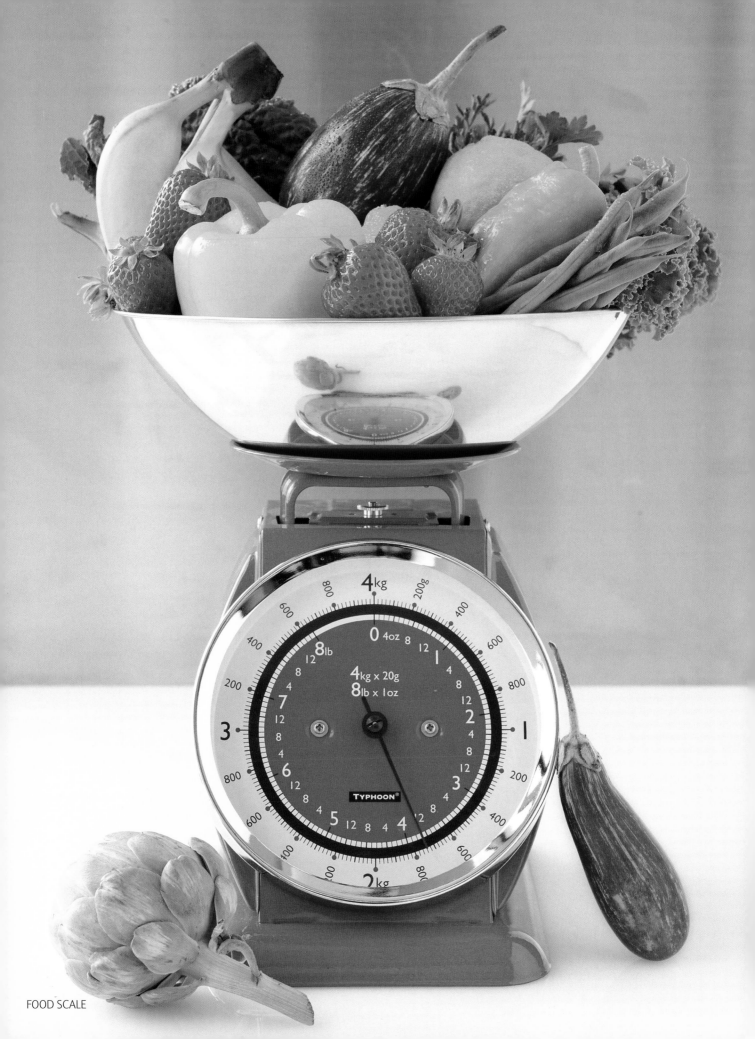

FOOD SCALE

CHAPTER 13

Diet Myths and Weight-Loss Facts

You're not alone if you find it confusing to sort through all the weight-loss hype. Dozens of diet books get published every year, and supplement-makers push magic pills that supposedly melt away pounds. Then, there's the seductive call for "fat acceptance," which encourages heavy women, in particular, to "embrace their curves"—often without mentioning the potentially dire health consequences of being overweight.

In this chapter, we explore common diet myths that could be sabotaging your weight-loss success. And we provide some weight-loss truths that help you shed unwanted pounds.

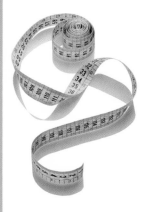

MYTH: High-protein foods like meat help you lose weight while fruits make you fat because they contain lots of carbohydrates and sugar.

FACT: Trendy low-carb, high-protein diets may deprive you of the protective benefits of foods like fruit, which is high in fiber and antioxidants.

Not only will you miss out on the healthy benefits from fruit, but piling on bacon and cheese for that high-protein diet may also increase the risk of a host of ailments, including gastrointestinal distress, heart disease and cancer. And because such diets allow an increase of saturated fat and cholesterol, researchers believe that they may increase the risk of cardiovascular disease. Research from Northwestern University also found that the more protein from meat a person consumes, the higher his or her weight tends to be.

MYTH: This country is overly concerned with obesity because we place too much emphasis on appearance.

FACT: Many obese people are unaware of the health risks of their situation.

The first and foremost obstacle in addressing the obesity epidemic is widespread lack of awareness and denial of the problem. A Cancer Research U.K. survey of 4,000 obese and overweight British men and women found that about half didn't believe that healthy eating could reduce cancer risk, and two-thirds didn't think that exercise could reduce cancer risk. Plus, more than one in four obese and overweight individuals said they did not want to lose weight. Given the burgeoning evidence of the link between obesity and the increased risk of serious ailments, including various cancers, these findings suggest that more explicit educational messages are necessary to help check the obesity epidemic.

Losing Weight Is Cheap

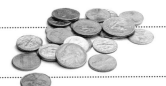

Some people think of losing weight as an expensive endeavor. But in reality, it can be quite affordable and can even save you money over the long run. You don't need to buy expensive equipment or premade meals. And keep in mind that the costs of not getting fit—including heart disease, diabetes and arthritis—are much higher than the costs of starting a weight-loss program.

MYTH: If your heart is healthy, it's okay to be pudgy.
FACT: Any amount of excess weight increases your heart disease risk.
Research shatters the myth that excess weight won't hurt you as long as your blood pressure and cholesterol levels are okay. Just having those extra pounds on your frame poses health risks, according to a three-decade study of 17,643 participants by the Chicago Heart Association Detection Project in Industry. Those who are obese but have normal blood pressure and healthy cholesterol have a 43 percent higher risk of dying of heart disease than those of normal weight.

MYTH: It's just a little baby fat; it doesn't matter if a child is chubby.
FACT: Parents are often in denial about their children's obesity.
Parents may look at their children through a forgiving lens, but their loving gaze is not so benign when it comes to childhood obesity. Nearly half of parents with an obese child believe that their child is "about the right weight"—an illusion that could doom these kids to a lifetime of weight problems and other health ailments.

A University of Michigan poll asked 1,400 parents their children's height and weight in order to calculate their body mass index, and then compared the numbers with the parents' characterization of their children's weight. Among parents of obese children, ages 6 to 11, almost 80 percent said that their kid was either "about the right weight" or "slightly overweight." Some even thought their obese child was "slightly underweight."

Similarly, researchers from the University of North Carolina at Chapel Hill, found that 68 percent of parents with obese children underestimated their kids' weight—even when the children were already showing signs of type 2 diabetes. What's worse, parents who demonstrate the least concern about their children's weight tend to have the heaviest kids, according to a Stanford University study.

MYTH: If you exercise regularly, extra pounds don't matter.
FACT: Fat cells negatively influence body chemistry, even if you exercise.
Many people carrying around excess pounds want to believe that exercise alone can neutralize the health risks. But research refutes this fantasy. A Harvard School of Public Health study tracked the body mass index, exercise patterns and incidence of heart disease in 38,987 women for nearly 11 years. Active, overweight women had a

DIET TIP
Can a sprinkle a day help keep weight gain away? Chicago researchers monitored subjects who sprinkled their food with calorie-free powders that smelled like high-flavor foods (including cocoa, banana and raspberry, plus savory flavors like taco, cheddar and horseradish). Test subjects lost an average of 5.6 pounds per month without making other changes in their diet, while a control group on a standard diet actually gained weight.

EXCERCISE CAN HELP YOU SHED UNWANTED POUNDS, BUT DIET ADJUSTMENTS ARE ESSENTIAL TOO.

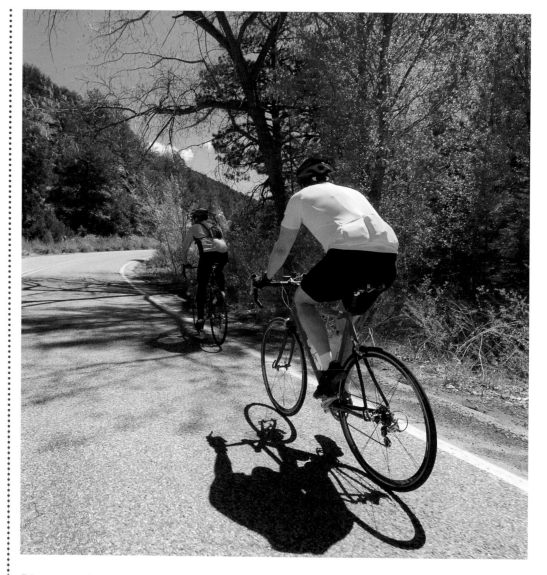

DIET TIP

Avoid talking on the phone while you are in the kitchen, as this can lead to unintentional, mindless grazing. For your next casual conversation, take your cordless around the house as you tidy up, or head outside with your cell phone while you take a brisk walk around the block instead.

54 percent higher risk of heart disease than active women of normal weight. And active, obese women faced an 87 percent higher risk. Exercise certainly helped: Subtract it, and the risk jumped to 88 percent for the inactive overweight and 250 percent for the inactive obese. Yet exercise itself clearly isn't enough to eliminate the dangers of being overweight.

MYTH: Your social life has little influence on your weight.
FACT: Overweight friends can be fattening.
We've all heard obesity described as an epidemic. Now, a Harvard Medical School study has characterized it as contagious. Researchers propose that obesity spreads, not through physical infection, but through the relaxation of social norms regarding appropriate body size. The study, published in the *New England Journal of Medicine*, analyzed data for more than 12,000 people from the multigenerational Framingham Heart Study and found that having an obese friend, spouse or sibling greatly increased a person's odds of becoming obese.

Lead researcher Nicholas Christakis, MD, MPH, PhD, believes that this acceptance of obesity spreads because people feel it's okay to be bigger when those around them are bigger. Among the study's findings: Those with an obese friend are 57 percent more likely to become obese; with an obese sibling, 40 percent; and with an obese spouse, 37 percent.

Connect-the-Dots Weight Maintenance

You can keep your weight on the straight and narrow by taking a piece of grid paper and making a simple graph (with pounds along the left side and days of the week along the bottom). By charting your weight on a daily basis, you will notice if your weight is trending up—and be able to make adjustments.

MYTH: It's better to be overweight than a yo-yo dieter.
FACT: Every bit of extra weight you lose is beneficial to your health.
Many people believe that it's better to make peace with extra pounds than risk the health perils of weight cycling, also called yo-yo dieting. But when compared to the health hazards of being overweight, any attempt to lose weight is worthwhile. In fact, just trying to lose weight lowers your mortality risk, according to a U.S. government health survey. While the study, published in the American College of Physicians' *Annals of Internal Medicine*, found the greatest longevity gains among those who succeed in losing weight, even those who tried and failed to drop pounds shrank their mortality rate by 19 percent. Researchers speculate that dieting might go hand in hand with other healthy behaviors, such as exercise and improved nutrition that ultimately lengthen life.

When trying to lose weight, don't let past failures—or fear of future ones—foil your resolve. It can take multiple attempts to win the battle of the bulge, according to researcher Diane Berry, PhD, who conducted a Yale University School of Nursing one-year weight-loss study. No one in the study of 20 women lost weight and kept it off the first time around. If you stray from your diet, forgive yourself and get back on track, instead of giving yourself permission to give over to overeating.

MYTH: Small, attainable goals will help you keep weight off.
FACT: The more ambitious the weight-loss goal, the better the odds of success.
Conventional wisdom warns against setting unrealistic goals, and yet research shows that dieters who go for the big numbers in weight loss shed more pounds than those with more modest expectations. A University of Minnesota study of 1,801 obese women found that those who aimed to lose more than the standard, "realistic" 10 percent of body weight lost the most. A 10-pound difference in goal weight was associated with 6 more pounds lost over the two-year period. So, for example, a woman with a goal weight 20 pounds lower than her friend's might expect to lose 12 pounds more than her friend, on average, over two years (all other factors being equal). Researchers believe that having higher weight-loss goals may help motivate people to make long-term changes, resulting in more weight loss.

DIET TIP

In this age of super-sized everything, dress sizes are inflating too. Women who would have been wearing a size 12 decades ago are now stepping into a "size 8." Don't let designers enable you into denial! Use a scale and a measuring tape—not a trip to the shopping mall—to keep an eye on your weight and size.

MYTH: Calcium-rich foods facilitate weight loss.

FACT: Overindulging in ice cream actually does make you fat. Sorry.

Headlines sometimes obscure the more subtle points of weight-loss research. For example, a University of Tennessee study found that high-calcium, particularly high-dairy, diets may enhance weight loss among obese individuals already following a low-calorie regimen. When the results were reported in the mainstream media, however, the "already following a low-calorie regimen" part often fell by the wayside, while the notion that ice cream, milk shakes and mozzarella might actually be diet foods took center stage. But, of course, dieters who disregard the fat and calorie content of their calcium sources are more apt to gain weight, not lose it.

GET YOUR CALCIUM
FROM PLANTS
LIKE KALE.

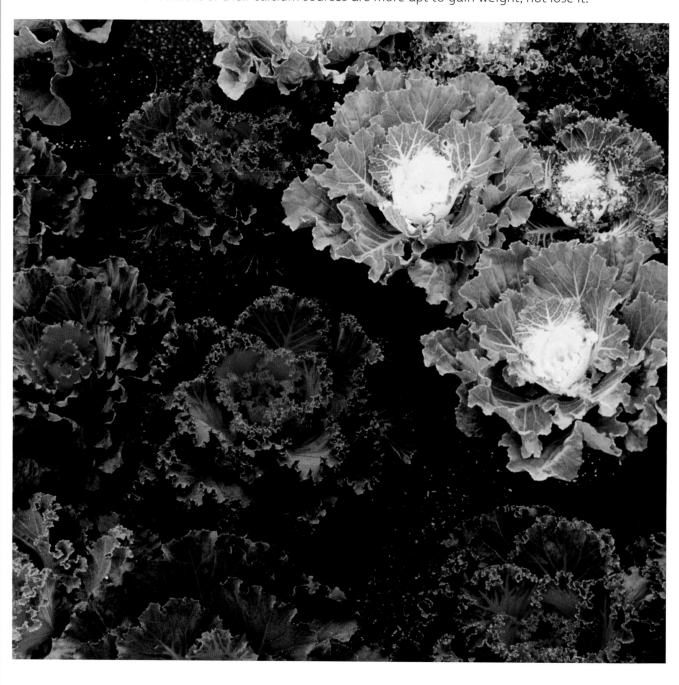

Savored Food Satisfies Longer

When people are stressed, they tend to gulp down their food—and eat more than if they savored every bite. A study conducted at Brazosport Memorial Hospital in Lake Jackson, Texas, found that when six women were asked to eat slowly, chew thoroughly and stop when their food no longer tasted as good as when they took their first bite, they lost, on average, 8 pounds. A control group averaged a 3 pound weight gain. Your body intuitively knows how many calories you need, and if you allow enough time for it to register what you've eaten as you eat, you'll know exactly when you've had enough and will be better able to stop eating at that point.

The calcium findings are part of a growing body of evidence of an association between nutrition deficiencies and obesity. In this case, a low-calcium diet increases blood levels of calcitriol (the active form of vitamin D), which stimulates calcium influx into the fat cells. That, in turn, stimulates lipogenic (or fat-creating) gene expression, leading the body to generate excess adipose, or fat. In other words, if you're calcium-deficient, your body is more disposed to create fat cells than when your calcium levels are adequate.

MYTH: Lifestyle changes have little impact on eating habits.
FACT: Marriage leads to weight gain.
The early years of wedlock are associated with a packing on of the pounds—6 to 8 in the first two years, according to a study in *Obesity*. Another study found that women gain an average of 24.7 pounds over 13 years of marriage, while men typically gain 19.4 pounds. One factor may lie between the sheets: Not getting enough sleep is a big diet saboteur. Not only does it sap your energy when it comes to exercise, but sleep loss affects appetite and fat-regulating hormones in a way that increases susceptibility to weight gain. Sleeping solo makes it more likely that you'll get the rest you need—nearly half of those who have a sleep partner report losing at least three hours of shut-eye per week due to a tossing, turning, snoring partner.

MYTH: Eating several small meals throughout the day supports weight loss.
FACT: Eating larger, planned meals helps keep calories under control.
Not only can small, unscheduled meals set you up to eat mindlessly without regard to how many calories you're consuming, it can be physiologically disadvantageous as well. In a study featured in the 2005 *American Journal of Clinical Nutrition,* when researchers had one group of women eat at regular, fixed times and another group spread their usual daily food intake into unscheduled meals throughout the day, they found that the women who ate larger, scheduled meals actually burned more calories during the three hours after they ate than those who ate unplanned meals. They produced less insulin, too, potentially lowering their odds of insulin resistance, which is linked to weight gain and obesity. The takeaway from this study: Figure out how many times a day you need to eat and stick to a schedule.

DIET TIP
If you're having trouble keeping weight down, try sitting up. Good posture will help you send satiety signals to the brain. Sitting upright lets food settle in the lower part of the stomach, allowing you to feel fuller faster.

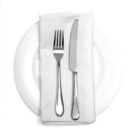

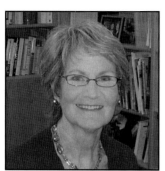

▶ Barbara J. Rolls

Barbara J. Rolls, PhD, is the endowed Helen A. Guthrie Chair in Nutritional Sciences at Pennsylvania State University. A veteran nutrition researcher, Dr. Rolls has focused on the study of hunger and obesity for more than 20 years. Her research examines the control of food and fluid intake, especially in terms of how they relate to obesity, eating disorders and aging.

Q: What is Volumetrics?

BR: Volumetrics is an eating plan based on research about how to control hunger while managing calories to lose or maintain weight. Satiety has been the missing ingredient in weight management. If you limit calories by simply eating less, you'll feel hungry and deprived. Volumetrics shows you how to make the right food choices to control hunger, so you can lose weight, keep it off and stay healthy. Feeling full and satisfied while eating foods you like is a critical part of this plan.

Q: What led you to develop the Volumetrics plan?

BR: Over the years, I kept noticing that the weight of foods people consumed was more consistent than the calories they consumed. Once you understand that the amount of foods people eat over a day or two is consistent, you have to start thinking about the impact of the density of calories in those portions. I also realized that we had ignored the impact of water on food intake. We really did not understand back then the importance of water in determining how much people were eating.

Q: Why do fad diets so often fail?

BR: Many popular diets are based on what people might want to hear, rather than on what research shows. I don't think people like the idea that it all boils down to calories in and calories out. They're looking for a way to magically melt pounds away while they keep eating the same amounts. Most popular diets overplay the relatively small metabolic effects produced by changing the proportions of fat, carbohydrates and protein. The idea that you have to manage overall calories gets lost.

Q: So, calorie reduction is more important than altering macronutrient distributions?

BR: Absolutely. I don't mean to say that your food choices can't affect your success. With Volumetrics, we show people how to choose foods to control hunger and enhance satiety while managing calories. It's based on science. We've done a number of practical studies to show how to implement this advice. You can modify your diet to include your favorite foods while eating healthy, balanced meals for weight management.

Q: You talk a lot about energy or calorie density—just what do those terms mean?

BR: These terms are interchangeable, and they refer to the energy content in a given weight of food, which is expressed in kilocalories per gram. Water is the component of food that has the biggest impact on energy density, because it adds weight to food without increasing calories, thereby decreasing energy density. Fiber also reduces energy density, but its influence is small compared with water's because most foods have more water than fiber. Conversely, fat increases energy density (9 kilocalories per gram versus 4 kilocalories per gram for carbohydrates and protein). Most fruits and vegetables are low in energy density because of their high water and low fat content. Adding fruits and vegetables to the diet reduces overall

> Many popular diets are based on what people want to hear, rather than what research shows.

energy density and increases the amount of food that can be consumed for a given level of calories. Personally, I eat lots of fruits and vegetables. I love them. We need to figure out ways to get people eating more fruits and vegetables, and that is now a focus of my research.

Q: Does Volumetrics work for everyone?

BR: If someone is eating for emotional reasons, they need to resolve those issues. I refer such people to a counselor.

Q: Doesn't a diet have to reduce fat intake to help someone lose weight?

BR: Oh, no. I don't advocate a really low-fat diet, because if you don't like the food, you're not going to keep eating it. I recommend up to 30 percent fat in a diet, but I think people need to cut any fat that they don't need. In the end, if you learn how to make the right choices to lower the calorie density, you'll be reducing fat and increasing water content.

Q: How is water content in food related to weight management?

BR: Just drinking water doesn't help enhance satiety. You have to have the water in the food. We've done four studies where we had people drinking water either before or during a meal, and it hasn't had any effect on food intake. But when you incorporate the water into the food, that's when you feel full. In one study, we compared the effects on 24 women consuming a casserole with low water content, the casserole along with a glass of water, or a soup with high water content. Each meal had the same calories, fat, carbohydrates and protein contents. The results showed that when the subjects consumed the soup, they ate less later and also reported less hunger.

DIET TIP

Whenever possible, eat fruits or vegetables with the peel left on. Many nutrients, like fiber and potassium, are concentrated in or just under the skin. For example, a medium-sized apple with skin has almost twice as much fiber as a peeled one. A potato with skin has 50 percent more potassium than a peeled one does. Just make sure to wash produce thoroughly before eating.

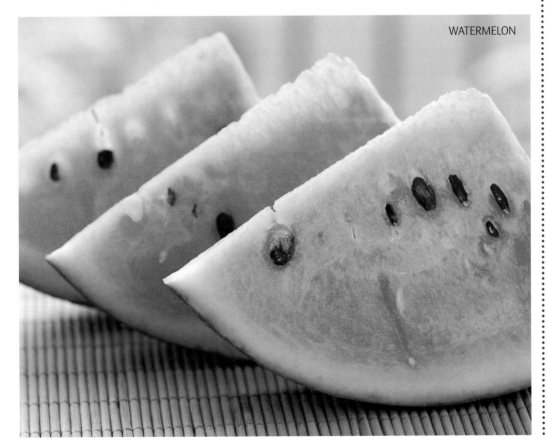

WATERMELON

EATING LOTS OF FRUITS AND VEGETABLES CAN HELP YOU FEEL FULLER LONGER AND PROVIDE ESSENTIAL NUTRIENTS.

Fad Diets Fail

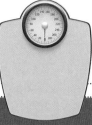

Crash diets and fad diets that emphasize one food over others can undermine your health, cause physical discomfort and thwart long-term weight-loss goals, according to the American Heart Association.

Diets that center on one or only a few specific foods disregard your need for a balanced diet made up of a variety of nutrient sources. If you restrict yourself to such an extreme diet for a few weeks, you're likely to develop nutrient deficiencies. Also, because these diets remove some of the pleasure from eating, it's nearly impossible to sustain them—and it's more tempting to overindulge in the aftermath.

The best way to lose weight includes maintaining a healthy diet with lots of fresh fruits and vegetables, whole grains, fish and nuts. Add regular exercise to the mix, and you'll be on the road to managing your weight.

DIET TIP
Since 1 pound of fat equates to 3,500 calories, you need to burn or cut an extra 500 calories per day to drop a pound per week. A 150-pound person can burn about 300 calories during an hour of brisk walking. This, plus filling up on low-cal, high-fiber fruit and vegetables, will help you reach your goal.

MYTH: Starvation-style diets are an effective way to lose weight.
FACT: Slow and steady weight loss is better in the long run.
While slashing calories before a wedding, reunion or other big event might sound like the fast track to weight loss, this strategy is likely to backfire. In fact, nutrition experts recommend that you don't dip below 1,200 to 1,500 calories per day. If you go on a crash diet for more than two weeks, your metabolism will temporarily slow down and your dieting efforts will result in less and less weight loss over time. The reason: Your body conserves energy to keep you from losing weight too quickly. And that's not all. When you drastically cut calories, you lose muscle along with fat—especially if you haven't been exercising. Because muscle is your body's calorie-burning furnace, this can slow down your metabolism, even long after your crash diet is done.

A better strategy is to aim to shed about a pound a week. Slow, steady weight loss ensures that you'll lose fat, not muscle. If you want to drop 10 pounds, get started 10 weeks before your goal, not four. You'll have a better chance of taking off the weight permanently. To drop a pound per week, shave 250 calories from your diet and burn an extra 250 calories through exercise each day.

MYTH: Healthy, all-natural foods can't make you fat.
FACT: Calories are calories, even when they come from healthy sources—so make portion control a priority.
People consistently underestimate the calories in nutritious foods such as yogurt, fish and baked chicken, according to researchers at Bowling Green State University who quizzed students on calorie counts. Just because a food is healthy doesn't mean you can eat big portions of it. For example, a handful of nuts can be 200 calories or more. And if you add that to your diet without cutting back elsewhere, it could be the reason you're gaining weight. So be vigilant about counting calories: Once you learn that half a cup of cereal can have as many as 200 calories or that there are about 220 calories in that single-serving bottle of orange juice, you'll be more prudent about how much you consume.

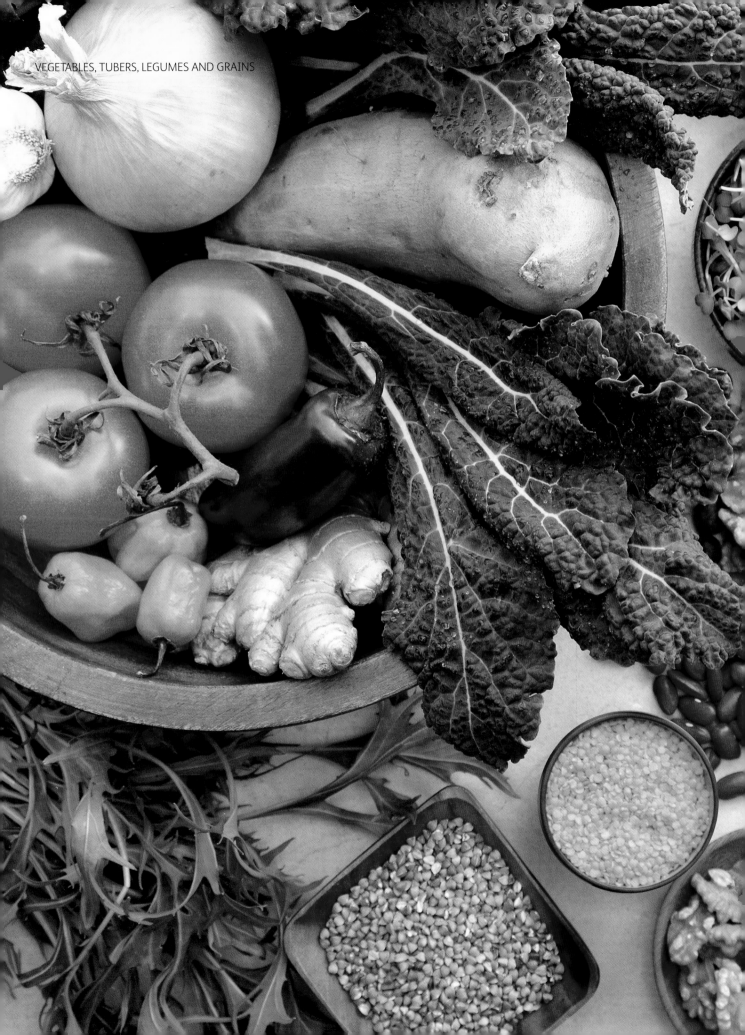

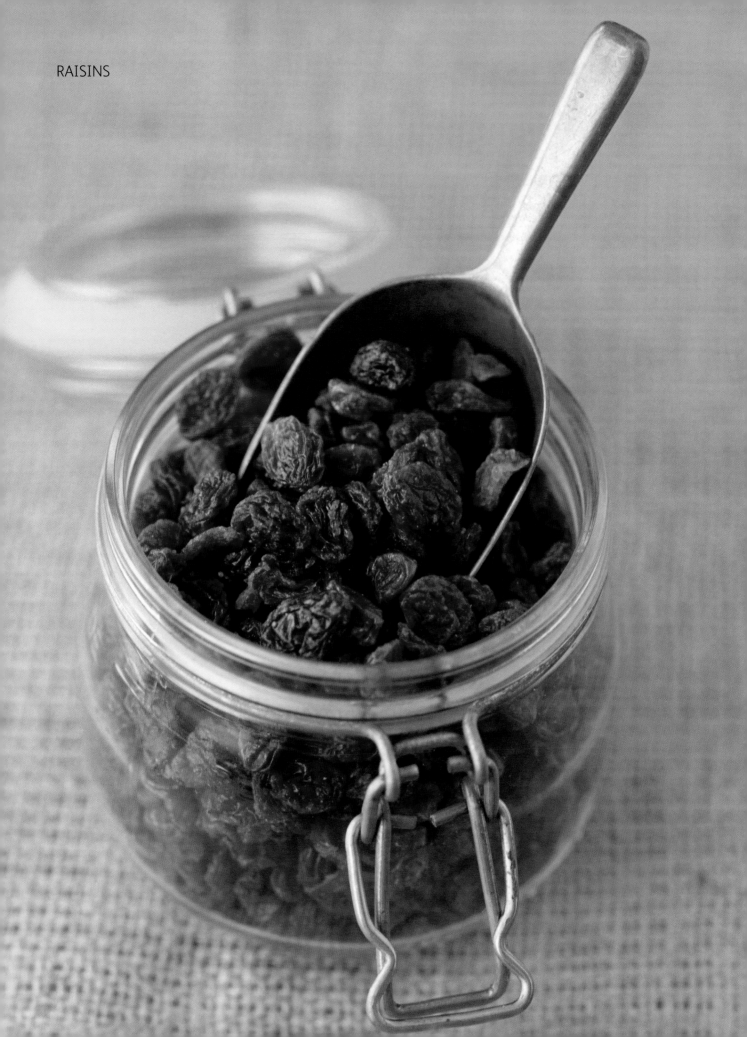

RAISINS

MYTH: Once you lose the weight, you can return to your old ways of eating.
FACT: Maintaining healthy eating habits after losing weight keeps you thin.
The National Weight Control Registry (NWCR) estimates that only 20 percent of dieters successfully keep off lost weight for more than a year. That's because after reaching a goal, many slide back into old eating habits. People who win at weight loss continue to eat intelligently even after they slim down. In fact, the NWCR found that people who maintain their healthy diet every single day are one-and-a-half times more likely to keep lost weight off in the long run than those who relax their diet on the weekend.

It helps to think of healthy eating as a work in progress, not as a "diet" with a beginning and an end. The key: Make small changes you can maintain so they become long-term habits. Start by creating a list of problem areas in your diet, and then tackle them one at a time. For example, if you snack on a handful of cookies every night before bed, substitute a bowl of fruit. Once you change that habit, pat yourself on the back and move on to your next goal.

MYTH: It's okay to splurge on low-fat and sugar-free foods.
FACT: People trick themselves into eating more of these foods than they should.
Research suggests that when a food is described as a diet food, we're subconsciously primed to eat more—even if it's actually as caloric as regular food. When Cornell University researchers offered the same M&M's candies labeled either regular or low-fat at a university open house, visitors ate 28 percent more of the low-fat snacks. While less fat does not necessarily mean fewer calories, people make the assumption that it does, which sets them up to overeat.

It's also important to check food labels, because so-called diet foods frequently don't actually save you calories. Smart low-fat snack alternatives include raisins, bananas and DOLE Fruit Cups.

Keep close tabs on portions, too. To downsize portions, use smaller plates, utensils and glasses. This simple trick will help you eat less. And note that portions tend to pile up when you're on the run. By taking the time to sit down and eat at a dinner table, you'll feel less inclined to eat more, according to a University of Toronto study. Mirrors in the dining area can help as well. And when you have to eat outside your home, immediately halve your entrée to take home for later.

Conclusion

The best way to keep from being fooled by diet and exercise falsehoods is to stay informed. Reliable sources, like the *Dole Nutrition News* (available at www.dole.com), are a good start. You might also try taking an inventory of your most cherished beliefs about what you eat and how much you exercise, and then do some research to test their validity. Once you're armed with nutrition facts and aware of dieting myths, you'll make better decisions and be primed to implement positive changes. Ask yourself: Do these beliefs help me maintain a healthy weight? Do they encourage me to be more fit? Or, have they become justifications for maintaining an unhealthy status quo? Being honest with yourself is a good first step toward a healthier life.

DIET TIP
Many restaurant side dishes can be calorie traps. Substitute steamed vegetables or salad in place of high-fat choices like French fries, mashed potatoes or creamed spinach. For example, replace an order of fries and ketchup (400 calories) with 2 cups of steamed broccoli seasoned with light soy sauce and pepper (only 100 calories).

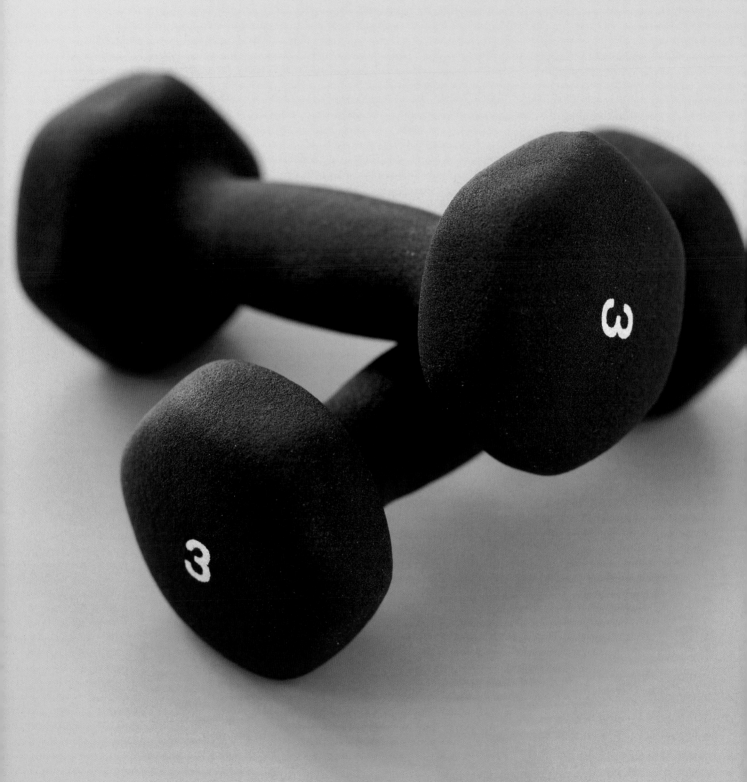

FREE WEIGHTS

CHAPTER 14

Exercise Your Health

Inactivity causes much of the fatigue, weakness, weight gain and other physical forms of decline usually blamed on aging. By engaging in regular exercise, you can maintain your stamina, strength, balance and flexibility throughout your life. It's never too late to reap the rewards of better health by starting an exercise plan today.

Exercise doesn't have to be a chore. Being active every day—doing something you enjoy that elevates your heart, gets your blood pumping and challenges your muscles—not only improves quality of life, but can also help you avoid injury or illness. Plus, exercising your way to better health helps you dodge medical expenses. Strive for a varied regimen that will yield the full range of fitness benefits.

FITNESS TIP
Women who do some vigorous physical activity most days of the week lower their risk of breast cancer, according to a study of 16,000 women in *Cancer Epidemiology, Biomarkers and Prevention*. These results applied only to women without a family history of the disease, but many studies have connected exercise to breast-health benefits.

Boost Activity, Live Longer, Age Better

By now, most folks know that good health requires regular exercise (even if they don't translate this knowledge into action).

Just to maintain your current weight, the Surgeon General recommends 30 minutes of moderate physical activity on most days of the week. This much exercise may also reduce your risk for some chronic diseases. To promote good health, bump that time up to 60 minutes of daily exercise, along with eating right and controlling calorie intake.

Often, when people think exercise, aerobic activities—such as walking, swimming or bicycling—come to mind. These types of exercise make you breathe hard and increase your heart rate, and any such activity will have benefits. But what may surprise you is that the more time you devote to exercise and the more intense your regular routine, the longer you are likely to live.

This connection between more intense exercise and longevity was revealed when researchers from Rush University examined the exercise stress tests of more than 5,000 women and found that those who couldn't exercise at higher levels were twice as likely to die of any cause during the eight-year study.

Fortunately, you can improve your exercise capacity. Exercise also builds strength and endurance over time, which means you'll feel fit and strong, even as you age. On the other hand, if you don't continue to regularly exercise, you'll lose fitness—at a rate that might startle you.

Beneficial exercise comes in many forms. You're probably familiar with aerobic-type exercises, including walking on treadmills, cycling or even dance class. This type of exercise is often called cardio training because it focuses on elevating your heart rate rather than on building muscles, such as your biceps or quads. Aerobic exercise helps burn calories and keep you trim.

However, one of the best ways to maintain and improve your fitness is through strength training, which entails using weights and working major muscle groups with resistance. The aim of strength training is to build muscles. The effects of such training can be weight loss and an improved physique. Neglect this type of exercise and you may be missing a great opportunity to feel stronger and younger, while warding off the effects of aging.

For example, one study found that women who skip weight lifting entirely will lose 5 pounds of muscle mass per decade—even if they regularly do cardio.

While most people gradually begin to lose muscle mass in their late 20s and early 30s, it doesn't become a potential health risk until they reach the age of 60. Strength training can guard against some of those health risks. For example, it can help lower blood pressure and ward off a host of ailments, including sarcopenia, a debilitating loss of muscle mass that can rob people of their mobility and affects an estimated 17 percent of people by the age of 75.

Lifting weights boosts muscle mass and strengthens bones—and gerontologists say it's never too late to start. Plus, seniors who start pumping iron are more likely to stay strong and independent.

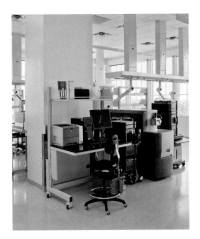

HIGH-TECH EQUIPMENT AT THE NORTH CAROLINA RESEARCH CAMPUS

▶ David C. Nieman

David Nieman, DrPH, FACSM, is a professor of health and exercise science, and director of the Human Performance Labs at Appalachian State University in Boone, North Carolina, and the North Carolina Research Campus in Kannapolis. Dr. Nieman has served two terms as president of the International Society of Exercise and Immunology and is currently vice president of the American College of Sports Medicine. He has run 58 marathons and ultramarathons, and was an acrobatic gymnast and coach for 10 years.

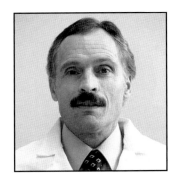

Q: Why is strength training important, and are there any groups of people it especially benefits?
DN: More than 600 muscles enable you to work out, play sports and accomplish your daily tasks. Your muscles are very responsive to use and disuse. Those muscles that are forcefully exercised become larger, a phenomenon called muscular hypertrophy. On the other hand, a muscle that is not used will atrophy or decrease in size and strength and become inflexible. According to government statistics, only one in five American adults performs physical activities that enhance and maintain strength and endurance two or more days per week.

Muscular fitness is more important for health than most people realize. Health benefits include increased bone density (which lowers the risk of osteoporosis or brittle bones in old age), muscle size, connective tissue strength and improved self-esteem.

You don't have to go to the weight room to improve muscular fitness.

DIET TIP

Weigh in to slim down. The National Weight Control Registry, the largest data bank of long-term losers—those who have successfully lost and kept off 30 pounds for at least a year—suggests that weight watchers who check the scale at least once a week have the best chance of maintaining their weight.

Muscle size and strength decrease by an average of 30 percent in adults between the ages of 30 and 70, often because of inactivity. This contributes to the weakness and frailty common in old age. According to other studies, elderly people who train with weights can recapture a good portion of their lost strength, enabling them to better perform the common daily activities of life. In fact, older adults have more to gain from building muscular fitness than any other age group.

There is little evidence to suggest that weight lifting reduces the risk for heart disease, cancer, diabetes, high blood pressure or high blood cholesterol. Also, training with weights does not increase aerobic fitness appreciably, primarily because the heart and lung system is not challenged sufficiently. For these reasons, make sure you have a "total fitness" program, with time and effort devoted to both resistance and aerobic training. Some activities, like rowing, for example, build up your chest, arms and legs while training your heart muscle.

Q: What are some other benefits of strength training?

DN: Low-back pain has been related to weak spinal and abdominal muscles and tight lower-back muscles. During certain types of lifting or exercise, weak trunk muscles may be unable to support the spine properly, leading to low-back pain. Intensive back-muscle exercise programs provide excellent therapy for low-back-pain sufferers, helping them reduce their pain and enabling them to return to work earlier than would otherwise be expected.

Individuals with osteoarthritis of the knee or hip joints have much to gain from weight training. Studies consistently show that strengthening the muscles around the joints reduces osteoarthritis symptoms, improves quality of life and enhances the capacity to accomplish the daily tasks of living.

Evidence supports the role of both weight training and aerobic exercise in improving insulin sensitivity, which means that blood-glucose levels stay under good control.

Q: How does strength training affect metabolism?

DN: Your metabolism, or specifically your resting metabolic rate (RMR), is the energy you expend each day to keep alive. Typically, the RMR is slightly less than 1 calorie per minute in women (or 1,200 to 1,500 calories per day), and somewhat more than 1 calorie per minute in men (or 1,600 to 1,900 calories per day). One calorie per minute equals the heat released by a burning candle or by a 75-watt lightbulb.

The RMR varies from one person to another, but nearly all of this is due to differences in body size, with the greatest RMR found in big people with high amounts of muscle and bone.

Weight lifting adds muscle, and every 4 to 5 pounds of muscle increases RMR by 28 to 50 calories a day. For weight training to have a large effect on muscle mass and RMR, more than one hour per day needs to be devoted to the weight room.

Q: What advice would you give someone who's looking to start a strength-training program?

DN: Muscular strength is the maximum one-effort force that you can generate against a resistance, while muscular endurance is the ability of the muscles to repeat a submaximal effort over and over. It takes muscular strength to bench-press a heavy weight once or twice before fatigue occurs, but it takes endurance to lift a lighter weight 15 to 20 times.

If you enjoy going to fitness clubs, I recommend a weight-training program. The minimum strength-training program is performing two to four sets of 8 to 12 repetitions of 8 to 10 exercises two to three times per week. Each repetition should be performed at 60 to 80 percent of the one repetition maximum (1RM, or the most you can lift just once). This is a basic program, however, and greater gains in muscular strength and power can be experienced using higher intensity (fewer repetitions with greater weight) with multiple sets—for example three sets of six reps to fatigue.

You don't have to go to the weight room, however, to improve muscular fitness. Muscle endurance and strength can also be developed through manual labor and calisthenics. Instead of heading to the weight room, simply do sit-ups, pull-ups, push-ups and leg squats. If you have the opportunity, cut, haul and split your own wood; lift hay bales; dig holes and ditches; and construct your own hiking trails. You'll build strength while doing some real work.

FITNESS TIP
Embrace weekly chores as an opportunity for increased physical activity. An hour of rigorous housework can burn well over 200 calories. Outdoor chores like raking leaves, stacking wood or washing the car all burn 150 to 300 calories in just 30 minutes.

Inactivity Ages You

While previous research has found that various kinds of exercise can slow aging by helping you maintain mental acuity, preserve aerobic capacity and ward off bone and muscle loss, research shows that regular activity actually helps rejuvenate your DNA. In a United Kingdom study of twins, the sibling who exercised least had DNA that measured 10 years older than the sibling who exercised about 45 minutes a day.

Vigorous aerobic exercise also naturally boosts human growth hormones, buffering the various, less-welcome consequences of age-related hormonal changes, such as thinning skin and expanding fat tissue.

Weights Whittle the Waist

Not only does strength training counteract the thinning of the bones in middle age, it can also help combat the thickening of the waist. All you need to do is hit the weights a couple of times a week.

Overweight women who began lifting weights twice weekly not only reduced overall body fat by nearly 4 percent, but they also significantly reduced the transfer of fat to their midsection, thus protecting themselves from the health risks associated with visceral fat deposited around their organs, according to University of Pennsylvania researcher Kathryn Schmitz, PhD, MPH.

The study divided 164 overweight and obese women, ages 24 to 44, into two groups. The first group attended twice-a-week strength training for four months, after which participants were told to continue lifting weights on their own. The second group received brochures recommending daily exercise. Participants of both groups were instructed to change their eating habits.

After two years, the strength trainers had not only continued with their weight-lifting regimen, but they had also reduced their overall body fat.

Why might this be? Perhaps because resistance work with weights beats cardiovascular exercise in terms of overall calorie expenditure. Even though weight training burns 8 to 10 calories versus cardio's 10 to 12 per minute, you continue to burn an additional 25 percent of the previous weight-lifting session's total well after you've tossed in the towel.

Plus, for every 3 pounds of muscle gained through weight training (a reasonable result for three months of weight lifting), you raise your resting metabolic rate by 120 calories per day.

Weight Training 101

You don't have to be preparing for a bodybuilding competition to pump iron. Beginning a strength-training program, whether it's with free weights or machines, is pretty easy.

At most gyms, trainers will help you get started. Plan on starting slowly, with two or three weight-training sessions each week. For the greatest calorie burn, aim for total-body workouts that target your arms, abdomen, legs and back, and go for moves that will incorporate several different muscle groups at a time—for example, squats, which call on muscles in both the front and back of your legs, as opposed to leg extensions, which isolate the quads.

For each exercise, try to do three sets of 10 to 12 repetitions with a weight heavy enough that by your last rep you can't eke out another one without compromising your form. To spark further muscle building, William Kraemer, PhD, a professor of kinesiology at the University of Connecticut, suggests alternating moderate-intensity workouts of 8 to 10 reps with lighter-weight 12 to 15 rep sets and superhard 3 to 5 rep sets.

FITNESS TIP

One difference between obese and lean women is how much they stand up. Compared with their lean counterparts, obese women tend to sit two-and-a-half hours more per day, states a study in the journal *Obesity*. That difference accounts for 315 fewer calories burned each day.

Go Longer for Heart Health

When you think about heart-friendly exercise, aerobic-type workouts like step classes and walking likely come to mind, and with good reason. Along with helping to strengthen your heart and burning lots of calories, aerobic exercise also helps lower your LDL (bad) cholesterol and increase the HDL (good) cholesterol. Such aerobic exercise can be done in short bursts of activity most days of the week to add up to the 30 minutes recommended by the Surgeon General.

Short bursts of exercise help your heart in many ways—keeping triglycerides, blood pressure and weight under control. But in a Japanese study, significant increases in HDL occurred only when exercise lasted longer than 30 minutes.

Amazingly, while frequency and intensity of physical activity did not impact HDL, every extra 10 minutes spent exercising yielded an increase in HDL. That's enough to reduce the risk for heart attack by roughly 3 percent, according to the analysis of 1,400 people of all ages, whose workout activities ranged from biking and brisk walking to swimming and skiing.

Stairway to a Longer Life

Take the stairs instead of the elevators and you'll dramatically increase your fitness levels. That's the conclusion of a Swiss study in which 69 university employees were banned from using elevators for three months at work. At the outset, this group could have been considered couch potatoes (with less than two hours of exercise a week). During the course of the experiment, they nearly quadrupled their use of stairs—to an average of 23 flights climbed and descended per day.

The result? A nearly 9 percent increase in aerobic capacity, which translates into a 15 percent drop in the chances of premature death. As the workers climbed up, their heart disease indicators crept down. Waist and fat mass shrunk nearly 2 percent, blood pressure dropped 2.3 percent and LDL decreased almost 4 percent. Impressive results, particularly as they were achieved so inexpensively.

It's easy to do something similar at your workplace. For example, the Dole Food Company posted plaques in their Westlake Village, California, headquarters encouraging employees to take the stairs. The signs are part of the Dole Nutrition Institute's award-winning Dole Employee Wellness program.

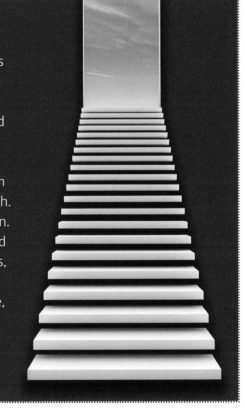

If longer exercise seems onerous, try mixing things up: One day, split exercise up into three or more 10-minute bursts; on other days, make exercise social—go hiking, surfing or even dancing with friends. Team sports, like soccer and volleyball, make longer workouts fun.

BALANCE EXERCISES CAN REDUCE THE RISK OF FALLS AND INJURIES.

Balance for Longevity

Falls are the leading cause of death due to injury among older adults in the United States, but balancing exercises can help prevent such mishaps and fend off disability as you age.

In 2005, 433,000 people age 65 and older were hospitalized for injuries related to unintentional falls, and 5,800 of those patients died from their injuries, according to the Centers for Disease Control and Prevention. The good news is that exercise can significantly improve your balance. Researchers at the University of Sydney in Australia found in a study of 9,603 participants that regular exercise can reduce the rate of falling by 17 percent.

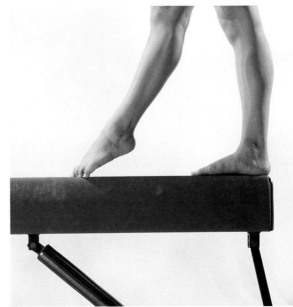

Four Exercises for Better Balance

Your balance can improve with some simple exercises. Add these four moves to your normal workout routine three days a week. Start by holding a chair or putting a hand to the wall for support and work up to balancing while exercising hands-free.

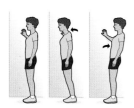

ROCK AND ROLL

Stand with your side to the wall within arm's reach. Your feet should be about hip-width apart. Without bending your knees, slowly shift your weight to your toes, leaning slightly forward as far as you can without tipping or letting your heels come off the floor. Then, shift your weight back to your heels, tilting backward without lifting your toes. Next, keeping your feet flat on the floor, sway to the left, and then to the right, as far as possible. For more of a challenge, bring your feet closer together, and then try this with your eyes closed.

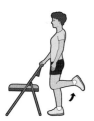

KICK YOUR BUTT

Stand straight, holding a table or chair for balance. Take three seconds to bend your left knee, bringing your calf as close to the back of your thigh as possible. Hold for a second or two, then slowly lower your leg over three seconds. Repeat with your right leg.

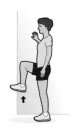

THE MARCH

Stand next to a wall for support and face sideways. Slowly (taking about 3 seconds) raise your right knee, bringing it as close to your chest as possible. Don't bend at the waist or hips. Hold for a second or two, then lower your leg, taking about three seconds. Repeat with your left leg.

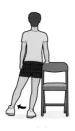

SCISSOR KICK

Stand straight, holding a table or chair for support. Slowly lift your left leg 6 to 12 inches to the side; do not bend your knee or upper body. Hold. Slowly lower, and repeat on your right side. Once you master this, hold the table with one hand—then with one finger, next with no hands, and finally with your eyes closed—to further improve your balance.

Five Stretches to Boost Flexibility

Add these moves to your postexercise routine, and you'll feel more supple in no time.

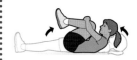

KNEE SQUEEZES (FOR UPPER-, MIDDLE- AND LOWER-BACK MUSCLES)

Lie on your back with your legs outstretched. Bend both knees and hold. Bring them toward your chest until you feel a stretch. Tuck your chin in, and slowly bring your head up to meet your knees. Stay relaxed. Hold for 20 to 30 seconds. Repeat four times.

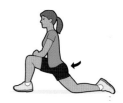

HIP FLEXOR STRETCHES (FOR MUSCLES IN THE FRONT OF HIPS AND THIGHS)

Begin by kneeling on the floor. Bring your right knee in front of you, and place your foot flat on the floor. Your left knee should be resting on the floor. Slowly lean forward to extend your left leg back, keeping your shin and knee on the floor. You should feel a stretch in the front of your right hip and thigh. Make sure your right knee isn't extending farther than your toes. (If it is, shift back until your knee is behind your toes.) Hold this stretch for 20 to 30 seconds; then switch sides. Repeat four times.

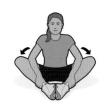

INNER THIGH AND GROIN STRETCHES (FOR INNER THIGHS AND GROIN)

Sit on the floor with your back straight. Place the heels of your feet together and drop your knees out to your sides. Clasp your hands around your ankles. Using your forearms, slowly press your knees toward the floor until you feel a stretch. Do not force your knees to the floor. Hold for 20 to 30 seconds. Repeat four times.

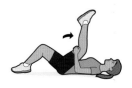

HAMSTRING STRETCHES (FOR BACKS OF THIGHS)

Lie on your back, keeping your lower back pressed against the floor. Bend both knees and keep your feet flat on the floor. Bring your hands to the back of your left thigh, and slowly straighten and raise your left leg. Gently pull your leg in toward your torso until you feel a stretch in the back of your leg. Hold for 20 to 30 seconds, then repeat with the other leg. Repeat four times with each leg. As this stretch becomes easier, keep the resting leg straight out in front of you, instead of bent, for more of a stretch.

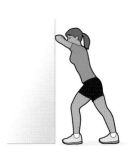

CALF STRETCHES (FOR BACKS AND SIDES OF CALVES AND THE ACHILLES TENDON)

Stand with your forearms against a wall and your right leg out in front of you with your knee slightly bent. Your knee shouldn't extend past your toes. Keep your left leg straight and your foot flat on the floor. Slowly lean forward on your right leg until you feel a stretch in the back of your calf. Hold for 20 to 30 seconds. This will stretch the upper part of your calf. Then slightly bend your left knee and repeat to stretch the lower part of your calf. Hold each stretch for 20 to 30 seconds; then switch sides. Repeat four times with each leg.

Fitness Breaks Boost Performance

Got a looming deadline? Take a break for fitness—and research says you'll increase your productivity.

It may sound risky to time-crunched professionals, but a study from the U.K.'s Leeds Metropolitan University and University of Bristol found that employees worked faster and more efficiently on days when they exercised during their lunch breaks. Researchers monitored more than 200 workers at three sites: a university, a life insurance firm and a computer company. Physical activity ranged in length from 30 to 60 minutes and in type from yoga to basketball.

Other research strengthens the link between exercise and productivity. Employees who exercised at least three days a week accomplish more and produce higher-quality work with less effort than their sedentary counterparts, according to a Minneapolis Center for Health Promotion survey of 683 workers. Lead researcher Nicolaas P. Pronk, PhD, suggests that fit workers have "greater endurance and are less likely to feel fatigue."

FITNESS TIP

No time for exercise? Try taking the stairs instead of the elevator, park on the perimeter of the lot when you go grocery shopping, meet friends for a hike rather than a meal or exercise while watching your favorite TV show.

Stretch *After* Exercise

Old ideas of stretching have been recently been turned upside down. Stretching before exercise might do more harm than good, according to a review of studies published in the *Clinical Journal of Sport Medicine* by Ian Shrier, MD, PhD. While cardio is a better way to warm up before a workout, stretching afterward is essential to maintaining flexibility. After exercise, muscles are more limber, and you'll have less chance of injury—so do your stretching postworkout.

Be Active, Stay Healthy

Upper respiratory infections are the most common illnesses in the world. The average person gets two to three such bouts a year. Dipping temperatures challenge immune function—and often the motivation to exercise as well. Researchers suspect that there's a causal relationship between reduced activity levels and immune system-related sickness.

This hypothesis is supported by research from professor David Nieman of Appalachian State University, whose study shows that regular, moderate exercise

Fitness Pays Off

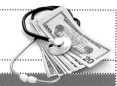

Want to pocket some extra cash? Get fit. Moderately to very physically active employees had on average $250 less in annual health care costs than their couch potato counterparts, according to a University of Michigan study. However, the savings were most profound among the obese, who cut $450 in annual health care costs when they exercised, adding up to an estimated 1.5 percent in health care savings for companies across the board.

boosts immunity. Thin, active, older women had T cells that functioned at a rate that was equal to women 40 years of age and 67 percent higher than other women. Another study found three times the number of colds among inactive, postmenopausal women, compared with those who walked for 45 minutes five days per week.

In addition to exercise, fortify your immune defenses by choosing superfoods like broccoli, spinach, cashews, guavas, plums and mangoes. These foods contain vitamins A and C, selenium, zinc and polyphenolic antioxidants—nutrients needed to maintain a healthy immune system. Other ways to optimize your immunity include getting vaccinations, washing your hands regularly, getting adequate sleep and meditating.

Reclaim Calcium

COLLARD GREENS

When you exercise hard enough to cause profuse perspiration, you lose calcium in addition to excess sodium through your sweat. And, it's best to rely on food sources over supplements to replenish calcium.

Although weight-bearing workouts fortify bones, women who exercised for an hour daily lost about 92 milligrams of calcium per day though sweat, a Purdue University study found. Most women are already short on this mineral, so even small losses increase their risk for osteoporosis. Eating leafy, green calcium-rich foods can offset this loss and further bolster bone strength.

Foods high in calcium that would be good to work into your diet include nonfat milk, collard greens and turnip greens.

Check Appetite with Exercise

If you truly want to curb your cravings, ditch the diet pills and hop on the treadmill. Contrary to the canard that says workouts make you eat more, a forthcoming Chilean study demonstrates that exercise actually suppresses appetite, naturally enabling you to eat 330 fewer calories a day.

Researchers had 15 overweight and obese men and women exercise (on a treadmill or bike) for 20 minutes, three days a week. After three months, the subjects had reduced caloric intake by an average of 16 percent, without even trying. The magic factor appears to be an exercise-induced 244 percent increase in a certain appetite-suppressing protein in the blood.

As a result of consuming fewer—and burning more—calories, all study participants enjoyed a dramatic drop in weight, blood pressure and body fat. Physical activity can help weight-loss efforts in other ways as well. Japanese researchers found that heavy exercise may dull your sweet tooth. Exercise builds muscle mass, which in turn increases your metabolic rate. Exercise plus diet appears to be the winning formula for weight loss: Study subjects who got active and ate less dropped 20 pounds, versus 15 pounds for those who only dieted.

FITNESS TIP

Forward march your way into a better mood. In one study by California State University, subjects were given pedometers and told to record both their moods and their mileage. Those who had the highest number of steps also had the highest energy levels.

Eat Yourself Back from Injury

Certain foods may be able to cut down your body's recovery time by providing the nutrient building blocks needed to repair stressed muscles or calm inflammation.

Here are some of the most common sports injuries, along with the mechanisms underlying the symptoms and suggested dietary recommendations to get you back in the game with minimal downtime.

For Bursitis, Tendonitis, Shin Splints

YOU NEED...	SO EAT...
Bromelain—reduces inflammation	Pineapples (Fresh or Frozen)
Omega-3 Fatty Acids—reduces inflammation	Wild Salmon, Walnuts, Flaxseeds
Vitamin C—linked to lower C-reactive protein levels	Red Bell Peppers, Kiwifruits, Oranges, Strawberries
Anthocyanins—reduces inflammation	Blueberries, Cherries, Blackberries

For a Pulled Hamstring

YOU NEED...	SO EAT...
Protein—relieves muscle soreness	Beans, Wild Salmon, Turkey Breast, Nuts
Potassium—necessary for building muscles	White Beans, Potatoes, Bananas
Vitamin E—reduces inflammation	Almonds, Sunflower Seeds, Pumpkin

For Muscle Cramps

YOU NEED...	SO EAT...
Water—maintains balance of electrolytes	Water, Fruits, Vegetables
Calcium—allows muscles to contract and relax	Nonfat Yogurt, Collard Greens, Sardines, Navy Beans
Magnesium—allows muscles to contract and relax	Oat Bran, Spinach, Artichokes, Soybeans
Potassium—allows muscles to contract and relax	White Beans, Potatoes, Bananas
Phosphorus—allows muscles to contract and relax	Lentils, Halibut, Salmon, Sunflower Seeds

For Bruising

YOU NEED...	SO EAT...
Bromelain—reduces swelling, speeds recovery	Pineapples
Vitamin K—helps with blood clotting	Collard Greens, Spinach, Broccoli
Vitamin C—spurs collagen synthesis	Red Bell Peppers, Kiwifruits, Oranges
Iron—helps oxygenate blood	Cooked Clams, Spinach, Green Peas
Protein—important for collagen formation	Beans, Wild Salmon
Copper—required for cross-linking collagen	Oysters, Shiitake Mushrooms, Cashews, Sunflower Seeds

For Cuts and Scrapes

YOU NEED…	SO EAT…
Vitamin A—fights infection	Sweet Potatoes, Butternut Squash, Carrots
Vitamin C—helps inactivate bacteria	Red Bell Peppers, Kiwifruits, Oranges
Manganese—required for collagen formation	Oats, Pineapples, Raspberries
Bromelain—digests dead cell matter	Pineapples (Fresh or Frozen)
Zinc—supports cell repair	Oysters, White Beans, Oats

For Sprains

YOU NEED…	SO EAT…
Vitamin C—spurs collagen synthesis	Red Bell Peppers, Kiwifruits, Oranges
Omega-3 Fatty Acids—reduces inflammation	Wild Salmon, Walnuts, Flaxseeds
Anthocyanins—reduces inflammation	Blueberries, Cherries, Blackberries
Bromelain—reduces swelling	Pineapples

For Fractures

YOU NEED…	SO EAT…
Calcium—required for bone formation	Nonfat Yogurt, Collard Greens, Sardines, Soybeans
Vitamin D—promotes calcium absorption	Oysters, DOLE Portobello Mushrooms, Sardines, Sunshine
Vitamin B12—linked to bone density	Clams, Oysters, Wild Salmon, Yellowfin Tuna
Potassium—reduces calcium excretion	White Beans, Potatoes, Bananas
Vitamin K—boosts mineral-binding capacity of bone proteins	Collard Greens, Spinach, Broccoli
Folate—counters homocysteine, linked to higher risk of fractures	Lentils/Beans, Spinach, Brussels Sprouts, Beets

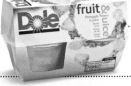

Grab Fruit for Sports Performance   DOLE FRUIT BOWLS

Don't throw away money on expensive sports gels—fruits such as raisins, bananas and figs deliver the same energy boost, and a much bigger nutritional bang, for a lot less money.

For example, when raisins were pitted against sports gels in a study in the *Journal of Strength and Conditioning Research*, the results proved that the fruit provides all the preworkout oomph you need.

An added bonus is that raisins provide what gels don't: vitamins, minerals and antioxidants, which all help minimize recovery time. The next time you're shopping, add these sports-friendly foods to your cart: **canned fruit, mandarin oranges, pineapples, mixed fruit, fruit bowls, dried fruit, dates, prunes and raisins.**

ALONG WITH BURNING
CALORIES, EXERCISE
HELPS SHED POUNDS
BY ACTIVATING
AN APPETITE-
SUPPRESSING PROTEIN.

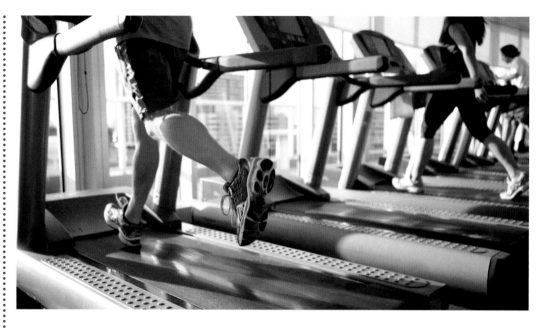

Workouts for Everyone

Starting an exercise program can be tough. First, it can be hard to tell if you're exercising long or hard enough to reap the healthy benefits. A good guideline: The Surgeon General recommends 30 minutes of exercise at least four days a week. But if your goal is to lose weight or to maintain your weight after already shedding some pounds, you should aim for 60 to 90 minutes a day.

An hour or more of exercise each day may sound like a lot, but here are three exercise plans that can help. The best part: You don't have to do your 60 minutes all at once. In fact, these workouts are designed to be 30 minutes or less to allow you to sneak them in during your day as you can. You can also combine the exercise plans with walking and everyday chores, such as raking leaves, to boost your minutes.

The following exercise plans are appropriate for various levels of fitness. If you haven't exercised in a while, begin with the walking plan, then move on to the others. If you already exercise, jump into the intermediate workouts for a new way to stay fit. As you build your fitness level, combine the workouts for even longer workouts and more variety; diversity, opposed to the intensity of a workout, can help preserve your brain health, according to researchers at Johns Hopkins University. Similar to the way exercise helps prevent heart disease, different workouts were found to protect the brain against the effects of dementia.

Quick Calorie Burn

Category: Interval training
Level: Intermediate to advanced
Time: 20 minutes
Frequency: Three times a week

Short bursts of vigorous activity can speed up weight loss and cut your workout time by up to half or more. This workout combines walking, marching and four easy-to-do exercises. Aside from a good pair of shoes, there's no additional equipment needed.

FITNESS TIP
During low-intensity portions of the Quick Calorie Burn workout, you should be able to easily carry on a conversation. When you kick into high gear, push yourself to the point that talking is nearly impossible.

JUMPING JACKS

Just like the ones you used to do in physical education class! Start with your feet together and arms at your sides. Jump your feet apart while raising your arms above the head. Go as fast as you can.

SPEED SKATER

Stand with your feet together, your arms at your sides. Jump to the right, leading with your right leg. Your left leg follows and crosses behind your right foot as you land. Simultaneously, reach your left arm across your body, as if trying to touch the floor. Repeat to the left. Jump side to side as quickly as possible.

HIGH KNEES

Run in place as fast as you can, lifting your knees out in front of you as high as possible. Swing your arms at your sides.

TWIST

Stand with your feet a few inches apart. Hop and rotate your knees to the right, as your arms go to the left, landing with your knees bent. Repeat, twisting in the opposite direction.

QUICK CALORIE BURN

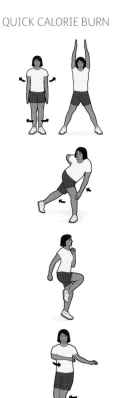

MINUTE BY MINUTE

At This Time...	Do This
0:00	Warm up by walking around or marching in place
2:00	Jumping Jacks
2:12	March in place
2:30	Speed Skater
2:42	March in place
3:00	High Knees
3:12	March in place
3:30	Twist
3:42	March in place
4:00	Repeat above intervals 7 more times in the order listed (minus the warm-up)
18:00	Cool down by walking or marching in place
20:00	Finish

FITNESS TIP

For First Steps Forward, choose softer surfaces; a smooth dirt trail or packed sand is your best bet. Squeeze your glutes with every step to reduce bouncing and jarring. And don't focus on speed yet—keep a comfortable pace throughout these workouts.

First Steps Forward

Category: Walking plan

Level: Beginner

Time: 10 minutes, twice a day; builds up to a 90-minute walk

This simple plan creates a baseline of fitness that's a good start for someone who hasn't exercised in a while and doesn't want to worry about equipment. By using mini-sessions to build up gradually, you'll burn more calories as you progress, while keeping the joints pain-free.

THREE-WEEK PLAN

Week 1: Walk for 10 minutes, twice a day, five times a week

Week 2: Walk for 15 minutes, twice a day, five times a week

Week 3: Keep on building. Increase the duration of your walks to 20 minutes, twice daily, five times a week.

Go a little faster. After three minutes of easy walking, pick it up to a brisk pace (as though you're late for an appointment) for as long as possible.

Inch up your endurance. Once a week, do one longer walk, adding five minutes each time, until you reach 60 to 90 minutes.

FITNESS TIP

To avoid injury in the Circuit of Fitness, allow at least three seconds to lift and three seconds to lower the weight for each repetition. Rest for no more than 15 seconds between exercises. It helps to have a clock with a second hand or a timer nearby. To keep the workout fresh and interesting, change the set order.

Circuit of Fitness

Category: Strength and circuit training

Level: Intermediate to advanced

Time: 30 minutes

This circuit-training routine includes a series of strength-training exercises that you perform back-to-back with little rest in between. Like traditional strength training, this type of circuit training builds muscle, which helps you burn more calories when you're not exercising. In addition, circuit training gives you a cardio workout. Because you move quickly from one exercise to the next, your heart rate stays up, and you burn more calories while you're lifting weights. The exercises are bunched into groups of three followed by a yoga stretch. These easy moves stretch your muscles, while also helping to further increase your strength.

Equipment: Exercise ball; yoga mat; sturdy chair; aerobic step (a stair step will work, too); dumbbells (should be heavy enough that the effort feels tough in the final 10 to 15 seconds of the exercise)

Frequency: Do the circuit exercises three times a week; build up to going through the circuit routine twice, which should take about an hour.

Repetitions: Perform each exercise for 60 seconds, unless otherwise noted.

WARM-UP

Five minutes of walking or, if you have a stationary bike, cycling.

Set 1

TWISTING CRUNCH ON A BALL

Sit on an exercise ball with your feet shoulder-width apart on the floor. Place your fingertips lightly behind your head. Lean back (the ball will roll slightly forward), so your rear and the small of your back are pressing against the ball. Using your abs, lift your shoulders up and forward, twisting your right shoulder toward your left side as you lift. Pause, then lower. Repeat, alternating sides.

DUMBBELL SQUAT

Stand with your back to a chair and your feet about shoulder-width apart. Hold the dumbbells at your shoulders, palms facing inward. Keeping your back straight, bend at the knees and hips as though you are sitting down. Don't let your knees move forward beyond your toes. Stop just shy of touching the chair; then stand back up.

CHEST PRESS

Lying on the floor (or a bench), hold the dumbbells end to end, just above chest height; your elbows should be pointing out. Press the dumbbells straight up, extending your arms. Hold; then lower.

STRETCH, COBRA

Lie facedown with your feet together, your toes pointed and your hands on the floor, with your palms down just in front of your shoulders. Pressing your hands into the floor, gently extend your arms, lifting your upper body off the floor as far as comfortably possible. If you feel any strain in your back, alter the pose so that you keep your elbows bent and your forearms on the floor. Hold for 15 seconds.

Set 2

REVERSE CURL

Lie with your arms at your sides, palms down. Bend your hips and knees, so that your legs are over your midsection and relaxed. Slowly contract your abdominal muscles, lifting your hips 2 to 4 inches off the floor. Hold, then slowly lower.

BICEPS CURL

Stand with your feet shoulder-width apart, holding dumbbells at your sides. Bending your elbows and turning your wrists upward, lift the dumbbells toward your shoulders. Don't move your upper arms. Stop when the dumbbells are at chest height, palms facing your body. Pause, then lower.

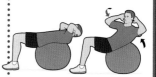
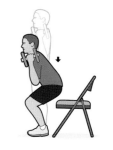
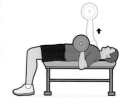
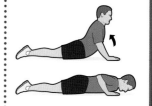
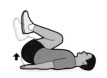
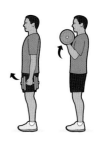

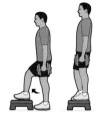

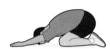

STEP UP

Stand facing an aerobic step or stair, holding dumbbells at your sides. Place your right foot on the step and lift yourself up. Tap your left foot on the top of the step, slowly lower your left foot to the floor and then step off with your right foot. Alternate feet.

STRETCH, PRAISE POSE

Kneel with your toes pointed behind you. Sit back onto your heels, and lower your chest to your thighs. Stretch your arms overhead, and rest your palms and forehead on the floor (or as close as comfortable). Hold for 15 seconds.

Set 3

CHEST LIFT

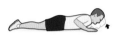

Lie facedown on the floor with your hands under your chin. Lift your head, chest and arms about 5 to 6 inches off the floor. Hold; then lower.

LUNGE

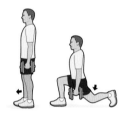

Standing with your feet together, hold dumbbells down at your sides, your palms facing inward. Take one big step forward with your left leg. Plant your left foot, then slowly lower your right knee toward the floor. Your left knee should be at a 90-degree angle, and your back should be straight. Press into your left foot, and push yourself back to the starting position. Repeat, alternating legs.

DIP

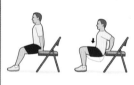

Sit on the edge of a sturdy chair, your hands grasping the seat on either side of your rear. Walk your feet out slightly, and inch your butt off the chair. Keeping your shoulders down and your back straight, bend your elbows back, and lower your butt toward the floor as far as comfortably possible. Slowly push back up.

STRETCH, DOWNWARD DOG

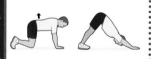

Position yourself on the floor on your hands and knees, with your feet flexed. Press your hands and feet into the floor, raising your hips toward the ceiling. Your body should look like an upside-down V. Keep lifting your tailbone toward the ceiling as you lower your heels to the floor. Hold for 15 seconds.

Set 4

CALF RAISE

Stand with your feet about hip-width apart, holding dumbbells at your sides. Slowly rise up onto your toes, keeping your torso and legs straight. Hold; then lower.

BACK FLY

Sit in a chair with your feet flat on the floor, about hip-width apart. Hold a dumbbell in each hand, so the weights are about chest level and about 12 inches from your body. Your palms should be facing each other with your elbows slightly bent, as if you were holding a beach ball. Bend forward from the hips about 3 to 5 inches. Keeping your back straight, squeeze your shoulder blades together, and pull your elbows back as far as comfortably possible. Pause; then return to start.

OVERHEAD PRESS

Sit in a chair with your feet flat on the floor. Hold dumbbells up at shoulder height, with your palms facing your ears. Press the dumbbells straight overhead, without locking your elbows. Hold; then lower.

STRETCH, WARRIOR

Stand with your feet hip-width apart. Take a step forward with your right foot, bending that knee. (Your knee shouldn't jut out over your toes.) Turn your left foot to the side, so your left arch faces the heel of your right foot. Raise your arms over your head, with your palms facing each other, and lift your chin slightly. Hold for 15 seconds; switch sides.

COOLDOWN

Five minutes of easy activity, such as walking or stationary cycling.

CIRCUIT OF FITNESS

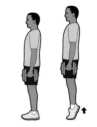
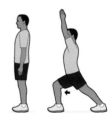
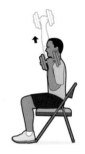
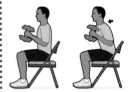

Sweat to Improve Your Mood

Your brain isn't a muscle. But like your quads and biceps, your mental state can be boosted by exercise. Working out may even make you happier. In a Pennsylvania State University and Harvard study of 16,000 men and women, those who rated themselves happiest also happened to be the most fit.

Regular exercise has been shown to be an effective stress reliever, and in another Harvard study, a 12-week strength-training program relieved the symptoms of clinical depression. The feel-good sensations from exercise may come from boosting the body's natural levels of anandamide.

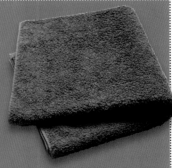

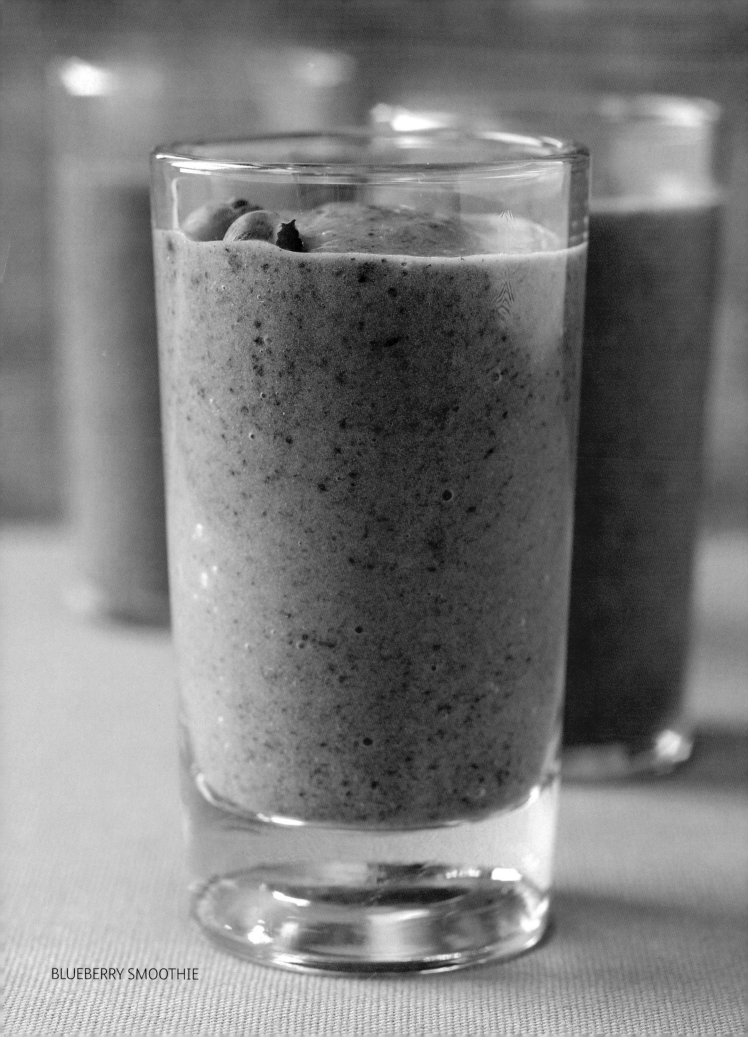

BLUEBERRY SMOOTHIE

CHAPTER 15

The Dole Diet:
A New Path to Weight Loss

It's common knowledge by now that consuming too many calories leads to weight gain and ultimately to obesity. As mentioned in previous chapters, researchers are finding increasing evidence that taking in too few nutrients also plays a role.

Consider some facts:

- Two-thirds of Americans are overweight or obese.

- One-third of the calories in our diet comes from junk food, alcohol and soda.

- Most Americans are deficient in potassium, fiber, magnesium and vitamins A and E.

- 60 percent of Americans don't get five servings of fruit and vegetables per day, let alone the 9 to 13 servings recommended by the USDA.

As Bruce Ames, PhD, director of the Nutrition and Metabolism Center at Children's Hospital, Oakland Research Institute, has observed: "If you sit down to a meal that doesn't give your body the nutrients it needs, your brain is likely to get the signal to go on eating until you get them." His theory inspired the development of the Dole Diet, which supports weight loss by providing 100 percent of your nutrient needs. (To see a day-by-day nutrient breakdown, check out page 342.)

In fact, the Dole Diet provides meal plans and recipes that can help you meet—and exceed—the high standards of the USDA Dietary Guidelines, while also losing weight. For example, the Dole Diet includes an average of 13 fruit and vegetable servings per day, while government guidelines recommend 9 to 13, depending on your weight range and target number of daily calories. While the guidelines recommend reducing saturated fat intake to less than 10 percent of total calories, the Dole Diet takes it down to 4 percent. Moreover, by reducing refined carbohydrates, the Dole Diet becomes a relatively low-carb plan, with 49 percent of calories coming from carbohydrates (compared with the government recommendation of 45 to 65 percent).

Government guidelines are based on 2,000 calories per day, but the Dole Diet averages about 1,600 calories per day—which puts most people on a fast and sustainable track for significant weight loss. If you have previously been consuming 2,000 calories a day, you could lose as much as 6 pounds over the course of the two-week Dole Diet. If you continue it over the course of two months, you will lose 24 pounds—and you'll be getting all the nutrients you need to promote health and feel satisfied.

USDA Dietary Guidelines for Americans 2005

Dietary Guidelines for Americans is published every five years by the U.S. Department of Health and Human Services (HHS) and the U.S. Department of Agriculture (USDA). The next update is slated for 2010.

	USDA	Dole Diet
Average calories per day	**2,000**	**1,600**
Calories from total fat	20–35%	31%
Calories from saturated fat	<10%	4%
Calories from carbohydrates	45–65%	49%
Fruit servings (½ cup) per day	4	6.2
Vegetable servings (½ cup) per day	5	6.4

Keep in mind that 2,000 calories is the target energy intake for the average normal-weight person. Larger, more athletic people need more calories, and smaller, less active folks need fewer calories. While this plan will lead to weight loss for most overweight people, the morbidly obese should seek medical advice.

Regardless of your weight, by following this diet, you will not only improve your health, you'll also stop starving your body of nutrients—and therefore, feel more satisfied. Paulette Lambert, RD, of the California Health and Longevity Institute, calls the Dole Diet, "an innovative approach in nutrition, focused on getting optimal nutrition from real, whole foods." Because each recipe has been selected to contribute to a two-week plan of well-balanced total nutrition, it's important not to make substitutions or take supplements while on the Dole Diet.

Week 1, Day 1: Monday 14 servings of fruits and vegetables

Breakfast	Snack	Lunch	Snack	Dinner
Blueberry Smoothie	DOLE Watermelon (1¼ cups, chunks)	Curried Apple and Butternut Squash Soup, plus salmon (6 oz)	Almonds (½ cup)	Caribbean Beans and Rice, plus DOLE Portobello Mushrooms (1 cup), added to recipe

Week 1, Day 2: Tuesday 15 servings of fruits and vegetables

Breakfast	Snack	Lunch	Snack	Dinner
Whole-grain cereal (¾ cup) with nonfat milk (1 cup), plus orange juice (1 cup)	DOLE Banana (1¼ cups, chunks)	Pineapple Gazpacho, plus Southwest Caesar Salad (6 oz)	DOLE Fruit Bowls (4 oz container)	Oysters Sautéed in Asian Sauce, plus wild rice (½ cup) and shiitake mushrooms (1 cup) added to recipe

Week 1, Day 3: Wednesday 14 servings of fruits and vegetables

Breakfast	Snack	Lunch	Snack	Dinner
Veggie Egg-White Omelet, plus a whole-grain English muffin	DOLE Apple	Broccoli and Pea Potage with Tarragon, plus Baby Spinach with Tender Reds (6 oz)	Almonds (½ cup)	Turkish Chicken with Spiced Dates, plus grilled DOLE Carrots (½ cup) and beets (½ cup) added to recipe

Week 1, Day 4: Thursday 12 servings of fruits and vegetables

Breakfast	Snack	Lunch	Snack	Dinner
Whole-grain cereal (¾ cup) with nonfat milk (1 cup), plus orange juice (1 cup)	DOLE Banana	Mixed Berry Gazpacho, plus Quinoa Salad	DOLE Fruit Bowls (4 oz container)	Yellowfin Tuna (6 oz), plus wild rice (½ cup) and wilted kale (1 cup)

Week 1, Day 5: Friday 16 servings of fruits and vegetables

Breakfast	Snack	Lunch	Snack	Dinner
Papaya Ginger Smoothie	DOLE Pineapple (¾ cup)	Roasted Red Pepper and Crab Chowder, plus Asian-Style Wilted Kale	DOLE Baby Carrots (8 carrots)	Portobello Turkey Loaf, plus DOLE Asparagus (½ cup) and roasted DOLE Sweet Potatoes (½ cup)

Week 1, Day 6: Saturday 12 servings of fruits and vegetables

Breakfast	Snack	Lunch	Snack	Dinner
Whole-grain cereal (¾ cup) with nonfat milk (1 cup), plus orange juice (1 cup)	DOLE Orange	Tuscan White Bean Soup, plus DOLE Italian Salad (3 oz)	Almonds (½ cup)	Pineapple Gazpacho, plus halibut (3 oz)

Week 1, Day 7: Sunday 9 servings of fruits and vegetables

Breakfast	Snack	Lunch	Snack	Dinner
Banana Almond Pancakes	DOLE Fruit Bowls (4 oz container)	Almond Turkey Salad with Cranberry Vinaigrette	DOLE Banana	Sweet Potato and Spinach Soup, plus salmon (6 oz)

Week 2, Day 1: Monday 11 servings of fruits and vegetables

Breakfast	Snack	Lunch	Snack	Dinner
Whole-grain cereal (¾ cup) with nonfat milk (1 cup), plus orange juice (1 cup)	Raspberries, blackberries or strawberries (1 cup)	Chicken Apple Almond Salad	DOLE Banana	Sesame Ginger Frittata with Broccoli and Shrimp

Week 2, Day 2: Tuesday 9 servings of fruits and vegetables

Breakfast	Snack	Lunch	Snack	Dinner
Porridge with Fruit, plus orange juice (1 cup)	Sweet potato sticks (1 cup)	Turkey, Avocado and Cheese Wrap	Peanuts (½ cup)	Chili non Carne, plus wild rice (3 oz)

Week 2, Day 3: Wednesday 14 servings of fruits and vegetables

Breakfast	Snack	Lunch	Snack	Dinner
Raspberry Smoothie	DOLE Mixed Berries (1 cup)	Roasted Red Pepper and Crab Chowder, plus Springtime Spinach Salad	Almonds (½ cup)	Curried Apple and Butternut Squash Soup, plus salmon (6 oz)

Week 2, Day 4: Thursday 8 servings of fruits and vegetables

Breakfast	Snack	Lunch	Snack	Dinner
Whole-grain cereal (¾ cup) with nonfat milk (1 cup), plus orange juice (1 cup)	DOLE Prunes (5)	Chili non Carne, plus wild rice (3 oz)	Kiwifruit with strawberries (½ cup)	Skillet-Blackened Salmon with Carrot Relish, plus wild rice (½ cup)

Week 2, Day 5: Friday 10 servings of fruits and vegetables

Breakfast	Snack	Lunch	Snack	Dinner
Porridge with Fruit, plus orange juice (1 cup)	Tangerine	Roasted Fennel Spinach Salad with Chicken	Almonds (½ cup)	Sweet Potato and Spinach Soup, plus halibut (6 oz)

Week 2, Day 6: Saturday 16 servings of fruits and vegetables

Breakfast	Snack	Lunch	Snack	Dinner
Denver Breakfast Sandwich, plus orange juice (1 cup)	DOLE Banana	Broccoli and Pea Potage with Tarragon, plus Apple and Walnut Salad	DOLE Orange	Bay Scallops with Green Beans

Week 2, Day 7: Sunday 17 servings of fruits and vegetables

Breakfast	Snack	Lunch	Snack	Dinner
Whole-grain cereal (¾ cup) with nonfat milk (1 cup), plus orange juice (1 cup)	DOLE Apple	Mixed Berry Gazpacho, plus DOLE European Blend Salad (3 oz)	Almonds (½ cup)	Wild Salmon and Bean Stew, plus DOLE Field Greens Salad (3 oz)

Eat More, Gain Less

Clinical studies have shown time and again that cutting calories is the key to losing weight. Yet the big question remains: When you reduce your caloric intake, how do you keep from being hungry all the time? By eating a lot, for one thing. It's simply a matter of choosing what you eat a lot of, wisely. Barbara J. Rolls, PhD, author of *The Volumetrics Weight-Control Plan,* has developed an approach that, just like the Dole Diet, emphasizes choosing more high-volume, high-fiber and high-water-content foods—such as fruits and vegetables—and fewer energy-dense foods that pack lots of calories into small portions—like butter, sugar and junk food.

Volumetrics grew out of research that found that healthy adults tend to eat the same volume of food each day. Dr. Rolls speculated that if that quantity was composed of fruits and vegetables, people would automatically reduce calories and curb cravings. Plus, they would take in more nutrients and lower disease risk.

Dr. Rolls has since investigated the weight-loss effects of unrestricted access to fruits and vegetables in several clinical trials. In one, researchers recruited 100 obese women, telling half of them to limit their fat intake and the other half to limit their fat intake but eat an unlimited amount of fruits and vegetables. After a year, the produce-unlimited women had lost 21 percent more weight (an average of 17 pounds versus 14 pounds) than the low-fat-only group. The fruit-and-veggie group actually consumed fewer calories—even though they were eating 25 percent more food by weight. By relying on fruits and vegetables—"heavy" because of water content, but "light" in terms of calories—the dieters naturally felt fuller, and they cut back on other more fattening foods.

This approach has shown promise in long-term weight loss, too. A six-year study found that women eating a Volumetrics-style, low-energy density diet reported significantly lower total calorie intakes; consumption of fewer servings of baked desserts, refined grains and fried vegetables; and more servings of vegetables, fruits and cereals. They also ate more meals at the table and fewer meals in front of the television. And, overall, the Volumetrics eaters reported less weight gain and lower body weight over time.

DOLE DIET TIP
Bone-helper vitamin D is another nutrient that's nearly impossible to get from whole foods alone. While many vitamin D sources are included in the Dole Diet, it is also recommended to enjoy an occasional meal in the sun to allow your skin to produce adequate amounts of vitamin D.

Blueberry Smoothie

Prep: 5 min. **Serves:** 3

1   *med. DOLE Banana*
1   *cup DOLE Frozen Tropical Gold Pineapple Chunks, partially thawed*
1   *cup DOLE Frozen Blueberries, partially thawed*
2   *containers (8 oz each) nonfat blueberry yogurt*
½   *cup (2 oz) soy protein or whey powder*

Combine banana, pineapple, blueberries, yogurt and soy protein in blender or food processor. Cover; blend until smooth.

Serving size (343g). Amount Per Serving: Calories 280, Calories from Fat 10, Total Fat 1g (2% DV), Saturated Fat 0g (0% DV), Trans Fat 0g, Cholesterol 5mg (2% DV), Sodium 270mg (11% DV), Potassium 480mg (14% DV), Total Carbohydrate 49g (16% DV), Dietary Fiber 4g (16% DV), Sugars 36g, Protein 21g, Vitamin A (2% DV), Vitamin C (20% DV), Calcium (30% DV), Iron (20% DV), Vitamin K (10% DV), Thiamin (10% DV), Riboflavin (15% DV), Vitamin B6 (15% DV), Folate (15% DV), Phosphorus (30% DV), Magnesium (10% DV), Copper (20% DV), Manganese (70% DV). Percent Daily Values (DV) are based on a 2,000 calorie diet.

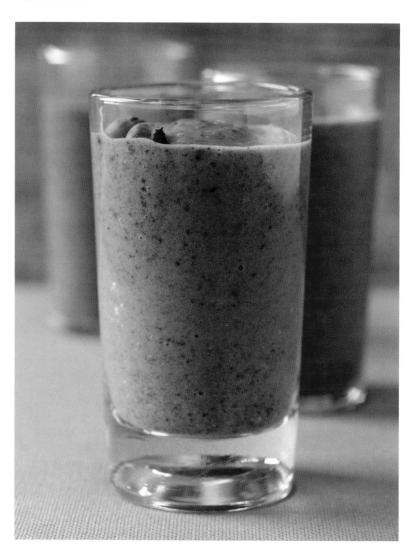

Curried Apple and Butternut Squash Soup

Prep: 20 min. **Cook:** 25 min. **Serves: 4**

1½   cups chopped DOLE Onions
⅓   cup chopped DOLE Carrots
⅓   cup chopped DOLE Celery
1   Tbsp almond oil
2½   cups peeled 1" pieces butternut squash
1   DOLE Apple, cored and diced, divided
1   Tbsp chopped DOLE Cilantro
1½   tsp curry powder
3   cups vegetable broth
¾   cup nonfat plain yogurt
¾   cup diced extra-firm tofu

Sauté onions, carrots and celery in oil in large stockpot over medium-high heat, stirring frequently, about 5 minutes.

Add squash, three-quarters of the apple, cilantro and curry powder. Cook 5 to 8 minutes; add broth and bring to a boil. Simmer an additional 10 minutes or until vegetables are tender. Cool slightly.

Place soup in batches in blender or food processor. Cover; blend until smooth. Return to stockpot.

Stir yogurt into the soup until blended. Add tofu and remaining apple; heat through.

Serving Size (509g). Amount Per Serving: Calories 210, Calories from Fat 60, Total Fat 6g (9% DV), Saturated Fat 0.5g (3% DV), Trans Fat 0g, Cholesterol 0mg (0% DV), Sodium 410mg (17% DV), Potassium 610mg (17% DV), Total Carbohydrate 34g (11% DV), Dietary Fiber 6g (24% DV), Sugars 17g, Protein 9g, Vitamin A (240% DV), Vitamin C (35% DV), Calcium (35% DV), Iron (20% DV), Vitamin E (15% DV), Vitamin K (15% DV), Thiamin (10% DV), Vitamin B6 (15% DV), Folate (15%), Phosphorus (10% DV), Magnesium (15% DV), Copper (10% DV), Manganese (30% DV), Molybdenum (10% DV). Percent Daily Values (DV) are based on a 2,000 calorie diet.

DOLE DIET TIP
To prepare fish, just broil or grill it, using cooking spray only, over medium heat 10 to 15 minutes, or until fish flakes easily with fork. Season with lemon pepper if desired.

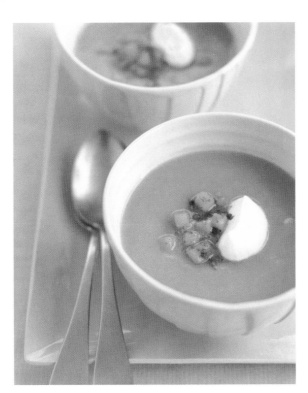

CURRIED APPLE AND BUTTERNUT SQUASH SOUP

FOOD PREP TIP

When you're making the wild rice for this recipe, or to serve as a side dish with other meals, follow the package directions but use water, not broth.

FOOD PREP TIP

To prepare the portobello mushrooms to serve with this meal or others, brush lightly with olive oil and fresh herbs of your choice. Broil or grill over medium heat 10 to 15 minutes, or until tender and lightly browned.

Caribbean Beans and Rice

Prep: 20 min. **Cook:** 20 min. **Serves:** 4

2	Tbsp almond or olive oil
1	med. DOLE Onion, chopped (1 cup)
1	cup sliced red bell pepper
1	cup sliced yellow bell pepper
3	cloves garlic, minced
2–3	tsp Cajun Creole or Jamaican Jerk Seasoning
½	tsp dried oregano, crushed
2	cans (15 oz each) black beans, rinsed and drained
1	cup vegetable broth
1	Tbsp lime juice
½	tsp salt
2	cups cooked wild or white rice

Heat oil over medium-high heat in large skillet.

Cook onion, bell peppers, garlic, seasoning and oregano until tender, about 8 minutes.

Add beans, broth, lime juice and salt. Bring to a boil; reduce heat and simmer, covered, 5 to 10 minutes.

Serve beans with rice.

Serving size (490g). Amount Per Serving: Calories 500, Calories from Fat 80, Total Fat 9g (14% DV), Saturated Fat 1g (5% DV), Trans Fat 0g, Cholesterol 0mg (0% DV), Sodium 560mg (23% DV), Potassium 1,030mg (29% DV), Total Carbohydrate 85g (28% DV), Dietary Fiber 22g (88% DV), Sugars 5g, Protein 23g, Vitamin A (20% DV), Vitamin C (170% DV), Calcium (10% DV), Iron (30% DV), Vitamin E (20% DV), Thiamin (45% DV), Riboflavin (10% DV), Niacin (15% DV), Vitamin B6 (30% DV), Folate (90% DV), Pantothenic Acid (10% DV), Phosphorus (40% DV), Magnesium (50% DV), Zinc (20% DV), Selenium (20% DV), Copper (30% DV), Manganese (110% DV), Molybdenum (220% DV). Percent Daily Values (DV) are based on a 2,000 calorie diet.

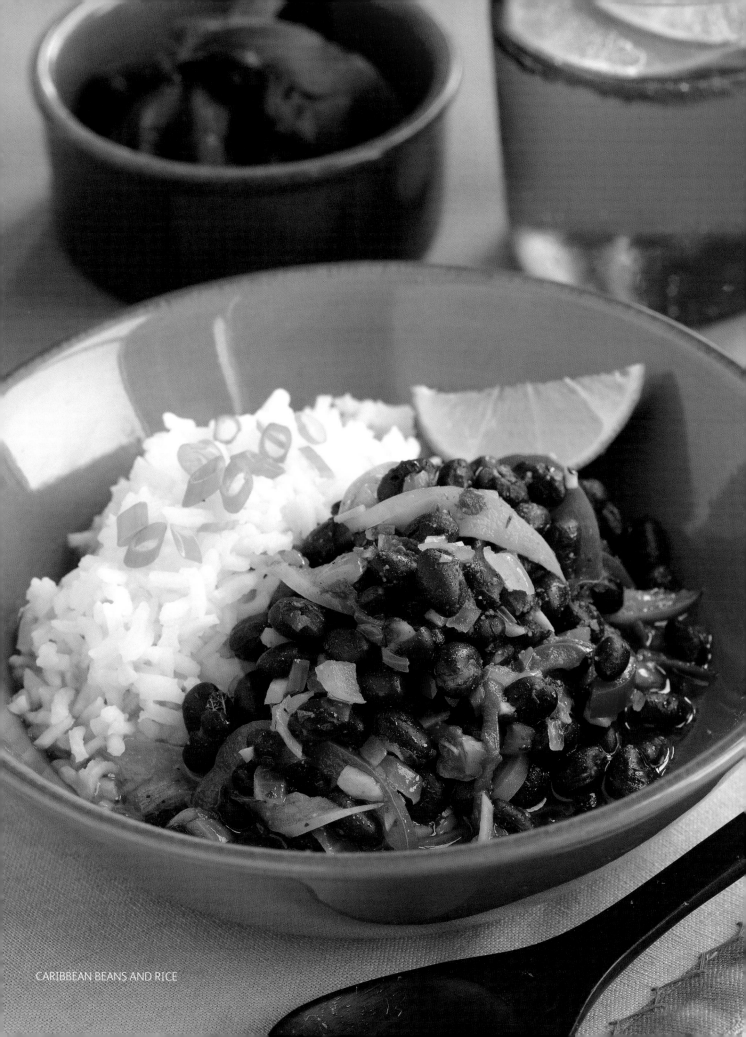

CARIBBEAN BEANS AND RICE

Pineapple Gazpacho

Prep: 25 min. **Chill:** 2 hr. **Serves:** 4

4	cups diced fresh DOLE Tropical Gold Pineapple, divided
1	large cucumber, peeled, seeded and chopped (2 cups), divided
1	cup chopped yellow bell pepper, divided
$^2/_3$	cup chopped DOLE Red Onion, divided
1¼	cups DOLE Pineapple Juice
3	Tbsp Italian salad dressing
2	Tbsp sugar or 4 tsp agave nectar*
2	Tbsp chopped DOLE Cilantro
1	tsp chopped jalapeño chili pepper

Mix 1 cup pineapple, ½ cup cucumber, ½ cup bell pepper and $^1/_3$ cup onion in medium bowl; set aside.

Combine remaining pineapple, cucumber, bell pepper, onion, pineapple juice, Italian dressing, sugar, cilantro and chili pepper in blender or food processor. Cover; blend until smooth. Stir into reserved pineapple mixture.

Cover; refrigerate 2 hours or until chilled.

*Agave nectar is a natural sugar alternative you can buy at natural food stores.

Serving Size (392g). Amount Per Serving: Calories 180, Calories from Fat 5, Total Fat 0.5g (1% DV), Saturated Fat 0g (0% DV), Trans Fat 0g, Cholesterol 0mg (0% DV), Sodium 135mg (6% DV), Potassium 540mg (15% DV), Total Carbohydrate 44g (16% DV), Dietary Fiber 4g (16% DV), Sugars 34g, Protein 2g, Vitamin A (6% DV), Vitamin C (280% DV), Calcium (6% DV), Iron (6% DV), Vitamin K (10% DV), Thiamin (15% DV), Vitamin B6 (20% DV), Folate (20% DV), Magnesium (10% DV), Copper (20% DV), Manganese (90% DV). Percent Daily Values (DV) are based on a 2,000 calorie diet.

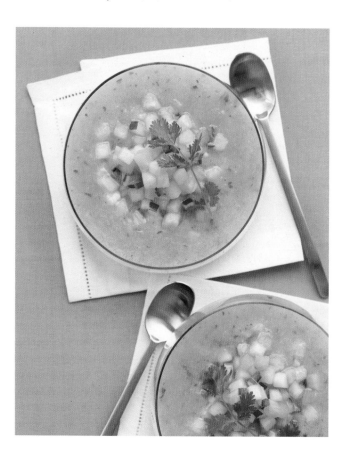

Southwest Caesar Salad

Prep: 10 min. **Serves:** 4

1   package (10 oz) DOLE Light Caesar Kit
1   can (14–16 oz) low-sodium kidney beans,
    rinsed and drained
1   can (8 oz) low-sodium whole-kernel corn,
    rinsed and drained
1   med. tomato, cut into wedges
1   med. red bell pepper, thinly sliced
½   med. DOLE Onion, thinly sliced

Combine romaine, croutons and Parmesan cheese from salad bag, beans, corn, tomato, pepper and onion in large serving bowl.

Pour dressing from packet over salad; toss to evenly coat.

Serving Size (275g). Amount Per Serving: Calories 190g, Calories from Fat 40g, Total Fat 4.5g (7% DV), Saturated Fat 1g (5% DV), Trans Fat 0g, Cholesterol 5mg (2% DV), Sodium 390mg (16% DV), Potassium 540mg (15% DV) Total Carbohydrate 32g (11% DV), Dietary Fiber 9g (36% DV), Sugars 5g, Protein 8g, Vitamin A (30% DV), Vitamin C (80% Vitamin), Calcium (6% DV), Iron (10% DV), Vitamin K (10% DV), Thiamin (10% DV), Riboflavin (10% DV), Vitamin B6 (10% DV), Folate (15% DV), Phosphorus (15% DV), Magnesium (10% DV), Zinc (15% DV), Copper (10% DV), Manganese (15% DV), Molybdenum (110% DV). Percent Daily Values (DV) are based on a 2,000 calorie diet.

DOLE DIET TIP

In order to meet the goal of providing 100 percent of nutrient needs, the Dole Diet incorporates some healthy fat to allow for maximum absorption of fat-soluble carotenoids (lycopene and beta-carotene) as well as vitamins A, D, E and K.

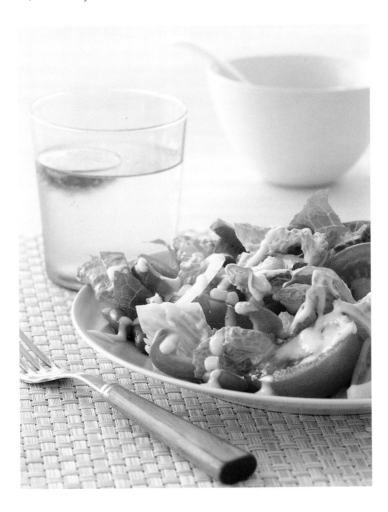

SOUTHWEST
CAESAR SALAD

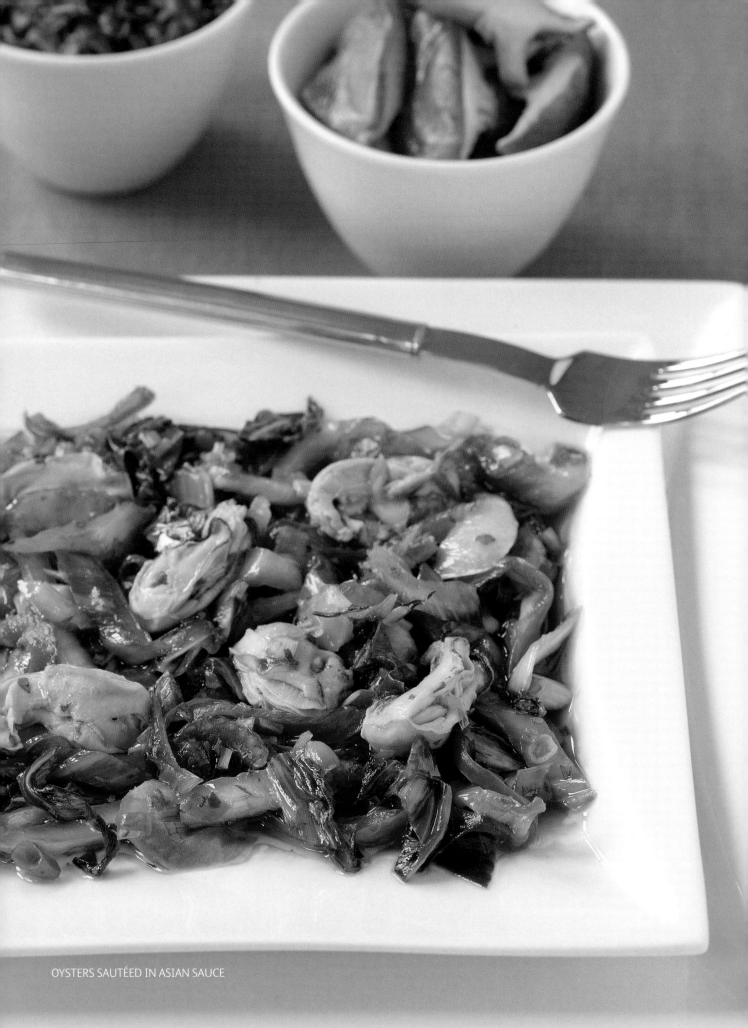

OYSTERS SAUTÉED IN ASIAN SAUCE

Oysters Sautéed in Asian Sauce

Prep: 20 min. **Cook:** 10 min. **Serves:** 5

2	pints fresh, shucked oysters, drained
2	Tbsp vegetable oil
3	baby bok choy (6–8 oz), diagonally sliced
2	ribs DOLE Celery, thinly sliced
1	cup sliced red bell pepper
½	cup chopped DOLE White Onion
1	Tbsp garlic, minced
1	tsp chopped lemongrass
2	Tbsp lemon juice
1	Tbsp sesame oil
1	Tbsp reduced-sodium soy sauce
2	DOLE Green Onions, chopped
1	Tbsp chopped DOLE Cilantro

Boil 1 quart of salted water in large saucepan. Add oysters and cook gently 2 to 3 minutes. Remove oysters from pan, drain, rinse and set aside.

Heat vegetable oil in large saucepan; add bok choy, celery, bell pepper, white onion, garlic and lemongrass. Sauté until just tender, about 5 minutes.

Add oysters, lemon juice, sesame oil and soy sauce; cook, stirring, just to heat through.

Stir in green onions and cilantro.

Serving Size (330g). Amount Per Serving: Calories 220, Calories from Fat 110, Total Fat 12g (18% DV), Saturated Fat 1.5g (8% DV), Trans Fat 0g, Cholesterol 70mg (23% DV), Sodium 330mg (14% DV), Potassium 510mg (15% DV), Total Carbohydrate 16g (5% DV), Dietary Fiber 3g (12% DV), Sugars 4g, Protein 12g, Vitamin A (60% DV), Vitamin C (90% DV), Calcium (10% DV), Iron (50% DV), Vitamin E (10% DV), Vitamin K (120% DV), Thiamin (15% DV), Riboflavin (15% DV), Niacin (10% DV), Vitamin B6 (15% DV), Folate (15% DV), Vitamin B12 (410% DV), Phosphorus (20% DV), Magnesium (20% DV), Zinc (790% DV), Selenium (70% DV), Copper (290% DV), Manganese (35% DV). Percent Daily Values (DV) are based on a 2,000 calorie diet.

FOOD PREP TIP

Getting 100 percent of your vitamin B5 needs using whole food sources can be challenging. Vitamin B5 simply isn't widely found, other than in fortified cereal and mushrooms—especially shiitake, portobello and white. That's why many meals include suggestions to add mushrooms, or to serve them as side dishes. To prepare the shiitake mushrooms served with this meal, first cook the sliced mushrooms with a small amount of water over medium heat 3 to 5 minutes, or until tender.

Veggie Egg-White Omelet

Prep: 15 min. **Cook:** 15 min. **Serves:** 8

2	tsp olive oil
¾	cup chopped DOLE Onion
½	cup chopped red bell pepper
2	cloves garlic, finely chopped
½	tsp dried oregano leaves, crushed
1	package (6 oz) DOLE Baby Portobello Mushrooms, sliced
½	tsp salt
½	tsp ground black pepper
1	package (6 oz) DOLE Baby Spinach
1½	cups egg whites or liquid egg substitute
¼	cup soy milk

Heat oil in large skillet over medium-high heat. Add onion, bell pepper, garlic and oregano. Cook 3 to 4 minutes, stirring occasionally.

Add mushrooms, salt and pepper; cook 3 minutes longer.

Stir in spinach; cook 3 minutes. Set aside.

Beat egg whites and soy milk in a large bowl.

Coat omelet pan with olive oil. Pour in eggs. With a spatula, lift edges of omelet, tilting pan to allow uncooked mixture to flow to bottom.

When omelet is set and slightly moist, spoon veggie mixture onto half of omelet, reserving ¼ cup for garnish if desired.

Slide omelet onto a large serving plate, folding omelet in half. Cut into 8 servings. Top with reserved ¼ cup veggie mixture as garnish.

Serving Size (122g). Amount Per Serving: Calories 60, Calories from Fat 10, Total Fat 1.5g (2% DV), Saturated Fat 0g (0% DV), Trans Fat 0g (0% DV), Cholesterol 0mg (0 % DV), Sodium 240mg (10% DV), Total Carbohydrate 5g (2% DV), Dietary Fiber 1g (4% DV), Sugars 1g, Protein 7g, Vitamin A (50% DV), Vitamin C (30% DV), Vitamin D (25% DV), Vitamin K (130% DV), Riboflavin (20% DV), Folate (10% DV), Iodine (15% DV), Selenium (20% DV), Manganese (15% DV). Percent Daily Values (DV) are based on a 2,000 calorie diet.

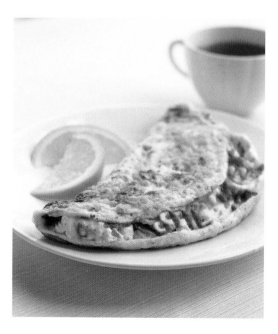

Broccoli and Pea Potage with Tarragon

Prep: 25 min. **Cook:** 25 min. **Serves:** 5

¼	cup chopped chives
3	Tbsp minced shallots
2	Tbsp olive oil
1	lb DOLE Broccoli, cut into florets
1	Tbsp chopped fresh tarragon
¼	tsp salt
¼	tsp ground black pepper
5½	cups vegetable broth
1½	cups frozen green peas, thawed
1½	cups cooked green lentils
4	cups sliced kale, blanched
⅔	lb halibut, cut into ¾" cubes, cooked

Sauté chives and shallots in oil in large stockpot over medium-high heat, stirring frequently, 3 to 5 minutes.

Add broccoli, tarragon, salt and pepper; sauté 5 minutes. Add broth and bring to a boil. Add peas and lentils. Cook additional 5 to 10 minutes, or until vegetables are tender. Cool slightly.

Place soup in batches in blender or food processor. Cover; blend until smooth. Return to stockpot. Add blanched kale and fish; heat through.

Serving Size (590g). Amount Per Serving: Calories 490, Calories from Fat 80, Total Fat 9g (14% DV), Saturated Fat 1g (5% DV), Trans Fat 0g, Cholesterol 25mg (8% DV), Sodium 750mg (31% DV), Potassium 1,540mg (44% DV), Total Carbohydrate 59g (20% DV), Dietary Fiber 25g (100% DV), Sugars 7g, Protein 40g, Vitamin A (270% DV), Vitamin C (260% DV), Calcium (25% DV), Iron (45% DV), Vitamin E (15% DV), Vitamin K (580% DV), Thiamin (50% DV), Riboflavin (25% DV), Niacin (40% DV), Vitamin B6 (45% DV), Folate (100% DV), Vitamin B12 (15% DV), Phosphorus (60% DV), Magnesium (50% DV), Zinc (25% DV), Selenium (50% DV), Copper (30% DV), Manganese (80% DV), Molybdenum (15% DV). Percent Daily Values (DV) are based on a 2,000 calorie diet.

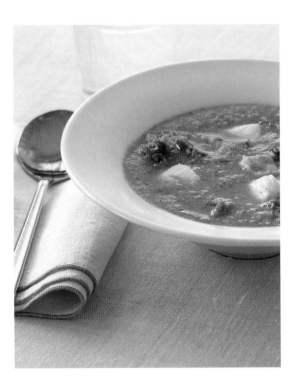

FOOD PREP TIP

To blanch kale, first cut the stems off by folding the leaves with a knife and cutting them crosswise into thin strips. Rinse well. Blanch in large pot of boiling water 5 minutes. Drain well.

FOOD PREP TIP

Cook the halibut in a few inches of simmering water for 5 minutes.

BROCCOLI AND PEA POTAGE WITH TARRAGON

Turkish Chicken with Spiced Dates, with Grilled Carrots and Beets

Prep: 5 min. **Cook:** 25 min. **Serves:** 6

6   boneless, skinless chicken breasts
1   cup vegetable broth
1   package (8 oz) DOLE Chopped Dates
½   cup chopped DOLE Onion
8   dried apricot halves, chopped
2   Tbsp apricot or peach fruit spread
½   tsp ground cinnamon

Coat large skillet with cooking spray. Cook chicken over medium-high heat 5 minutes on each side or until chicken is no longer pink in center. Remove from heat; cover and keep warm.

Add broth, dates, onion and apricots to skillet. Bring to a boil, stirring occasionally. Reduce heat to low; cook until liquid is reduced by half (8 to 10 minutes).

Stir apricot spread and cinnamon into sauce until blended; spoon over chicken.

Serving Size (389g). Amount Per Serving: Calories 380, Calories from Fat 35, Total Fat 4g (6% DV), Saturated Fat 1g (5% DV), Trans Fat 0g, Cholesterol 70mg (23% DV), Sodium 140mg (6% DV), Potassium 1,020mg (29% DV), Total Carbohydrate 59g (20% DV), Dietary Fiber 7g (28% DV), Sugars 49g, Protein 31g, Vitamin A (80% DV), Vitamin C (35% DV), Calcium (6% DV), Iron (10% DV), Vitamin E (10% DV), Riboflavin (10% DV), Niacin (10% DV), Vitamin B6 (30% DV), Pantothenic Acid (15% DV), Phosphorus (25% DV), Magnesium (10% DV), Selenium (35% DV), Copper (10% DV), Manganese (10% DV). Percent Daily Values (DV) are based on a 2,000 calorie diet.

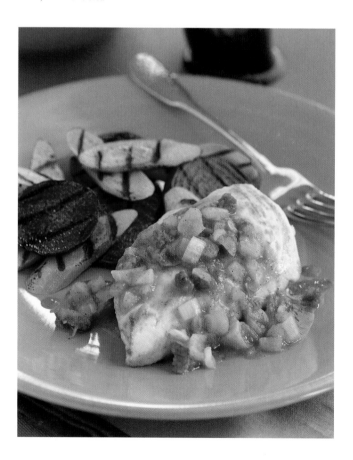

TURKISH CHICKEN WITH SPICED DATES, WITH GRILLED CARROTS AND BEETS

Mixed Berry Gazpacho

Prep: 20 min. **Chill**: 2 hr. **Serves**: 4

1	cup fresh or frozen DOLE Blueberries, thawed, divided
2	cups fresh or frozen DOLE Raspberries, thawed
2	cups fresh or frozen DOLE Blackberries, thawed
1½	cups DOLE Pineapple Juice
1	cup apple juice
2	containers (8 oz each) nonfat mixed-berry yogurt
1	orange, peeled, seeded and diced
1	DOLE Apple, cored and diced
⅓	cup chopped Brazil nuts

Reserve ½ cup blueberries. Combine remaining blueberries, raspberries, blackberries, pineapple juice and apple juice in blender or food processor. Cover; blend until smooth.

Stir in yogurt until blended. Stir in reserved blueberries, orange and apple. Or leave unstirred for garnish. Cover; refrigerate 2 hours, or until chilled. Garnish with nuts and serve.

Serving Size (1,368g). Amount Per Serving: Calories 770, Calories from Fat 80, Total Fat 9g (14% DV), Saturated Fat 2g (10% DV), Cholesterol 20mg (7% DV), Sodium 450mg (19% DV), Potassium 1,960mg (56% DV), Total Carbohydrate 135g (45% DV), Dietary Fiber 11g (44% DV), Sugars 95g, Protein 33g, Vitamin A (6% DV), Vitamin C (130% DV), Calcium (150% DV), Iron (10% DV), Vitamin E (10% DV), Vitamin K (35% DV), Thiamin (15% DV), Riboflavin (70% DV), Vitamin B6 (10% DV), Folate (20% DV), Phosphorus (90% DV), Magnesium (40% DV), Selenium (300% DV), Copper (25% DV), Manganese (80% DV). Percent Daily Values (DV) are based on a 2,000 calorie diet.

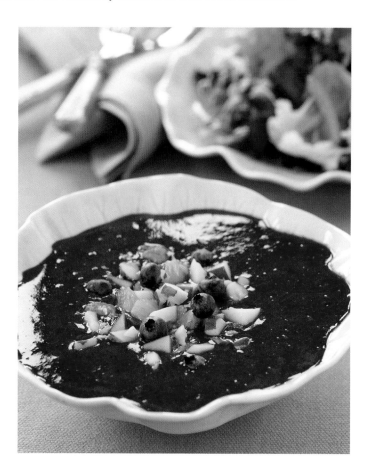

DOLE DIET TIP

The Dole Diet provides an average of 13 fruit and vegetable servings per day (easily meeting the USDA's recommended 9 to 13). Considering that one serving is actually half a cup, this is not as hard as it sounds. For example, one large banana actually counts as two fruit servings (since it's roughly a full cup).

MIXED BERRY
GAZPACHO

DOLE DIET TIP

Choosing whole-grain, high-fiber breads, cereals and rice in place of white flour doubles your chances of keeping trim, according to a Harvard study of 74,000 women. Those who ate more than two daily servings of whole grains were almost 50 percent less likely to be overweight than their refined-grain-eating peers.

Quinoa Salad

Prep: 15 min. **Cook:** 30 min. **Chill:** 1 hr. **Serves:** 6

1	cup quinoa
½	lb DOLE Asparagus, cooked and cut into 1" pieces
2	cups chopped red or green bell peppers
1	med. tomato, chopped
½	cup chopped DOLE Celery
½	cup sliced almonds
⅓	cup fat-free or light Italian dressing
1	tsp grated lemon peel

Boil 1 quart of water in medium saucepan. Stir in quinoa and bring to a boil again.

Cover and reduce to simmer. Cook 12 minutes. Let stand 15 minutes or until quinoa absorbs almost all of water. Fluff with fork. Drain if necessary. Cool slightly.

Combine quinoa with asparagus, bell peppers, tomato, celery, almonds, dressing and lemon peel in large bowl. Chill 1 hour to blend flavors.

Serving Size (165g). Amount Per Serving: Calories 180, Calories from Fat 50, Total Fat 6g (9% DV), Saturated Fat 0.5g (3% DV), Cholesterol 0mg (0% DV), Sodium 260mg (11% DV), Potassium 420mg (12% DV), Total Carbohydrate 25g (8% DV), Dietary Fiber 4g (16% DV), Sugars 3g, Protein 7g, Vitamin A (45% DV), Vitamin C (40% DV), Calcium (6% DV), Iron (15% DV), Vitamin E (20% DV), Vitamin K (30% DV), Thiamin (15% DV), Riboflavin (15% DV), Vitamin B6 (15% DV), Folate (30% DV), Phosphorus (20% DV), Magnesium (20% DV), Zinc (10% DV), Copper (20% DV), Manganese (45% DV). Percent Daily Values (DV) are based on a 2,000 calorie diet.

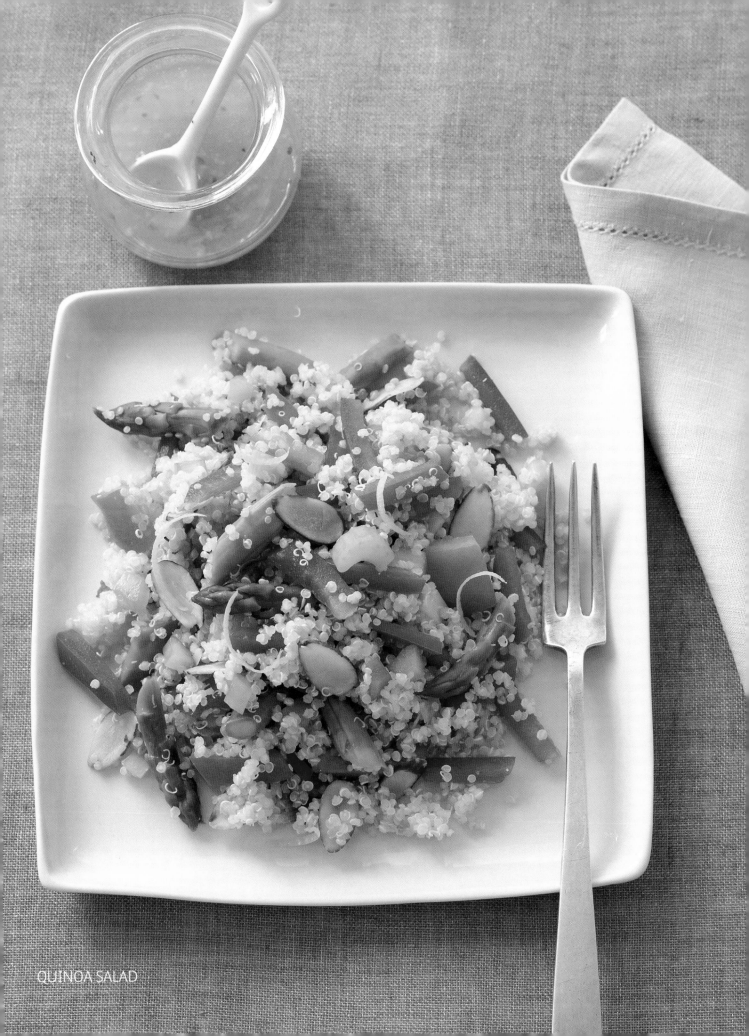

QUINOA SALAD

DOLE DIET TIP
Bananas boost fat-burning. They contain resistant starch, a fiber with digestive by-products that block the conversion of some carbohydrates into fuel, forcing your body to rely on its fat stores instead.

Papaya Ginger Smoothie

Prep: 5 min. **Serves:** 2

1	cup fresh or frozen papaya chunks
½	cup calcium-fortified vanilla soy milk
1	medium DOLE Banana
2	Tbsp peppermint leaves
½	tsp ground ginger

Combine papaya, soy milk, banana, peppermint leaves and ginger in blender or food processor. Cover; blend until smooth.

Serving Size (191g). Amount Per Serving: Calories 120, Calories from Fat 10, Total Fat 1g (2% DV), Saturated Fat 0g (0% DV), Trans Fat 0g, Cholesterol 0mg (0% DV), Sodium 25mg (1% DV), Potassium 480mg (14% DV), Total Carbohydrate 26g (9% DV), Dietary Fiber 3g (12% DV), Sugars 15g, Protein 3g, Vitamin A (25% DV), Vitamin C (80% DV), Calcium (8% DV), Iron (4% DV), Vitamin E (10% DV), Vitamin B6 (15% DV), Folate (10% DV), Vitamin B12 (15% DV), Selenium (2% DV), Manganese (15% DV). Percent Daily Values (DV) are based on a 2,000 calorie diet.

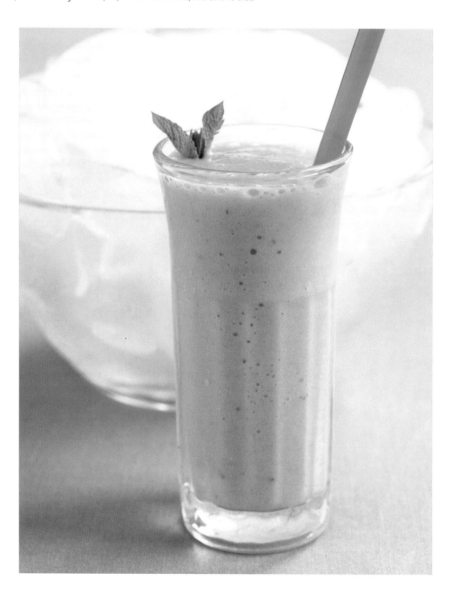

Roasted Red Pepper and Crab Chowder

Prep: 20 min. **Cook:** 35 min. **Serves:** 4

2	large red bell peppers, cut into ¾" cubes
2	cups thickly sliced DOLE White Mushrooms
1	Tbsp almond oil
2	cans (14½ oz each) vegetable broth
1	can (14½ oz) diced tomatoes with basil, garlic and oregano
2	cups sliced collard greens, stem center removed
1	cup water
⅓	cup oat bran
1	tsp grated orange peel
1	tsp dried herbes de Provence
½	tsp fennel seed, crushed
½	lb fresh shucked oysters, chopped
½	lb cooked crabmeat

Preheat oven to 450°F.

Mix bell peppers and mushrooms in 15" x 10" jelly roll pan. Drizzle with oil; toss to coat. Spread in single layer in pan. Roast 15 to 20 minutes or until crisp-tender and lightly browned, stirring after 10 minutes.

Combine roasted peppers and mushrooms with broth, tomatoes, collard greens, water, oat bran, orange peel, herbs and fennel seed in large stockpot. Bring to a boil. Reduce heat and simmer 5 minutes. Add oysters and cook 5 minutes longer. Add crabmeat; heat through.

Serving Size (643g). Amount Per Serving: Calories 230, Calories from Fat 60, Total Fat 6g (9 % DV), Saturated Fat 0.5g (3 % DV), Trans Fat 0g, Cholesterol 70mg (23 % DV), Sodium 1,320mg (55 % DV), Potassium 560mg (16 % DV), Total Carbohydrate 24g (8 % DV), Dietary Fiber 5g (20 % DV), Sugars 8g, Protein 23g, Vitamin A (100 % DV), Vitamin C (220 % DV), Calcium (10 % DV), Iron (25 % DV), Vitamin E (20 % DV), Vitamin K (120 % DV), Thiamin (15 % DV), Riboflavin (30 % DV), Niacin (20 % DV), Vitamin B6 (15 % DV), Folate (20 % DV), Vitamin B12 (150 % DV), Pantothenic Acid (15 % DV), Phosphorus (25 % DV), Magnesium (10 % DV), Selenium (80 % DV), Copper (60 % DV), Manganese (50 % DV). Percent Daily Values (DV) are based on a 2,000 calorie diet.

DOLE DIET TIP

The premise of the Dole Diet is that meeting nutrient requirements will help you lose weight. When obese study subjects significantly increased their vitamin C intake, they were able to burn 40 percent more fat than a control group during exercise. Kiwifruits, papayas, red bell peppers and strawberries all contain more than 100 percent vitamin C per serving.

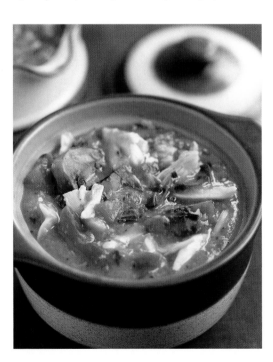

ROASTED RED PEPPER
AND CRAB CHOWDER

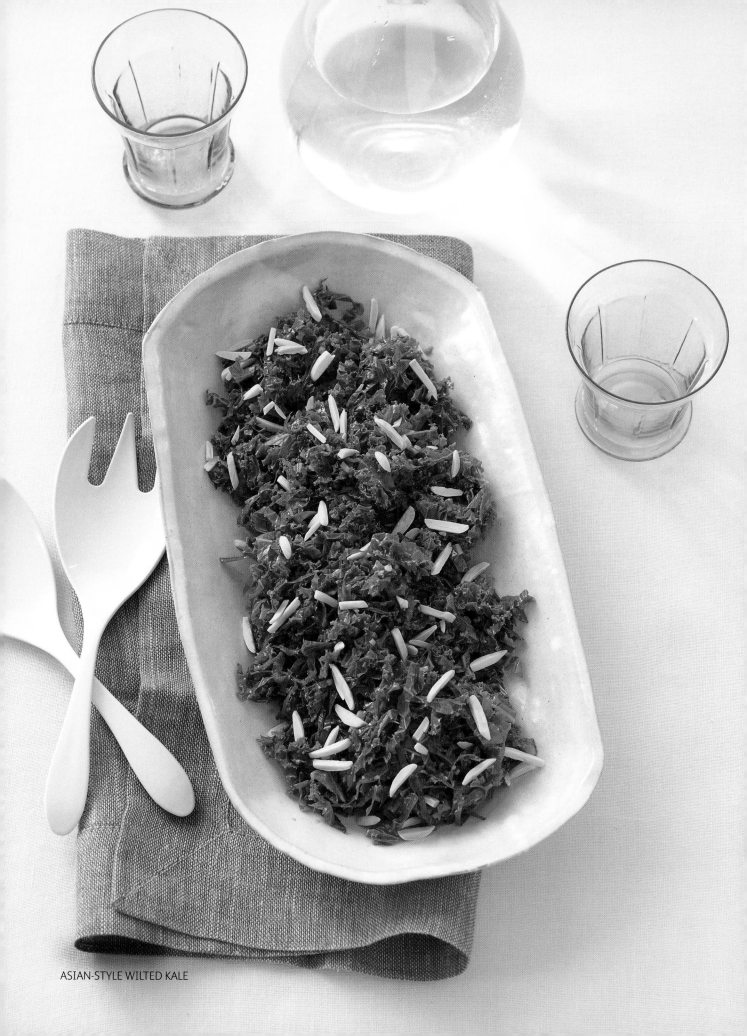

ASIAN-STYLE WILTED KALE

Asian-Style Wilted Kale

Prep: 10 min. **Cook:** 10 min. **Serves:** 2

1	bunch (¾ lb) curly kale
2	tsp olive or canola oil
2	cloves garlic, minced
1	tsp minced ginger
⅓	tsp red pepper flakes (optional)
2	tsp light soy sauce or liquid aminos (soy substitute)
1	tsp sesame oil (optional)
¼	cup slivered almonds, toasted

Cut stems off kale leaves with knife. Cut leaves crosswise into thin threads. Rinse well. Blanch in large pot of boiling water 2 to 3 minutes. Drain well.

Heat olive oil in nonstick skillet over medium-high heat. Add garlic, ginger and red pepper flakes, if using; cook over low heat, stirring, 1 to 2 minutes. Add blanched kale and soy sauce to pan.

Cook, stirring, 5 to 7 minutes or until heated through.

Stir in sesame oil, if using, just before serving. Sprinkle with almonds.

Serving Size (207g). Amount Per Serving: Calories 200, Calories from Fat 130, Total Fat 14g (22% DV), Saturated Fat 1.5g (8% DV), Trans Fat 0g, Cholesterol 0mg (0% DV), Sodium 340mg (14% DV), Potassium 540mg (15% DV), Total Carbohydrate 16g (5% DV), Dietary Fiber 5g (20% DV), Sugars 3g, Protein 7g, Vitamin A (470% DV), Vitamin C (120% DV), Calcium (20% DV), Iron (15% DV), Vitamin E (30% DV), Vitamin K (1,740% DV), Thiamin (10% DV), Riboflavin (15% DV), Vitamin B6 (20% DV), Phosphorus (15% DV), Magnesium (20% DV), Copper (20% DV), Manganese (70% DV). Percent Daily Values (DV) are based on a 2,000 calorie diet.

DOLE DIET TIP

Always rinse kale well. And be sure to remove the stems from leaves. For a basic wilted kale, cover the leaves in boiling water, cook for 2 to 3 minutes and drain. Then sauté the kale in a skillet with olive oil 5 to 7 minutes, or until tender.

FOOD PREP TIP

Place asparagus stalks in a saucepan of boiling water and cook 3 to 5 minutes or until tender.

FOOD PREP TIP

To prepare the roasted sweet potatoes, lightly brush potato pieces with olive oil and a fresh herb of your choice. Bake at 375°F 30 minutes, or until tender.

Portobello Turkey Loaf

Prep: 20 min. **Bake:** 50 min. **Serves:** 6

1½	lbs raw ground lean turkey
1½	cups finely chopped DOLE Portobello Mushrooms
¾	cup finely chopped DOLE Onions
¾	cup plain bread crumbs
1½	tsp salt
1	tsp ground black pepper
¾	cup liquid egg substitute

Preheat oven to 375°F.

Stir turkey, mushrooms, onions, bread crumbs, salt, pepper and egg substitute until thoroughly mixed.

Form into loaf in 13" x 9" pan.

Bake 40 to 50 minutes or until meat reaches 160°F internal temperature.

Serving Size (211g). Amount Per Serving: Calories 370, Calories from Fat 150, Total Fat 17g (26% DV), Saturated Fat 4.5g (23% DV), Trans Fat 0g, Cholesterol 115mg (38% DV), Sodium 870mg (36% DV), Potassium 600mg (17% DV), Total Carbohydrate 14g (5% DV), Dietary Fiber 2g (8% DV), Sugars 2g, Protein 38g, Vitamin A (2% DV), Vitamin C (2% DV), Calcium (8% DV), Iron (20% DV), Riboflavin (25% DV), Niacin (35% DV), Vitamin B6 (25% DV), Pantothenic Acid (25% DV), Phosphorus (30% DV), Magnesium (10% DV), Zinc (25% DV), Selenium (80% DV), Copper (15% DV). Percent Daily Values (DV) are based on a 2,000 calorie diet.

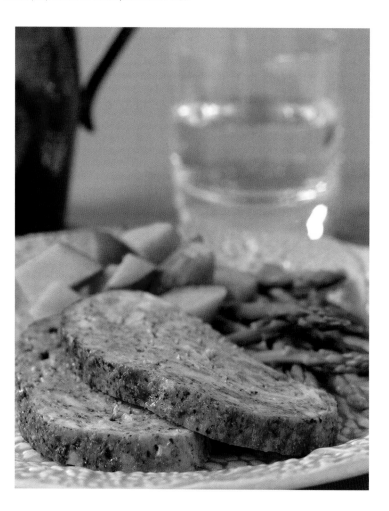

Tuscan White Bean Soup

Prep: 15 min. **Cook:** 45 min. **Serves:** 7

1	med. DOLE Onion, chopped (1 cup)
1	large leek, white part, chopped (½ cup)
3	cloves garlic, chopped
1	Tbsp olive oil
3–4	sprigs fresh rosemary or 1 tsp dried rosemary
2–3	sprigs fresh thyme or ½ tsp dried thyme
2	quarts vegetable broth
3	cans (15 oz each) cannellini or great northern beans, rinsed and drained
½	tsp salt
¼	tsp ground white pepper

Sauté onion, leek and garlic in oil in large stockpot over medium heat, stirring frequently until translucent, about 10 minutes. Add rosemary and thyme. Cook 5 minutes longer.

Add broth, beans, salt and pepper. Bring to a boil; reduce heat and simmer, covered, 15 to 20 minutes.

Remove rosemary and thyme sprigs. Pour two-thirds of beans into blender or food processor. Cover; blend until pureed. Stir beans back into soup; heat through.

Serving Size (446g). Amount Per Serving: Calories 670, Calories from Fat 35, Total Fat 4g (6% DV), Saturated Fat 1g (5% DV), Trans Fat 0g, Cholesterol 0mg (0% DV), Sodium 1,270mg (53% DV), Potassium 2,590mg (74% DV), Total Carbohydrate 122g (41% DV), Dietary Fiber 38g (152% DV), Sugars 8g, Protein 40g, Vitamin A (15% DV), Vitamin C (25% DV), Calcium (35% DV), Iron (60% DV), Vitamin K (20% DV), Thiamin (80% DV), Riboflavin (25% DV), Niacin (20% DV), Vitamin B6 (45% DV), Folate (220% DV), Pantothenic Acid (20% DV), Phosphorus (80% DV), Magnesium (90% DV), Zinc (30% DV), Selenium (35% DV), Copper (80% DV), Manganese (140% DV). Percent Daily Values (DV) are based on a 2,000 calorie diet.

DOLE DIET TIP

Why does the Dole Diet serve up so much soup? Diners consume fewer calories overall when they start with soup. Research also links regular soup consumption with higher levels of vitamin C, folate and beta-carotene. By filling you up and helping you meet nutrient needs, you'll feel more satisfied with fewer calories.

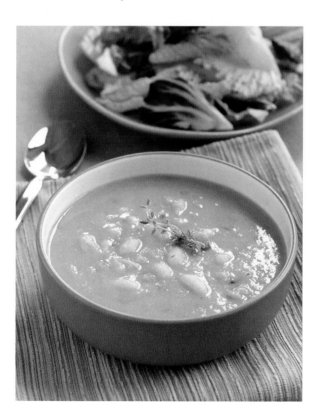

TUSCAN WHITE
BEAN SOUP

Vitamin E, an antioxidant and immunity booster, is another nutrient with limited food sources. Its importance accounts for the abundance of almond garnishes and snacks and the creative use of almond flour in some of our recipes. Sunflower seeds are another top source of vitamin E; a quarter cup of them provides nearly 60 percent of your daily needs.

Banana Almond Pancakes

Prep: 15 min. **Serves:** 3

1½ cups pancake and waffle mix
¼ cup almond flour
1 cup nonfat milk
2 Tbsp canola oil
1 egg
1 large DOLE Banana, diced

Whisk pancake mix, flour, milk, oil and egg. Stir in banana. Cook per package directions.

Serving Size (247g). Amount Per Serving: Calories 470, Calories from Fat, Total Fat 19g (29% DV), Saturated Fat 2g (10% DV), Trans Fat 0g, Cholesterol 85mg (28% DV), Sodium 270mg (11% DV), Total Carbohydrate 62g (21% DV), Dietary Fiber 13g (52% DV), Sugars 15g, Protein 19g, Vitamin A (10% DV), Vitamin C (8% DV), Calcium (45% DV), Iron (20% DV), Vitamin E (20% DV), Thiamin (30% DV), Riboflavin (40% DV), Niacin (30% DV), Vitamin B6 (40% DV), Folate (30% DV), Vitamin B12 (50% DV), Phosphorus (15% DV), Iodine (10% DV), Magnesium (40% DV), Zinc (45% DV), Selenium (10% DV). Percent Daily Values (DV) are based on a 2,000 calorie diet.

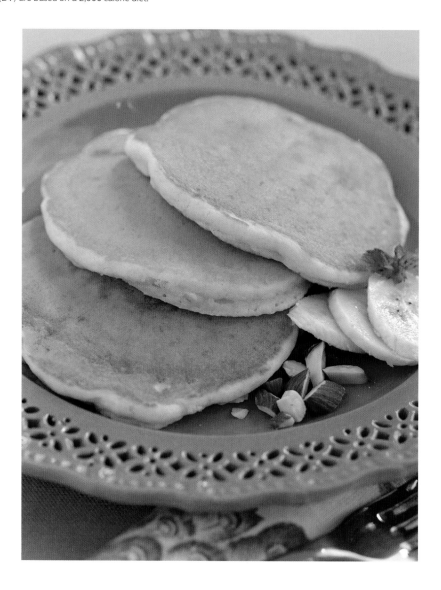

Almond Turkey Salad with Cranberry Vinaigrette

Prep: 20 min. **Serves:** 4

Vinaigrette
¾   cup DOLE Fresh or Frozen Cranberries
1   cup orange juice
2   Tbsp honey
¼   cup balsamic vinegar
2   Tbsp chopped fresh mixed herbs

Salad
1   package (16 oz) DOLE Classic Iceberg Salad
1   lb cooked turkey breast, chopped
½   cup toasted, slivered almonds
¾–1 cup fat-free Cranberry Vinaigrette

For the vinaigrette, first cook cranberries with juice, in small saucepan, until skins burst. Cool.

Combine cooked cranberries with honey, vinegar and herbs in blender or food processor. Cover; blend until smooth. Makes 1⅔ cups. Set aside.

Combine salad, turkey and almonds in large salad bowl.

Pour ¾ to 1 cup Cranberry Vinaigrette over salad. Toss gently to coat evenly.

Serving Size (287g). Amount Per Serving: Calories 370, Calories from Fat 180, Total Fat 20g (31% DV), Saturated Fat 1g (5% DV), Trans Fat 0g, Cholesterol 95mg (32% DV), Sodium 420mg, (18% DV), Potassium 590mg (17% DV), Total Carbohydrate 11g (4% DV), Dietary Fiber 3g (12% DV), Sugars 6g, Protein 38g, Vitamin A (10% DV), Vitamin C (6% DV), Calcium (6% DV), Iron (15% DV), Vitamin E (20% DV), Vitamin K (35% DV), Riboflavin (20% DV), Niacin (45% DV), Vitamin B6 (35% DV), Folate (10% DV), Pantothenic Acid (10% DV), Phosphorus (35% DV), Magnesium (20% DV), Zinc (15% DV), Selenium (50% DV), Copper (10% DV), Manganese (25% DV), Molybdenum (20% DV). Percent Daily Values (DV) are based on a 2,000 calorie diet.

DOLE DIET TIP
Cranberries help prevent urinary-tract infections because they contain compounds that inhibit bacteria from sticking to bladder walls. Bonus: New research has linked cranberry juice consumption with an increase in HDL (good) cholesterol.

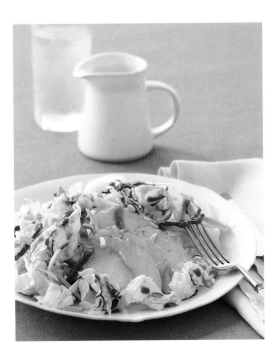

ALMOND TURKEY SALAD
WITH CRANBERRY
VINAIGRETTE

Sweet Potato and Spinach Soup

Prep: 15 min. **Cook:** 30 min. **Serves:** 5

2	tsp olive oil
1	cup chopped DOLE Onion
½	cup chopped DOLE Carrots
1	tsp curry powder
½	tsp seasoned salt
½	tsp freshly ground black pepper
5	cups vegetable broth, divided
1	large (12 oz) DOLE Sweet Potato, peeled and cubed
1	DOLE Apple, cored and chopped
1	package (14 oz) soft tofu, drained
2	Tbsp cornstarch
1	package (6 oz) DOLE Baby Spinach

Heat oil over medium-high heat in large stockpot. Add onion, carrots, curry powder, salt and pepper. Cook 4 to 5 minutes, stirring occasionally.

Stir in 4 cups of the broth, sweet potato and apple. Bring to a boil; reduce heat and simmer 20 minutes, or until sweet potato is tender. Cool slightly.

Combine tofu, cornstarch and remaining 1 cup broth in blender or food processor. Cover; blend until smooth. Remove from container; set aside.

Process sweet potato mixture in batches in blender or food processor until smooth. Pour into stockpot; add tofu mixture.

Heat over medium heat until bubbles appear around edge. Add spinach; cook until spinach wilts, about 5 minutes. Do not boil.

Serving Size (413g). Amount Per Serving: Calories 170, Calories from Fat 35, Total Fat 4g (6% DV), Saturated Fat 0.5g (3% DV), Trans Fat 0g, Cholesterol 0mg (0% DV), Sodium 1,020mg (43% DV), Potassium 570mg (16% DV), Total Carbohydrate 28g (9% DV), Dietary Fiber 5g (20% DV), Sugars 11g, Protein 6g, Vitamin A (150% DV), Vitamin C (20% DV), Calcium (8% DV), Iron (10% DV), Magnesium (10% DV), Copper (10% DV). Percent Daily Values (DV) are based on a 2,000 calorie diet.

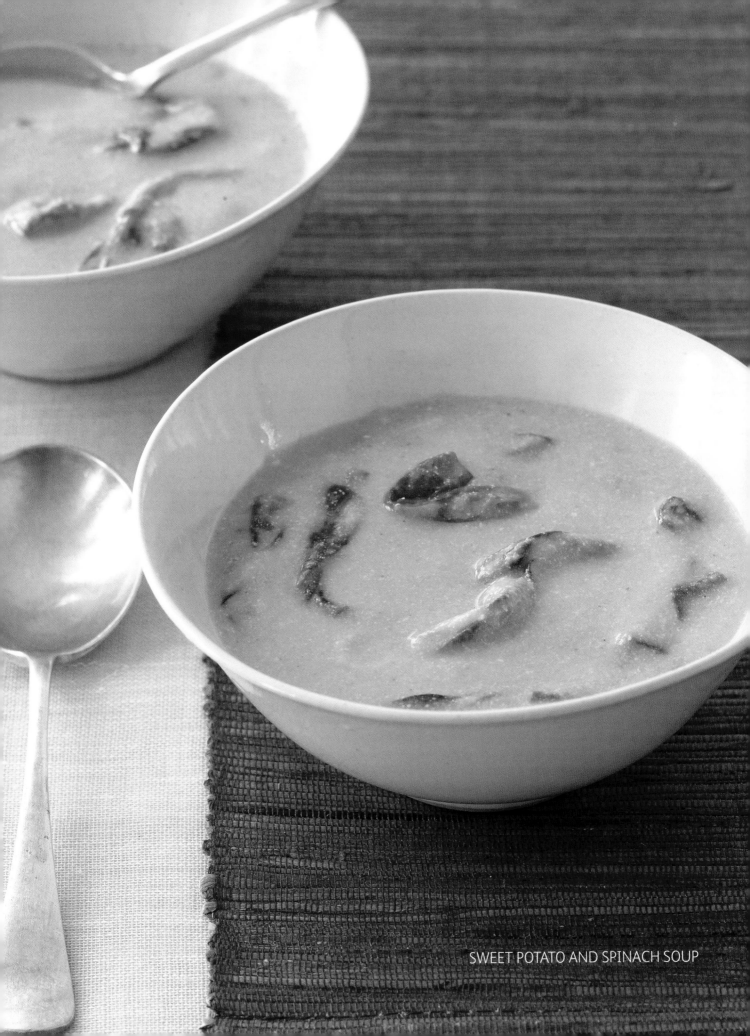

SWEET POTATO AND SPINACH SOUP

DOLE DIET TIP
Researchers in Brazil found that women who ate 300 grams of apples or pears daily (the equivalent of one large piece of fruit) lost more weight compared with nonfruit eaters. Since both groups of women followed low-calorie diets, it may be that the fiber content of the apples and pears helped the women feel full longer.

Chicken Apple Almond Salad

Prep: 20 min. **Serves:** 4

12	oz boneless, skinless cooked chicken breast, chopped
½	cup diced DOLE Celery
⅓	cup DOLE Seedless Raisins
⅓	cup soy mayonnaise
1	tsp lemon juice
1	package (10 oz) DOLE Classic Iceberg Lettuce
2	DOLE Apples, cored and sliced
1	cup cubed DOLE Cantaloupe
¼	cup slivered almonds, toasted

Combine chicken, celery, raisins, mayonnaise and lemon juice in large bowl. Mix well; cover and refrigerate until needed.

Arrange lettuce on each serving plate.

Spoon refrigerated mixture in center of lettuce; arrange apples and cantaloupe around mixture. Sprinkle with almonds.

Serving Size (321g). Amount Per Serving: Calories 350, Calories from Fat 120, Total Fat 13g (20% DV), Saturated Fat 2g (10% DV), Trans Fat 0g, Cholesterol 80mg (27% DV), Sodium 250mg (10% DV), Potassium 700mg (20% DV), Sugars 23g, Protein 30g, Vitamin A (35% DV), Vitamin C (35% DV), Calcium (6% DV), Iron (10% DV), Vitamin E (15% DV), Vitamin K (70% DV), Riboflavin (15% DV), Niacin (60% DV), Vitamin B6 (30% DV), Folate (10% DV), Pantothenic Acid (10% DV), Phosphorus (25% DV), Magnesium (15% DV), Selenium (35% DV), Manganese (15% DV), Molybdenum (10% DV). Percent Daily Values (DV) are based on a 2,000 calorie diet.

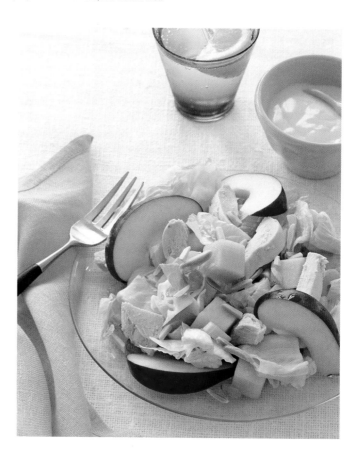

Sesame Ginger Frittata with Broccoli and Shrimp

Prep: 20 min. **Cook:** 15 min. **Serves:** 4

2	cups DOLE Broccoli ½" florets, cooked just until tender
1	cup finely chopped DOLE Red Onion
2–3	DOLE Green Onions, finely chopped
5	oz peeled, cooked shrimp, cut into ½" pieces
½	tsp sesame oil
3	large eggs
4	large egg whites
2	Tbsp all-purpose flour
1	Tbsp cornstarch
1	Tbsp DOLE Pineapple Juice
½	cup vegetable broth
1	Tbsp reduced-sodium soy sauce
1	clove garlic, minced
½	tsp grated, peeled fresh ginger

Combine broccoli, red onion, green onions, shrimp and oil in large bowl.

Whisk eggs, egg whites and flour in another bowl until well-blended. Pour over vegetable mixture; mix well and set aside.

Stir together cornstarch and pineapple juice in small saucepan. Add broth, soy sauce, garlic and ginger. Bring to a boil over medium heat, stirring constantly.

Continue cooking 2 to 3 minutes, until thickened. Keep sauce warm.

Coat large, ovenproof, nonstick skillet with cooking spray. Heat skillet over medium-low heat. Stir in egg and vegetable mixture, and pour into skillet, smoothing mixture into even layer. Cover and cook 6 to 8 minutes, or until eggs are set and bottom is browned.

Place skillet under broiler about 2 minutes, until eggs are cooked through. Loosen frittata from skillet with spatula. Cut frittata into quarters. Serve with warm sauce.

Serving Size (439g). Amount Per Serving: Calories 260, Calories from Fat 50, Total Fat 6g (9% DV), Saturated Fat 1.5g (8% DV), Trans Fat 0g, Cholesterol 260mg (87% DV), Sodium 660mg (28% DV), Potassium 600mg (17% DV), Total Carbohydrate 19g (6% DV), Dietary Fiber 2g (8% DV), Sugars 8g, Protein 32g, Vitamin A (35% DV), Vitamin C (120% DV), Calcium (10% DV), Iron (30% DV), Riboflavin (60% DV), Niacin (10% DV), Vitamin B6 (15% DV), Folate (20% DV), Vitamin B12 (20% DV), Pantothenic Acid (15% DV), Phosphorus (20% DV), Iodine (70% DV), Magnesium (15% DV), Zinc (10% DV), Selenium (90% DV), Copper (10% DV), Manganese (20% DV), Molybdenum (15% DV). Percent Daily Values (DV) are based on a 2,000 calorie diet.

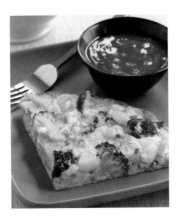

DOLE DIET TIP

Nutrition scientist Nicholas Gillitt, PhD, says: "Steaming or light boiling can reduce the nutrition value of some foods, though only by 10 to 12 percent. In some cases, cooking actually increases the nutrition value of foods, such as carrots and tomatoes." Bottom line: If cooking makes veggies more palatable, then by all means prepare according to taste.

SESAME GINGER FRITTATA WITH BROCCOLI AND SHRIMP

DOLE DIET TIP

Thirst is sometimes mistaken for hunger, so drink plenty of water to avoid this common diet pitfall. Drinking water may also elevate your metabolic rate, according to German researchers. Plus, adequate hydration can help enhance exercise endurance.

Porridge with Fruit

Prep: 10 min. **Cook:** 10 min. **Serves:** 7

1½	cups old-fashioned oatmeal
⅔	cup almond flour
½	cup oat bran
3	cups water
2	cups soy milk
¾	cup DOLE Seedless Raisins
⅓	cup chopped DOLE Pitted Prunes
⅓	cup chopped almonds

Agave nectar or brown sugar (optional)

Combine oatmeal, flour, bran, water, milk and raisins in large saucepan and bring to a boil. Reduce heat and cook, uncovered, about 5 minutes, stirring occasionally.

Stir in prunes and almonds, and serve immediately. Sprinkle with agave nectar or brown sugar, if desired.

Serving Size (235g). Amount Per Serving: Calories 280, Calories from Fat 90, Total Fat 10g (15% DV), Saturated Fat 1g (5% DV), Trans Fat 0g, Cholesterol 0mg (0% DV), Sodium 50mg (2% DV), Potassium 400mg (11% DV), Total Carbohydrate 42g (14% DV), Dietary Fiber 6g (24% DV), Sugars 19g, Protein 10g, Vitamin A (2% DV), Vitamin C (0% DV), Calcium (8% DV), Iron (15% DV), Vitamin E (20% DV), Thiamin (15% DV), Phosphorus (20% DV), Magnesium (25% DV), Selenium (15% DV), Copper (10% DV), Manganese (60% DV). Percent Daily Values (DV) are based on a 2,000 calorie diet.

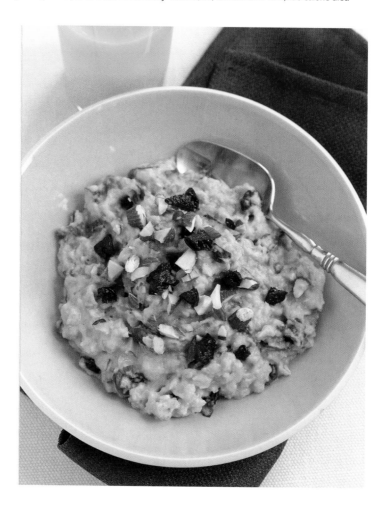

Turkey, Avocado and Cheese Wrap

Prep: 20 min. **Serves:** 4

4	*fat-free whole wheat tortillas, burrito-size*
2	*cups DOLE Hearts of Romaine Salad, divided*
1	*lb cooked turkey breast, chopped, divided*
1	*DOLE Avocado, diced, divided*
1	*tomato, chopped, divided*
½	*cup low-fat shredded cheddar cheese, divided*

Warm tortilla in large nonstick skillet or griddle coated with cooking spray. Layer one-quarter romaine, turkey, avocado, tomato and cheese on tortilla. Fold in sides and roll up. Repeat for each wrap.

Serving Size (282g). Amount Per Serving: Calories 530, Calories from Fat 200, Total Fat 23g (35% DV), Saturated Fat 6g (30% DV), Trans Fat 0g, Cholesterol 120mg (40% DV), Sodium 770mg (32% DV), Potassium 440mg (13% DV), Total Carbohydrate 38g (13% DV), Dietary Fiber 2g (8% DV), Sugars 3g, Protein 41g, Vitamin A (25% DV), Vitamin C (20% DV), Calcium (25% DV), Iron (DV 25%), Riboflavin (15% DV), Niacin (30% DV), Vitamin B6 (25% DV), Pantothenic Acid (10% DV), Phosphorus (30% DV), Zinc (25% DV), Selenium (60% DV). Percent Daily Values (DV) are based on a 2,000 calorie diet.

DOLE DIET TIP

Middle age doesn't have to mean a thicker middle. University of Pennsylvania researchers have found that overweight women who began lifting weights twice weekly not only reduced overall body fat by nearly 4 percent, but also significantly reduced the transfer of fat to the midsection. So bench-press to beat belly fat.

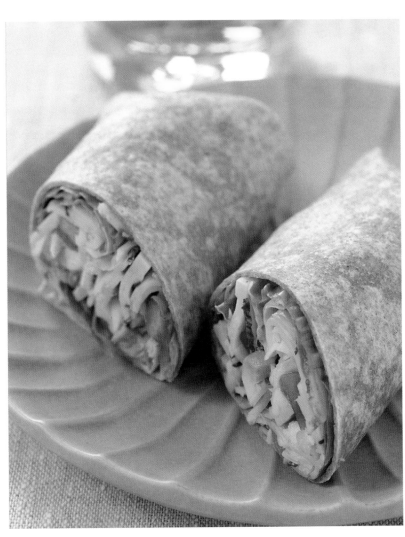

TURKEY, AVOCADO AND CHEESE WRAP

Chili non Carne

Prep: 20 min. **Cook:** 30 min. **Serves:** 6

1	Tbsp olive oil
¼	tsp crushed red pepper
2	cups diced DOLE Mushrooms
1½	cups diced DOLE Carrots
¾	cup chopped DOLE Onion
¾	cup chopped green bell pepper
1	medium zucchini, chopped
4	cloves garlic, chopped
1	tsp dried Mexican oregano
1	tsp ground cumin
½	tsp chili powder
½	tsp dried thyme leaves
1	package (14 oz) vegetarian ground beef, crumbled
1	can (15 oz) chili beans
1	can (14½ oz) diced tomatoes with jalapeño chili peppers
2	Tbsp chopped DOLE Cilantro

Heat oil and red pepper over medium-high heat in large nonstick saucepan for 1 minute. Add mushrooms, carrots, onion, bell pepper, zucchini, garlic, oregano, cumin, chili powder and thyme; sauté 5 to 8 minutes, stirring frequently.

Add vegetarian beef, beans and tomatoes. Lower heat to simmer. Cook, uncovered, 20 minutes, stirring occasionally. Stir in cilantro.

Serving Size (338g), Amount Per Serving: Calories 220, Calories from Fat 35, Total Fat 4g (6% DV), Saturated Fat 0.5g (3% DV), Trans Fat 0g, Cholesterol 0mg (0% DV), Sodium 880mg (37% DV), Potassium 530mg (15% DV), Total Carbohydrate 31g (10% DV), Dietary Fiber 11g (44% DV), Sugars 3g, Protein 22g, Vitamin A (120% DV), Vitamin C (50% DV), Calcium (15% DV), Iron (20% DV), Vitamin K (10% DV), Riboflavin (15% DV), Niacin (15% DV), Vitamin B6 (15% DV), Pantothenic Acid (10% DV), Phosphorus (10% DV), Selenium (10% DV), Copper (15% DV), Manganese (20% DV). Percent Daily Values (DV) are based on a 2,000 calorie diet.

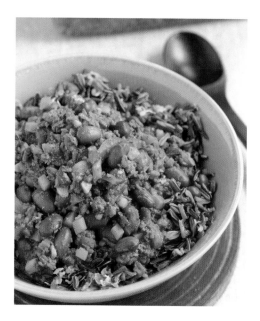

Raspberry Smoothie

Prep: 5 min **Serves**: 3

1   medium DOLE Banana
1   cup DOLE Frozen Tropical Gold Pineapple Chunks,
      partially thawed
1   cup DOLE Frozen Raspberries, partially thawed
2   containers (8 oz each) nonfat raspberry yogurt
½   cup (2 oz) soy protein or whey powder

Combine banana, pineapple, raspberries, yogurt and soy protein in blender or food processor. Cover; blend until smooth.

Serving Size (374g). Amount Per Serving: Calories 390, Calories from Fat 10, Total Fat 1g (2% DV), Saturated Fat 0g (0% DV), Trans Fat 0g, Cholesterol 5mg (2% DV), Sodium 290mg (12% DV), Potassium 630mg (18% DV), Total Carbohydrate 78g (26% DV), Dietary 7g (28% DV), Sugars 63g, Protein 23g, Vitamin A (2% DV), Vitamin C (45% DV), Calcium (25% DV), Iron (20% DV), Thiamin (10% DV), Vitamin B6 (15% DV), Folate (20% DV), Phosphorus (15% DV), Magnesium (10% DV), Copper (25% DV), Manganese (90% DV). Percent Daily Values (DV) are based on a 2,000 calorie diet.

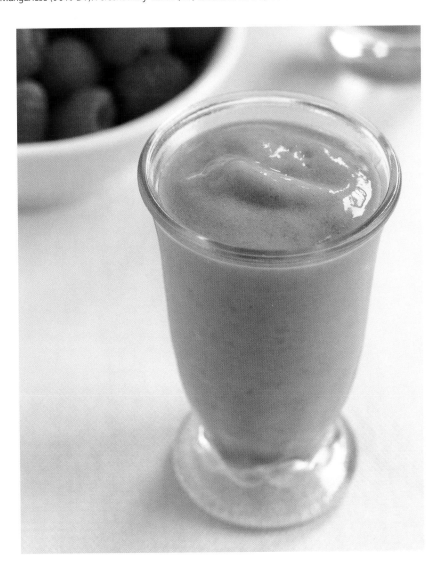

DOLE DIET TIP

Fiber fights breast cancer! A University of Leeds study found that premenopausal women with the highest fiber intake had half the breast cancer risk of those who ate the least amount. Get the recommended 25 grams of fiber from a cup of black beans, a cup of raspberries, a pear and a banana.

Springtime Spinach Salad

Prep: 15 min. **Serves:** 6

½	lb fresh DOLE Asparagus or 1 package (10 oz) frozen asparagus tips
¼	cup water
1	package (6 oz) DOLE Baby Spinach
1	pint fresh DOLE Strawberries, sliced
1	cup julienne-sliced DOLE Red Onion
⅔	cup crumbled feta or blue cheese
½	cup bottled raspberry vinaigrette or red wine vinaigrette

Break off woody ends of fresh asparagus (the bottom 1" to 1½") and discard. Cut asparagus into 1" lengths. Place in microwavable dish with water. Microwave on high 3 minutes. Immediately rinse asparagus under cold water 1 minute; drain well. Place asparagus, spinach, strawberries, onion and cheese in large bowl. Toss ingredients well with salad dressing; serve immediately.

Serving size (191g). Amount Per Serving: Calories 140, Calories from Fat 80, Total Fat 9g (14% DV), Saturated Fat 2.5g (13% DV), Trans Fat 0g, Cholesterol 15mg (5% DV), Sodium 390mg (16% DV), Total Carbohydrate 14g (5% DV), Dietary Fiber 4g (16% DV), Sugars 6g, Protein 4g, Vitamin A (25% DV), Vitamin C (60% DV), Calcium (15% DV), Iron (10% DV), Vitamin K (20% DV), Riboflavin (10% DV), Folate (10% DV), Phosphorus (10% DV), Manganese (15% DV). Percent Daily Values (DV) are based on a 2,000 calorie diet.

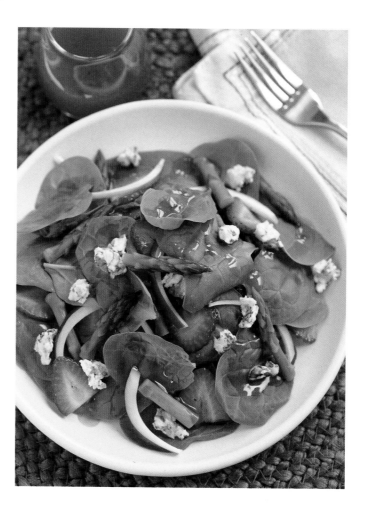

Skillet-Blackened Salmon with Carrot Relish

Prep: 20 min. **Bake:** 15 min. **Serves:** 6

3	cups shredded DOLE Carrots
⅓	cup white wine vinegar
3	Tbsp honey
3	Tbsp chopped DOLE Green Onions
3	Tbsp diced red or green bell pepper
¾	tsp ground mustard
¼	tsp celery seed
1	tsp brown mustard
2	tsp olive oil
2¼	lb salmon fillets (6 pieces)
¾	cup salsa

Preheat oven to 375°F.

Stir carrots, vinegar, honey, onions, bell pepper, mustard and celery seed in medium glass or stainless steel bowl. Set aside.

Mix together brown mustard and oil. Brush on salmon. Sear in hot sauté pan or griddle.

Spoon salsa over salmon. Finish cooking in oven 10 to 15 minutes or until salmon is cooked through. Serve carrot relish over salmon.

Serving Size (299g). Amount Per Serving: Calories 390, Calories from Fat 140, Total Fat 16g (25% DV), Saturated Fat 2.5g (13% DV), Trans Fat 0g. Cholesterol 120mg (40% DV), Sodium 270mg (11% DV), Potassium 1,350mg, Total Carbohydrate 17g (6% DV), Dietary Fiber 2g (8% DV), Sugars 13g, Protein 44g, Vitamin A (220% DV), Vitamin C (20% DV), Calcium (6% DV), Iron (10% DV), Vitamin D (120% DV), Vitamin E (15% DV), Vitamin K (20% DV), Thiamin (35% DV), Riboflavin (50% DV), Niacin (90% DV), Vitamin B6 (90% DV), Folate (15% DV), Vitamin B12 (90% DV), Pantothenic Acid (35% DV), Phosphorus (45% DV), Magnesium (20% DV), Zinc (10% DV), Selenium (110% DV), Copper (30% DV), Molybdenum (10% DV). Percent Daily Values (DV) are based on a 2,000 calorie diet.

DOLE DIET TIP

Not only does fish have roughly half the calories and less than a tenth the saturated fat of beef, research suggests that it helps you feel full longer. Plus, lab studies found that the omega-3 fatty acids in fish prevented fat-cell growth.

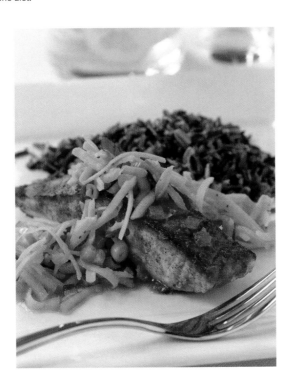

SKILLET-BLACKENED
SALMON WITH
CARROT RELISH

FOOD PREP TIP

For the Mango Vinaigrette, place ¾ cup DOLE Frozen Mango Chunks, thawed; ⅓ cup DOLE Frozen Raspberries, thawed; ¾ cup orange juice; 2½ Tbsp rice vinegar; and 1½ Tbsp honey in blender or food processor. Cover; blend until smooth. Makes 1¾ cup.

Roasted Fennel Spinach Salad with Chicken

Prep: 20 min. **Bake:** 1 hr. **Serves:** 6

¾	lb fennel, cut in half
1	package (6 oz) DOLE Baby Spinach
1½	lb grilled chicken breast, cut into chunks
1	can (14 oz) artichoke hearts, quartered and drained
1	jar (6 oz) marinated artichoke hearts, drained
⅔	cup shredded DOLE Carrots
1⅓	cups fat-free Mango Vinaigrette
⅓	cup slivered almonds, toasted

Preheat oven to 375°F.

Place fennel on baking sheet coated with cooking spray.

Bake 45 to 60 minutes or until tender. Cool slightly; cut into cubes.

Combine fennel, spinach, chicken, artichoke hearts and carrots in large bowl. Pour Mango Vinaigrette (see Food Prep Tip at left) over salad. Toss to coat. Sprinkle with almonds.

Serving Size (368g). Amount Per Serving: Calories 420, Calories from Fat 200, Total Fat 22g (34% DV), Saturated Fat 2g (10% DV), Trans Fat 0g, Cholesterol 60mg (20% DV), Sodium 1,310mg (55% DV), Potassium 510mg (15% DV), Total Carbohydrate 29g (10% DV), Dietary Fiber 11g (44% DV), Sugars 7g, Protein 32g, Vitamin A (70% DV), Vitamin C (40% DV), Calcium (8% DV), Iron (20% DV), Vitamin K (15% DV), Folate (20% DV), Phosphorus (10% DV), Magnesium (15% DV), Copper (10% DV), Manganese (20% DV). Percent Daily Values (DV) are based on a 2,000 calorie diet.

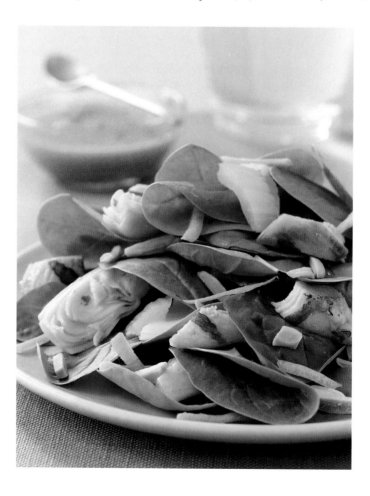

Denver Breakfast Sandwich

Prep: 20 min. **Cook:** 12 min. **Serves:** 4

1	cup chopped tomatoes
⅔	cup chopped red or green bell pepper
⅓	cup chopped DOLE Onion
2	cups liquid egg substitute
¼	tsp ground black pepper
8	slices whole grain bread, toasted

Sauté tomatoes, bell pepper and onion until tender in large nonstick skillet coated with cooking spray, about 5 minutes.

Add egg substitute and black pepper; cook, stirring often, until just set.

Place about 1 cup egg mixture on 1 slice of toast and top with another slice. Cut in half diagonally. Repeat for each sandwich.

Serving Size (276g). Amount Per Serving: Calories 270, Calories from Fat 60, Total Fat 6g (9 % DV), Saturated Fat 1.5g (8 % DV), Trans Fat 0g, Cholesterol 0mg (0 % DV), Sodium 540mg (23 % DV), Potassium 610mg (17 % DV), Total Carbohydrate 29g (10 % DV), Dietary Fiber 5g (20 % DV), Sugars 8g, Protein 23g, Vitamin A (25 % DV), Vitamin C (50 % DV), Calcium (15 % DV), Iron (25 % DV), Thiamin (20 % DV), Riboflavin (30 % DV), Niacin (10 % DV), Vitamin B6 (10 % DV), Folate (20 % DV), Pantothenic Acid (35 % DV), Phosphorus (30 % DV), Magnesium (15 % DV), Zinc (15 % DV), Selenium (70 % DV), Copper (10 % DV), Manganese (60 % DV). Percent Daily Values (DV) are based on a 2,000 calorie diet.

DOLE DIET TIP

Research shows breakfast eaters burn an extra 200 to 300 calories per day. Perhaps that's why a study in the *Journal of Epidemiology* found that those who skip breakfast are 4.5 times more likely to be obese than those who eat a morning meal.

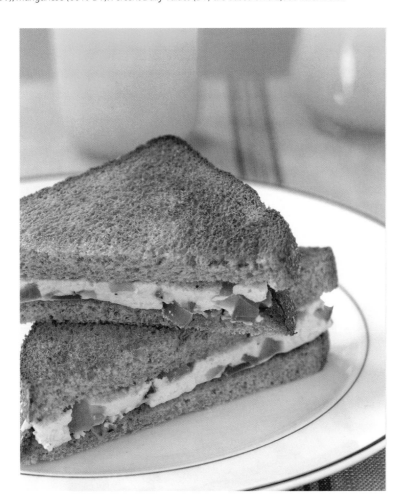

DENVER BREAKFAST
SANDWICH

FOOD PREP TIP

If desired, substitute ⅓ cup bottled balsamic vinaigrette for the dressing in the Apple and Walnut Salad recipe.

Apple and Walnut Salad

Prep: 10 min. **Serves**: 4

1	*package (10 oz) DOLE Very Veggie Salad*
1	*DOLE Apple, cored and thinly sliced*
1	*DOLE Green Apple, cored and thinly sliced*
¼	*cup crumbled blue cheese*
½	*cup chopped walnuts, toasted*
¼	*cup olive oil*
4	*tsp balsamic or red wine vinegar*
1	*Tbsp finely chopped shallot*
1	*tsp Dijon mustard*

Toss salad, apples, blue cheese and walnuts in large bowl.

Stir oil, vinegar, shallot and mustard until blended in a separate bowl.

Pour dressing over salad; toss to coat.

Serving Size (177g). Amount Per Serving: Calories 300, Calories from Fat 230, Total Fat 26g (40% DV), Saturated 4.5g (23% DV), Trans Fat 0g, Cholesterol 5mg (2% DV), Sodium 160mg (7% DV), Total Carbohydrate 15g (5% DV), Dietary Fiber 3g (12% DV), Sugars 10g, Protein 5g, Vitamin A (60% DV), Vitamin C (25% DV), Calcium (8% DV), Iron (8% DV), Vitamin E (10% DV), Vitamin K (15% DV), Phosphorus (10% DV), Copper (15% DV), Manganese (25% DV). Percent Daily Values (DV) are based on a 2,000 calorie diet.

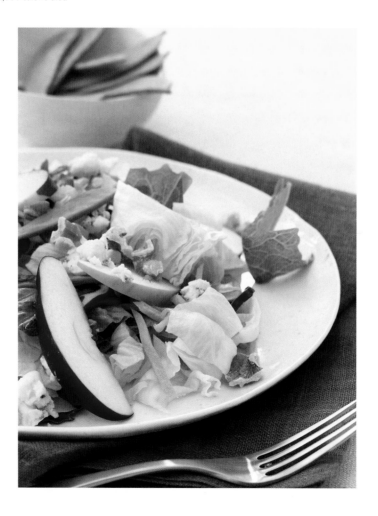

Bay Scallops with Green Beans

Prep: 20 min. **Cook:** 15 min. **Serves:** 4

3   cups 1" pieces green beans
1   cup chunked red bell pepper
1   jalapeño chili pepper, finely chopped (1 Tbsp)
2   cloves garlic, minced
2   Tbsp olive oil
1   lb bay scallops
1   Tbsp prepared pesto sauce
1   Tbsp chopped DOLE Cilantro

Sauté green beans, bell pepper, chili pepper and garlic in oil in large nonstick skillet over medium-high heat until just tender, 8 to 10 minutes.

Add scallops and pesto sauce. Continue cooking, stirring occasionally, until scallops are just cooked through, about 5 minutes. Stir in cilantro.

Serving Size (248g). Amount per Serving: Calories 360, Calories from Fat 190, Total Fat 21g (32% DV), Saturated Fat 4.5g (23% DV), Trans Fat 0g, Cholesterol 70mg (23% DV), Sodium 640mg (27% DV), Potassium 610mg (17% DV), Total Carbohydrate 20g (7% DV), Dietary Fiber 3g (12% DV), Sugars 2g, Protein 23g, Vitamin A (40% DV), Vitamin C (60% DV), Calcium (10% DV), Iron (10% DV), Vitamin E (20% DV), Vitamin K (25% DV), Thiamin (10% DV), Riboflavin (15% DV), Niacin (15% DV), Vitamin B6 (15% DV), Folate (20% DV), Vitamin B12 (25% DV), Phosphorus (35% DV), Magnesium (25% DV), Zinc (10% DV), Selenium (45% DV), Copper (10% DV), Manganese (25% DV). Percent Daily Values (DV) are based on a 2,000 calorie diet.

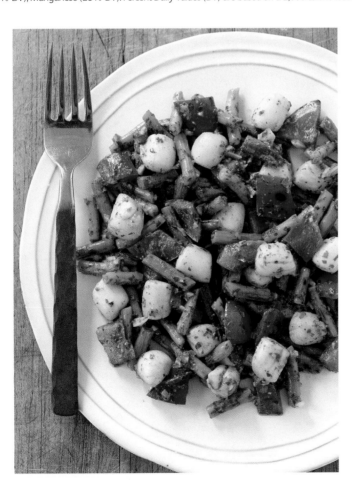

DOLE DIET TIP

University of Wisconsin researchers found that the body burns unsaturated fats more efficiently than saturated fats after exercising. Unsaturated fats include avocado, olive oil, nuts and fatty fish, while saturated sources include whole milk, butter and red meat.

BAY SCALLOPS WITH GREEN BEANS

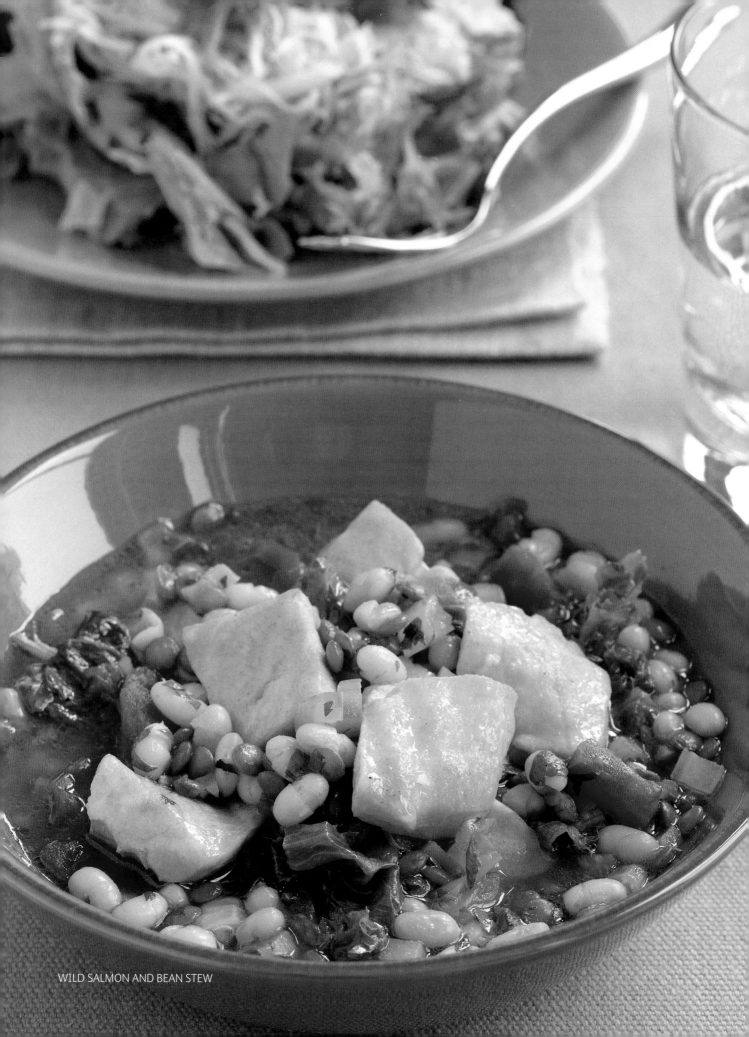

WILD SALMON AND BEAN STEW

Wild Salmon and Bean Stew

Prep: 25 min. **Cook:** 20 min. **Serves:** 8

1½	cups chopped DOLE Celery
1½	cups chopped DOLE Carrots
¾	cup chopped DOLE Onion
2	cloves garlic, minced
1½	tsp ground cumin
2	Tbsp almond oil
⅓	cup unsweetened soy or whey protein powder
6	cups vegetable broth
1	can (14½ oz) diced tomatoes with mild green chilies
3	cups canned navy beans, rinsed and drained
1	cup cooked brown lentils
1	lb wild salmon fillet, cut into 1" cubes
3	cup bite-size pieces chicory
2	Tbsp chopped DOLE Cilantro

Sauté celery, carrots, onion, garlic and cumin in oil in large stockpot over medium-high heat, stirring frequently, 5 to 10 minutes. Stir in protein powder until blended.

Add broth, tomatoes, beans and lentils; bring to a boil. Add salmon, chicory and cilantro; simmer 8 to 10 minutes, or until salmon is cooked through.

Serving Size (473g). Amount Per Serving: Calories 470, Calories from Fat 90, Total Fat 10g (15 % DV), Saturated Fat 1g (5 % DV), Trans Fat 0g, Cholesterol 40mg (13 % DV), Sodium 1,340mg (56 % DV), Potassium 1,650mg (47 % DV), Total Carbohydrate 63g (21 % DV), Dietary Fiber 23g (92 % DV), Sugars 7g, Protein 36g, Vitamin A (110 % DV), Vitamin C (20 % DV), Calcium (20 % DV), Iron (35 % DV), Vitamin D (40 % DV), Vitamin E (15 % DV), Vitamin K (60 % DV), Thiamin (60 % DV), Riboflavin (30 % DV), Niacin (45 % DV), Vitamin B6 (50 % DV), Folate (90 % DV), Vitamin B12 (30 % DV), Pantothenic Acid (20 % DV), Phosphorus (60 % DV), Magnesium (45 % DV), Zinc (25 % DV), Selenium (50 % DV), Copper (50 % DV), Manganese (80 % DV), Molybdenum (30 % DV). Percent Daily Values (DV) are based on a 2,000 calorie diet.

DOLE DIET TIP

It's best to get nutrients from food, not supplements. The Dole Diet provides 100 percent of your nutrition needs mainly from whole foods, in which nutrients work synergistically. Supplements pose vitamin-toxicity risks, and may even interfere with your body's ability to naturally absorb nutrients from food.

Dole Diet Two-Week Summary

Nutrient	Mon.	Tue.	Wed.	Thur.	Fri.	Sat.	Sun.	Mon.
	Day 1/1	Day 1/2	Day 1/3	Day 1/4	Day 1/5	Day 1/6	Day 1/7	Day 2/1
Calories	1,990	1,510	1,670	1,490	1,570	1,580	1,620	1,490
Calories from Fat	710	320	660	310	280	540	500	630
Total Fat/g	79	35	74	34	32	61	56	65
Saturated Fat/g	9.0	4.5	8.0	6.0	4.0	6.0	7.0	8.0
Trans Fat/g	0	0	0	0	0	0	0	0
Cholesterol/mg	75	90	240	95	90	75	275	170
Carbohydrates/g	386	267	176	234	167	189	157	146
Protein/g	144	54	96	78	95	89	129	98
Sodium	107%	57%	103%	36%	116%	108%	78%	53%
Potassium	208%	112%	117%	97%	134%	127%	125%	110%
Dietary Fiber	288%	140%	164%	128%	168%	120%	136%	100%
Vitamin A	170%	220%	470%	40%	820%	270%	220%	300%
Vitamin C	400%	830%	470%	380%	750%	740%	380%	180%
Calcium	110%	110%	90%	50%	100%	140%	70%	110%
Iron	150%	200%	100%	70%	110%	180%	90%	160%
Vitamin D	252%	150%	40%	8%	56%	35%	130%	130%
Vitamin E	140%	80%	130%	60%	80%	140%	80%	150%
Vitamin K	370%	170%	1,510%	80%	1,850%	290%	730%	80%
Vitamin B1—Thiamin	200%	200%	100%	60%	120%	200%	110%	180%
Vitamin B2—Riboflavin	170%	200%	90%	70%	100%	180%	130%	230%
Vitamin B3—Niacin	160%	170%	60%	140%	90%	200%	180%	260%
Vitamin B6	140%	210%	90%	100%	130%	200%	190%	260%
Folic Acid	350%	230%	180%	60%	200%	250%	130%	150%
Vitamin B12	240%	570%	25%	70%	300%	160%	110%	210%
Vitamin B5	140%	190%	45%	35%	60%	140%	70%	160%
Phosphorus	250%	120%	130%	130%	130%	150%	170%	160%
Magnesium	260%	100%	140%	110%	110%	160%	110%	120%
Zinc	240%	340%	60%	50%	140%	150%	60%	150%
Selenium	220%	260%	100%	450%	170%	140%	230%	160%
Copper	380%	280%	120%	90%	180%	110%	90%	100%

Tue.	Wed.	Thur.	Fri.	Sat.	Sun.	Nutrient	Diet
Day 2/2	Day 2/3	Day 2/4	Day 2/5	Day 2/6	Day 2/7		Daily Average
1,900	1,500	1,810	1,260	1,200	1,600	Average Calories/day	1,585
710	340	700	220	430	580	% Calories from Total Fat	25%
79	38	78	25	48	64	Total Fat/g	55
13.0	6.0	9.0	4.0	7.0	10.0	% Calories from Saturated Fat	3%
0	0	0	0	0	0	Trans Fat/g	0
100	205	130	180	45	125	Cholesterol/mg	135
182	103	182	155	159	195	% Calories from Carbohydrates	39%
129	92	114	115	49	80	Protein/g	195%
93%	63%	71%	81%	68%	63%	Sodium	78%
125%	97%	144%	125%	87%	109%	Potassium	123%
168%	80%	164%	96%	100%	144%	Dietary Fiber	143%
260%	590%	340%	540%	430%	500%	Vitamin A	369%
380%	210%	540%	380%	410%	380%	Vitamin C	459%
100%	45%	130%	150%	110%	140%	Calcium	104%
110%	50%	180%	180%	70%	170%	Iron	130%
25%	120%	160%	35%	35%	35%	Vitamin D	87%
80%	50%	180%	70%	50%	140%	Vitamin E	102%
110%	280%	80%	510%	300%	170%	Vitamin K	466%
200%	70%	280%	170%	70%	190%	Vitamin B1—Thiamin	154%
150%	100%	300%	180%	50%	210%	Vitamin B2—Riboflavin	154%
210%	170%	300%	280%	35%	180%	Vitamin B3—Niacin	174%
180%	150%	320%	220%	80%	180%	Vitamin B6	175%
170%	90%	210%	190%	90%	170%	Folic Acid	176%
80%	100%	270%	140%	45%	130%	Vitamin B12	175%
90%	80%	160%	140%	35%	150%	Vitamin B5	107%
180%	110%	210%	160%	90%	140%	Phosphorus	152%
110%	70%	140%	130%	90%	120%	Magnesium	126%
90%	40%	170%	140%	30%	170%	Zinc	131%
180%	190%	150%	190%	70%	370%	Selenium	206%
150%	70%	170%	60%	60%	110%	Copper	141%

Underscored page references indicate sidebars, tables, and marginal tips.

A

Abdominal fat
    health risks from, 245–46, 245
    strength training reducing, 257, 331
Aerobic exercise, 159, 279, 280, 281, 282–83
Age-related macular degeneration (AMD), 72, 163, 164, 166, 167, 169
Aging
    chromosome breakdown with, 17
    exercise slowing, 281
    factors affecting, 4
    high blood pressure and, 152
    immune function and, 30, 231–32
    loss of muscle mass with, 279, 280
    mental decline with
        cause of, 187
        preventing, 188–97
    obesity and, 246, 250
Alcohol, effects on
    bone health, 217, 226
    brain health, 194
    breast-feeding, 180
    heart health, 156
Almonds
    Almond Turkey Salad with Cranberry Vinaigrette, 325
    Banana Almond Pancakes, 324
    Chicken Apple Almond Salad, 328
    for immunity, 235
    as superfood, 116
    vitamin E in, 324
Alpha-carotene, 70, 155
Alzheimer's disease
    incidence of, 189
    obesity and, 188
    preventing, with
        blueberries, 190
        choline, 39
        fish, 91, 193
        fruit and vegetable juice, 193
        green tea, 76
        niacin, 27, 194
        quercetin, 80, 190
        vitamin E, 43, 193
    vitamin B12 deficiency with, 35
AMD. See Age-related macular degeneration
American diet, problems with, 128
Ames, Bruce, 15, 16–17, 298
Amish, activity levels of, 246
Anderson, John, 217–18
Anemia, 16, 49
Antacids, affecting phosphorus intake, 52
Anthocyanins, 74–75, 132, 138, 151, 158
Antioxidants
    anthocyanins, 74–75, 132, 138, 151, 158

anti-aging effects of, 4
for bone health, 218
carotenoids, 69–72, 129–30, 133, 151, 163
flavanols, 75–77, 138, 154
flavones, 78
flavonoids, 73–74, 130, 133, 141
flavonols, 80–81
from foods vs. supplements, 134, 140–41, 146, 187
for immunity, 235
isoflavones, 79
for joint health, 202–3
for leukemia prevention, 178
for lowering LDL cholesterol, 151
neutralizing free radicals, 73, 133, 135, 135, 137, 138, 138, 163, 202
ORAC scores of, 73, 74, 133, 135, 137
overview of, 133–34, 135, 137–38
for preventing free-radical damage, 187
sources of, 74, 133, 150, 187 (see also specific foods)
synergistic effects of, 15
Apples
    antioxidants in, 132, 135, 137
    Apple and Walnut Salad, 338
    Chicken Apple Almond Salad, 328
    Curried Apple and Butternut Squash Soup, 305
    for preventing Alzheimer's disease, 190
    quercetin in, 132, 190, 232, 233
    as superfood, 102
    for weight loss, 328
Arthritis. See Joint health; Osteoarthritis; Rheumatoid arthritis
Artichokes, as superfood, 111
Arugula, as superfood, 106
Asparagus, as superfood, 107
Astronauts, antioxidant protection for, 135
Atherosclerosis, 145, 146, 147
Atrial fibrillation, 147
Avocado
    Turkey, Avocado and Cheese Wrap, 331

B

Balance, for preventing falls, 283
Bananas
    Banana Almond Pancakes, 324
    fat-burning from, 318
    for immunity, 236
    influencing gender of baby, 60, 177
    nutrients in, 135, 137
    as superfood, 93
Beans
    Caribbean Beans and Wild Rice, 306
    Chili non Carne, 332
    nutrients in, 90, 137
    as superfood, 120–21
    Tuscan White Bean Soup, 323
    Wild Salmon and Bean Stew, 341
Beets

Turkish Chicken with Spiced Dates, with Grilled Carrots and Beets, 314
Belly fat. See Abdominal fat
Berries. See also specific berries
    for immunity, 235
    Mixed Berry Gazpacho, 315
    for protecting astronauts, 135
    quercetin in, 232, 233, 235
Beta-carotene
    health benefits from, 69
        for bones, 226
        for eyes, 163, 167
        reduced CRP, 69, 155
    vitamin A and, 163
Beta-carotene supplements, 72, 140
Beta-cryptoxanthin, 70, 155
Betaine, for pregnancy health, 175
Betanin, for lowering LDL cholesterol, 151
Bioavailability, of food constituents, 132
Biotin, overview of, 31–32
Birth control failure, obesity and, 178, 180
Birth defects
    choline deficiency and, 39
    folate preventing, 32, 33, 175
Black beans
    Caribbean Beans and Wild Rice, 306
    as superfood, 120
Blackberries, as superfood, 97
Black cod, as superfood, 115
Bladder cancer, vitamin E preventing, 42
Blood-brain barrier, diet protecting, 194
Blood pressure control. See also High blood pressure
    chocolate for, 154
    vegetarian protein for, 89
Blood sugar
    chromium reducing, 48
    exercise controlling, 280
Blueberries
    Blueberry Smoothie, 304
    health benefits from, 75, 75
    ORAC score of, 75, 133, 137
    for preventing Alzheimer's disease, 190
    quercetin in, 80, 190, 232
    as superfood, 93
BMI, 247, 255
Body fat, 245–46, 257, 281–82
Body mass index (BMI), 247, 255
Bone health
    antioxidants for, 218
    exercise for, 219, 227, 227
    foods to avoid for, 217, 223, 226
    fruits and vegetables for, 88, 218, 219, 253, 253
    LDL cholesterol and, 226
    nutrients for
        calcium, 46, 217, 220, 220, 227
        copper, 50
        fluoride, 49
        folate, 32, 224
        magnesium, 217, 220

manganese, 57
potassium, 60, 61, 217, 223
vitamin B12, 35, 223
vitamin C, 36, 217, 224
vitamin D, 40, 217, 223
vitamin K, 45, 224
zinc, 217
prebiotic fiber for, 225
weight-bearing exercise for, 219, 253, 257
Bone loss. *See also* Osteoporosis
causes of, 218, 252–53
Brain health
alcohol and, 194
anthocyanins for, 132
foods for, 189–94
heart health and, 196
meditation for, 197
mind exercise for, 189
nutrients for
choline, 39
magnesium, 56
manganese, 57
niacin, 27, 194
selenium, 61
vitamin B12, 35
vitamin E, 43, 193
zinc, 65
obesity and, 188
physical activity for, 196–97
quercetin for, 80
Brazil nuts
for joint health, 210
selenium in, 61, 65, 210
as superfood, 116
Bread, whole-wheat, as superfood, 123
Breakfast
calorie burning from, 337
improving brain function, 190
for preventing overeating, 248
for weight loss, 261
Breast cancer
preventing, with
choline, 39
fiber, 20
vitamin D, 41
soy isoflavones and, 79
Breast-feeding, 180, 181, 182–83
British paradox, 140
Broccoli
anticancer benefits of, 82, 83
Broccoli and Pea Potage with Tarragon, 313
for eye health, 167
for joint health, 209
Sesame Ginger Frittata with Broccoli and Shrimp, 329
as superfood, 104
Bromelain, 83, 85, 203, 205
Brown rice, as superfood, 123
Brussels sprouts, as superfood, 110

Butternut squash
Curried Apple and Butternut Squash Soup, 305
for immunity, 238
for joint health, 205
as superfood, 107

C
Cabbage
anticancer benefits of, 82–83
red, 138
as superfood, 111
Caesar salad
Southwest Caesar Salad, 309
Calcium
for bone health, 47, 217, 220, 220, 227
loss of, in perspiration, 226, 287
overview of, 46–47
for pregnancy health, 177
role of, in plants and animals, 129
in supplements, 141
vs. food, 47, 220
for weight loss, 268–69
Calorie burning
from breakfast, 337
in cold weather, 153
from walking, 232
for weight loss, 272
Calorie density of food, 270–71
Calories, overconsumption of, 14, 298
Cancer. *See also specific types of cancer*
deaths from, 15
folate and, 33
magnesium deficiency and, 16, 17
micronutrient supplementation and, 15
obesity linked to, 248–50
preventing, with
anthocyanins, 75
calcium, 46
carotenoids, 69, 70
flavones, 78
glucosinolates, 82–83
green tea, 76–77
magnesium, 55
quercetin, 80, 81, 233
selenium, 61
vitamin B6, 31, 31
vitamin D, 41
vitamin K, 45
zeaxanthin, 72
soy isoflavones and, 79
vitamin D deficiency and, 16, 17
Cantaloupe
for eye health, 167
as superfood, 98
Carbohydrates
diets restricting, 19, 264
function of, 18
good vs. bad, 18, 18
limiting, for heart health, 145
Cardiovascular disease. *See also* Heart

disease
preventing, with
beta-carotene, 69
fiber, 20
tomatoes, 70
reducing death risk from, 70
Cardiovascular health. *See also* Heart health
anthocyanins for, 75
flavanols for, 76, 76
Carotenoids, 69–72, 129–30, 133, 151, 163
Carrots
Skillet-Blackened Salmon with Carrot Relish, 335
as superfood, 108
Turkish Chicken with Spiced Dates, with Grilled Carrots and Beets, 314
vitamin A in, 25
Cashews, as superfood, 116
Cataracts, 26, 72, 164, 166, 167, 169
Catfish, as superfood, 115
Cauliflower
anticancer benefits of, 82, 83
as superfood, 106
Celery, nutrients in, 81
Cereals, fortified, 27, 34
Cervical cancer, preventing, 89
Cheese
Turkey, Avocado and Cheese Wrap, 331
Cherries
for joint health, 205
as superfood, 102
Chicken
Chicken Apple Almond Salad, 328
Roasted Fennel Spinach Salad with Chicken, 336
Turkish Chicken with Spiced Dates, with Grilled Carrots and Beets, 314
Chicory, as superfood, 105
Children
obesity in (*see* Obesity, in children)
osteoporosis in, 219
Chili
Chili non Carne, 332
Chlorophyll, in plants, 129
Chocolate
flavanols in, 75
for heart health, 154
Cholesterol
cinnamon lowering, 73
diet affecting, 145, 148
function and production of, 147–48
HDL
chocolate and, 154
exercise increasing, 282
function of, 145, 148
obesity lowering, 248
heart disease risk from, 145, 147, 148
LDL
atherosclerosis from, 145

bone health and, 226
exercise lowering, 282
foods lowering, 150–51, 154
function of, 148
vitamin C and, 36
vitamin E supplements and, 43, 141
niacin for, 27
obesity and, 147, 248, 250
Choline
for improving memory, 39, 173, 175
overview of, 38–39
for pregnancy health, 39, 173, 175
Chondroitin, 203
Chromium, overview of, 48
Cinnamon, antioxidant rating of, 73
Citrus fruits, flavanones in, 77, 77
Cloves, antioxidant rating of, 73
Cocoa
for heart health, 154
ORAC score of, 133
Cod, black, as superfood, 115
Colas, effect on bones, 223
Colds, preventing, 232, 235, 238, 286–87
Cold weather
calorie-burning activities during, 153
heart attacks and, 153
Collard greens, as superfood, 103
Colon cancer. See also Colorectal cancer
folate fortification and, 33
obesity and, 249
preventing, with
blueberries, 75
fiber, 20
quercetin, 233
vitamin D, 41
Colorectal cancer. See also Colon cancer
folate and, 33
preventing, with
fiber, 20
flavonols, 81
selenium, 61
red meat and, 24
vitamin B6 deficiency and, 31
Commercials, exercising during, 159
Conrad, Andrew, 4–5
Copper
deficiency of, 47, 49
overview of, 49–50
for pregnancy health, 50, 177
zinc affecting absorption of, 50, 65
Crab
Roasted Red Pepper and Crab Chowder, 319
Cranberries
health benefits from, 75, 325
as superfood, 101
Cravings
during pregnancy, 174
reducing
with exercise, 79, 287
with fruits and vegetables, 89

time needed for, 156
C-reactive protein (CRP)
eye disease and, 166
as heart disease predictor, 155–56
reducing, 69, 155–56
vitamin C and, 36
Cruciferous vegetables. See also specific cruciferous vegetables
anticancer benefits of, 82–83
antioxidants in, 138
C3G, fat burning from, 249
Cycling, osteopenia from, 227

D
Dates
Deglet Noor, as superfood, 100
Turkish Chicken with Spiced Dates, with Grilled Carrots and Beets, 314
Dehydration, 255
Dementia. See also Alzheimer's disease
incidence of, 189
obesity and, 188
preventing, 189, 197
Dental health, nutrients for, 40, 48, 49, 49
Depression
nutrient deficiencies with, 33, 35, 41
relieving, with
exercise, 295
music, 35
omega-3 fatty acids, 193
Diabetes
cinnamon for, 73
gestational, 174, 178, 180
obesity and, 147, 248, 252
preventing, 31, 56, 261, 326
selenium and, 61
vitamin D deficiency with, 41
Dietary Reference Intakes (DRIs), 90
Diet foods, overeating, 275
Diet myths, 264–75
Diets
bad
changing, 17
characteristics of, 16
fad, 270, 272, 272
low-carb, dangers of, 19, 264
Disease, factors influencing, 4, 5, 17
DNA damage
cancer from, 17
causes of, 5, 16
DNA repair, 4, 5, 31
Dole, scientific research of, 4–5, 8–9
Dole Diet
description of, 298–99
meal plans for, 300–303
philosophy behind, 9
recipes for
Almond Turkey Salad with Cranberry Vinaigrette, 325
Apple and Walnut Salad, 338
Asian-Style Wilted Kale, 321

Banana Almond Pancakes, 324
Bay Scallops with Green Beans, 339
Blueberry Smoothie, 304
Broccoli and Pea Potage with Tarragon, 313
Caribbean Beans and Rice, 306
Chicken Apple Almond Salad, 328
Chili non Carne, 332
Curried Apple and Butternut Squash Soup, 305
Denver Breakfast Sandwich, 337
Egg-White Veggie Omelet, 312
Mixed Berry Gazpacho, 315
Oysters Sautéed in Asian Sauce, 311
Papaya Ginger Smoothie, 318
Pineapple Gazpacho, 308
Porridge with Fruit, 330
Portobello Turkey Loaf, 322
Quinoa Salad, 316
Raspberry Smoothie, 333
Roasted Fennel Spinach Salad with Chicken, 336
Roasted Red Pepper and Crab Chowder, 319
Sesame Ginger Frittata with Broccoli and Shrimp, 329
Skillet-Blackened Salmon with Carrot Relish, 335
Southwest Caesar Salad, 309
Springtime Spinach Salad, 334
Sweet Potato and Spinach Soup, 326
Turkey, Avocado and Cheese Wrap, 331
Turkish Chicken with Spiced Dates, with Grilled Carrots and Beets, 314
Tuscan White Bean Soup, 323
Wild Salmon and Bean Stew, 341
2-week summary of, 342–43
DOLE Portobello Mushrooms. See Mushrooms, DOLE Portobello
Dress sizes, downsizing of, 267
DRIs, 90
Dyslexia, zinc deficiency with, 65

E
Eating out
overeating when, 249, 341
substitutions when, 275
Eggs
Denver Breakfast Sandwich, 337
Egg-White Veggie Omelet, 312
Sesame Ginger Frittata with Broccoli and Shrimp, 329
Energy density of food, 270–71
Epilepsy, manganese deficiency and, 57
Erikson, Keith, 128, 133–34
Esophageal cancer, obesity and, 249, 250
Exercise(s)
aerobic, 159, 279, 280, 281, 282–83
benefits of, 278

anti-aging, 4, 7, 8, <u>281</u>
blood pressure reduction, 153
brain health, 189, 196–97
diabetes prevention, <u>261</u>
gestational diabetes prevention, <u>178</u>
heart health, <u>151</u>, 158–59, 282–83
improved balance, 283, 284
improved immunity, 233, <u>235</u>, 239,
    286–87
improved mood, <u>287</u>, <u>295</u>
improved productivity, <u>286</u>
joint health, 202, <u>213</u>
longevity, 7, 8, 278
osteoporosis prevention, <u>219</u>, <u>220</u>
reduced cravings, <u>79</u>
reduced CRP, 156
reduced health care costs, <u>286</u>
stress relief, <u>147</u>
weight loss, 258, 261, <u>272</u>, 287, <u>308</u>
wound healing, <u>154</u>
during commercials, <u>159</u>
fat burning after, <u>339</u>
finding opportunities for, <u>286</u>
foods for recovery from, <u>288–89</u>
household chores as, <u>281</u>
iron needs with, 54
lack of, obesity from, 254
morning vs. afternoon, <u>180</u>
myth about, 265–66
nutrient deficiencies and, 26, <u>26</u>
recommended amount of, 17, 278, 290
stair climbing as, <u>283</u>
strength-training (see Strength training)
stretching, 285, 286
weight-bearing, increasing bone density,
    <u>219</u>, 253, 257
workouts for
    Circuit of Fitness, 292–95
    First Steps Forward, 292
    Quick Calorie Burn, 290–91
Eye health
    conditions affecting, 166
    nutrients for
        beta-carotene, 163, 167
        lutein, 72, 163, 166–67
        riboflavin, 26, 167
        selenium, 167
        vitamin A, 24, 163
        vitamin C, 167
        vitamin E, 167
        zeaxanthin, 72, 163, 167
        zinc, 169

F
Fad diets, 270, 272, <u>272</u>
Falls, preventing, 283
Fast food, <u>41</u>, 155–56, 250, 254
Fat, body, 245–46, 257, 281–82
Fat burning
    from bananas, <u>318</u>
    from vitamin C, <u>36</u>, <u>319</u>

Fats, dietary
    bone health and, 226
    in Dole Diet, <u>309</u>
    effect on blood-cholesterol levels, 148
    function of, 22
    good vs. bad sources of, 22, <u>22</u>, <u>23</u>, <u>245</u>
        (see also Saturated fats; Trans
        fats; Unsaturated fats)
    heart health and, 145
    immunity and, <u>239</u>
    increased consumption of, 14
    joint health and, 213
    reducing intake of, 271
Fennel
    Roasted Fennel Spinach Salad with
        Chicken, 336
Fetal brain development, choline for, 173
Fiber
    health benefits from, 20, <u>20</u>, 89, <u>148</u>,
        150
    prebiotic, for bone health, 225
    soluble vs. insoluble, 19, 150
    sources of, <u>19</u>
Figs, dried, as superfood, <u>98</u>
Fish
    for heart health, 145
    for joint health, 203, 213
    mercury contamination from, 91, <u>175</u>
    nutrients in, 90–91
    omega-3 fatty acids in, <u>23</u>, 91, 193, 203,
        210, 213, <u>335</u>
    for preventing
        Alzheimer's disease, 91, 193
        eye diseases, 164
    for rheumatoid arthritis, 210
    satiety from, <u>24</u>, 91, <u>335</u>
    as superfood, <u>113–15</u>
Fitness, definition of, 258
Flavanols, 75–77, <u>138</u>, <u>154</u>
Flavanones, 77, <u>77</u>
Flavones, 78
Flavonoids, 73–74, 130, 133, 141
Flavonols, 80–81
Flounder, as superfood, <u>114</u>
Flu, 233, 235, 238
Fluoride, overview of, 48–49
Folate
    for bone health, 32, 224
    overview of, 32–33
    for reducing homocysteine, 32, 146, 224
    vitamin B6 and, <u>31</u>
Folate deficiency, increasing
    homocysteine, 145
Folic acid. See Folate
Food labels
    RDAs on, <u>90</u>
    serving size on, <u>91</u>
Food safety precautions, <u>238</u>
Food variety, for maximizing health
    benefits, 132
Fortified foods, 27, 33, <u>33</u>, <u>34</u>

Fractures
    alcohol and, 226
    homocysteine and, 35, 224
    from osteoporosis, 218
    preventing, with
        calcium, 46, 217
        potassium, 223
        vitamin D, 40, 223
        vitamin K, 45, 224
    vitamin B12 deficiency and, 35
Free radicals
    antioxidants neutralizing, 73, 133, 135,
        <u>135</u>, 137, 138, <u>138</u>, 163, 202
    declining brain function from, 187
    description of, 187
French paradox, <u>76</u>, <u>140</u>
Fried foods, avoiding, 145, <u>148</u>
Fruit enzymes, 83, 85
Fruit juice
    grape, for heart health, 156, 158
    grapefruit, effects on medications, <u>77</u>
    for preventing Alzheimer's disease, 193
Fruits. See also specific fruits
    antioxidants in, 133
    in Dole Diet, <u>315</u>
    health benefits from, 88–89
        anti-aging, 4, 7, 8, 88
        for bones, 253, <u>253</u>
        for brain, 189, 190
        for heart, 145, <u>150</u>, 159
        for joints, 202–3
        longevity, 7, 8
        obesity prevention, 8, 159, <u>250</u>
        weight loss, 89, 128
    inadequate consumption of, 14
    increasing intake of, <u>140</u>
    low energy density of, 270–71
    nutrients in peel of, <u>271</u>
    pectin in, for weight loss, <u>256</u>
    recommended servings of, 298, 299
    vs. sports gels, <u>289</u>
    as superfoods, <u>93–102</u>
    washing, <u>141</u>

G
Gallstone prevention
    fiber for, 20
    magnesium for, <u>56</u>
    nuts for, 90
Garlic, for immunity, 236
Gastroesophageal reflux disease, <u>259</u>
Gastrointestinal cancer, beta-carotene
    supplements and, 140
Gastrointestinal distress, from obesity, 261
Genetic code, nutrition affecting, 4
Genetics, role of, in eye diseases, 164
Gestational diabetes, 174, <u>178</u>, 180
Ginger, for morning sickness, <u>175</u>
Glucosamine, 203
Glucosinolates, 82–83, 138, <u>138</u>
Glutathione, for eye health, 167

GPCS, for bone health, 225
Grapefruit, as superfood, 99
Grapefruit juice, effects on medications, 77
Grape juice, for heart health, 156, 158
Green beans
    Bay Scallops with Green Beans, 339
Green tea
    antioxidants in, 138
    health benefits from, 76–77
Grocery shopping, self-checkout and, 258
Guava, as superfood, 95

H
Hair health, vitamin B5 and, 29
Halibut, as superfood, 113
Hand washing, for preventing colds and
    flu, 235, 238
Hazelnuts, as superfood, 117
Headaches, riboflavin reducing, 26
Head injury, diet and, 194
Health awareness, of men, 45
Hearing loss, folate and, 33
Heart attacks
    cold weather and, 153
    CRP level predicting, 154, 155
    deaths from, 146
    preventing, 146, 154, 159, 282
    recovery after, 159
    risk factors for
        high blood pressure, 248
        high cholesterol, 148
        obesity, 250, 252
        stress, 158
Heart disease. *See also* Cardiovascular
    disease
    antioxidant supplements and, 141
    deaths from, 15
    incidence of, 146
    magnesium levels and, 16
    preventing, with
        diet, 145, 146, 148, 150–51
        quercetin, 233
        vegetarian protein, 89–90
    risk factors for
        chronic inflammation, 154–55
        high blood pressure, 152–53
        high cholesterol, 145, 147, 148
        high homocysteine, 145–46
        obesity, 146, 147, 246, 248, 265, 266
        smoking, 146
        snoring, 151
        stress, 146, 158
Heart health. *See also* Cardiovascular
    health
    brain health and, 196
    exercise for, 151, 158–59, 282–83
    foods for, 89, 145, 148, 150, 154, 155,
        156, 158
    foods to avoid for, 145
    nutrients for
        choline, 38

folate, 33
lycopene, 70
magnesium, 55
niacin, 27
potassium, 59
quercetin, 80
vegetable proteins, 23
vitamin B6, 30
vitamin B12, 35
vitamin C, 36, 205
vitamin D, 40
zinc, 64
    water drinking for, 155
High blood pressure. *See also* Blood
    pressure control
    in children, 250
    effects of, 152
    from excess sodium, 63, 152, 152
    heart disease and, 152–53
    incidence of, 152
    obesity and, 147, 248
    preventing, with
        exercise, 153
        folate, 33
        magnesium, 55, 153
        potassium, 59, 153
        salt restriction, 62
        tea, 152
        vegetarian protein, 23, 153
        vitamin C, 153
        vitamin D, 40
High-fructose corn syrup, 217, 246
High-protein diets, problems with, 19, 264
Homocysteine
    bone fractures and, 35, 224
    heart disease and, 145–46
    nutrients lowering
        choline, 38
        folate, 32, 146, 224
        vitamin B6, 30, 146
        vitamin B12, 35, 223
Hunger control. *See also* Satiety
    soup for, 257, 271, 323
Hypertension. *See* Blood pressure control;
    High blood pressure

I
Immunity
    aging and, 231–32
    challenges to, 233
    exercise for, 233, 235, 239, 286–87
    habits protecting, 238–39
    malnutrition and obesity affecting, 231
    meditation for, 236
    nutrients for
        quercetin, 232–33, 235
        selenium, 62
        sulfur, 236
        vitamin A, 25, 238
        vitamin B6, 30
        vitamin C, 236

vitamin D, 42
vitamin E, 43, 235
zinc, 64, 238
    prebiotic fiber for, 236
    stress and, 238
Infection, obesity and, 253
Inflammation. *See also* C-reactive protein
    (CRP)
    bromelain for, 83, 85
    eye disease and, 166
    as heart disease risk factor, 154–55
    lowering, 155–56
Intelligence, of vegetarians, 190
Interval training workout, 290–91
Inulin, for calcium absorption, 46
Iodine
    overview of, 50–51
    for pregnancy health, 178
Iron
    in Dole Diet, 312
    functions of, 16
    overview of, 52, 54
Iron deficiency, 16, 52, 52, 54, 312
Isoflavones, 79

J
Joint health. *See also* Osteoarthritis;
    Rheumatoid arthritis
    diet for, 202–3, 205–10, 213
    exercise for, 202, 213
    nutrients for
        potassium, 61
        vitamin C, 36, 203, 205, 206
        vitamin D, 40
    turmeric tea for, 212
    weight control for, 212
Joseph, James, 187

K
Kale
    Asian-Style Wilted Kale, 321
    as superfood, 103
Kidney beans, red, as superfood, 120
Kidney stones, contributors to, 63, 226
Kipp, Deborah E., 202–3
Kiwifruits, as superfood, 95
Kuna Indians, cardiovascular health of, 76

L
Lead poisoning, iron deficiency and, 54
Leath, Steven, 128, 129–30
Lettuce, as superfood, 105, 110, 164
Leukemia, antioxidants preventing, 178
Lila, Mary Ann, 9, 128, 130, 132
Lima beans, as superfood, 121
Liver cancer, preventing, 45, 61, 224
Liver disease, manganese toxicity and, 57
Longevity
    factors increasing, 7, 8, 267, 278
    obesity and, 255
Lovelady, Cheryl, 254–55, 257–58

Low-back pain, 280
Low-carb diets, dangers of, 19, 264
Lung cancer
    beta-carotene supplements and, 72, 140
    preventing, with
        quercetin, 81, 233
        selenium, 61
    red meat and, 24
Lung health, vitamin C for, 36
Lutein
    for eye health, 72, 163, 166–67
    food preparation and, 70
    sources of, 72, 164
Lycopene, 70, 155

M
Macadamia nuts, as superfood, 117
Macronutrients, 16. *See also*
        Carbohydrates; Fats, dietary;
        Protein(s)
Macular degeneration. *See* Age-related
        macular degeneration (AMD)
Magnesium
    for blood pressure control, 55, 153
    for bone health, 217, 220
    overview of, 54–56
    zinc supplements and, 65
Magnesium deficiency, 16, 17
Malnutrition
    impairing immunity, 231
    obesity and, 312
Manganese, overview of, 56–57
Mangoes, as superfood, 99
Marriage, weight gain during, 269
Massage, for osteoarthritis relief, 205
McIntosh, Michael, 163–64
Meal planning and frequency, 269
Meat
    avoiding, for bone health, 226
    increased consumption of, 14
    lean, for heart health, 145
    overweight and, 261
    red
        cancer risk from, 24
        eye disease and, 169
        rheumatoid arthritis and, 213
Meditation
    for brain health, 197
    for immunity, 236
Melanoma, zinc preventing, 64
Memory, choline improving, 39, 173, 175
Mental health. *See also* Depression; Mood
    thiamin for, 25
    vegetables for, 89
    vitamin D for, 41
Mercury contamination, from fish, 91, 175
Metabolism, effects on
    crash diets, 272
    green tea, 77
    muscle, 280, 282
    riboflavin, 26

Micronutrients. *See also specific vitamins
        and minerals*
    deficiencies of, 16–17 *(see also specific
        micronutrient deficiencies)*
    functions of, 16
Migraines
    magnesium for, 56
    riboflavin preventing, 26
Milk
    effect on antioxidants in tea, 140
    increasing multiple births, 182
Miscarriage, overweight increasing, 180
Mitochondrial damage, manganese
        preventing, 56
Molecule nutrients, 16
Molybdenum, overview of, 47
Monounsaturated fats, 22, 151, 245
Mood, exercise improving, 287, 295
Morning sickness, 175
Mortality
    nutrients and, 42, 55
    sodium restriction and, 63
Multiple births, milk consumption
        increasing, 182
Multiple sclerosis, vitamin D deficiency
        and, 41
Murdock, David H., 7–9, 88
Muscle mass
    loss of
        with aging, 279, 280
        from dieting, 258
    metabolism increased by, 280, 282
    potassium preserving, 59
Mushrooms
    DOLE Portobello
        for bone health, 223
        for joint health, 210
        Portobello Turkey Loaf, 322
        vitamin D in, 41, 210, 223
    for immunity, 233
    vitamin B5 in, 311
Music, benefits of, 35, 196–97

N
Nail strength, biotin for, 32
Navy beans, as superfood, 120
Nectarines, as superfood, 102
Neonatal hyperthyroidism, iodine
        preventing, 178
NES (Night Eating Syndrome), 188
Neural tube defects
    nutrients preventing, 33, 175
    from zinc deficiency, 178
Newby, L. Kristin, 145–46
Niacin
    for brain health, 27, 194
    overview of, 27
Niacin supplements, 27
Nieman, David C., 9, 231–33, 279–81,
        286–87
Night Eating Syndrome (NES), 188

Nutraceuticals
    benefits of, 130
    from foods vs. supplements, 130, 132
Nutrients. *See also* Macronutrients;
        Micronutrients
    deficiencies of, 14, 16, 52, 269, 272,
        298 *(see also specific nutrient
        deficiencies)*
    definition of, 130
    in foods vs. supplements, 15, 187, 333
    in superfoods *(see* Superfoods*)*
    types of, 16
Nutrition, advantages of understanding,
        33
Nuts. *See also specific nuts*
    choosing, 209
    health benefits from, 90, 238
    as superfood, 116–19

O
Oatmeal
    Porridge with Fruit, 330
    as superfood, 122
Obesity. *See also* Overweight
    BMI determining, 247, 255
    breakfast skipping and, 337
    in children
        aging circulatory system, 159, 250
        brain health and, 188
        health risks of, 250, 252
        high blood pressure from, 152
        parental denial of, 265
        pregnancy diet influencing, 183
        preventing, 181, 250, 252
    contributors to, 245, 254, 266–67, 282,
        298
    diabetes and, 147, 248, 252
    foods preventing, 8, 9, 250
    health effects of, 244, 245–46, 255
        on bones, 218–19, 252–53
        on brain, 188
        cancer, 248–50
        eye disease, 166
        gastrointestinal distress, 261
        heart disease, 146, 147, 246, 248,
            265, 266
        impaired immunity, 231
        inconclusive radiology tests, 252
        infection, 253
        unawareness of, 264
    increase in, 244, 261
    longevity and, 255
    malnutrition and, 312
    in men vs. women, 245
    nutrient deficiencies with, 16, 52, 269,
        298
    osteoarthritis and, 202, 206, 212
    during pregnancy, 174
    rates of, in U.S. states, 248
    reproductive health and, 178, 180
    workplace effects of, 252, 253

Omega-3 fatty acids
  for bone health, 217
  for eye health, 164
  in fish, 23, 91, 193, 203, 210, 213, 335
  for heart health, 145, 146, 150
  for joint health, 203, 213
  for mental state, 193
  for rheumatoid arthritis, 210
  for weight management, 23
Onions
  for osteoporosis prevention, 225
  quercetin in, 190, 232, 233
ORAC scores, of antioxidants, 73, 74, 133, 135, 137
Oranges, navel, as superfood, 97
Osteoarthritis. See also Joint health; Rheumatoid arthritis
  bromelain and papain for, 203
  cause of, 201, 202
  massage for, 205
  nutrients preventing
    selenium, 61, 210
    vitamin C, 206
  obesity and, 202, 206, 212
  strength training and, 280
  symptoms of, 201, 202
Osteopenia, 226, 227
Osteoporosis
  alcohol and, 217
  from calcium loss, 287
  in children, 219
  incidence of, 218
  magnesium for treating, 220
  preventing, with
    exercise, 219, 220
    muscular fitness, 279
    onions, 225
    vitamin K, 224
  vitamin B12 deficiency and, 35, 223
Ovarian cancer, preventing, 41
Overeating
  breakfast preventing, 248
  of diet foods, 275
  from eating out, 249, 341
  reflux from, 259
Overweight. See also Obesity
  BMI determining, 247, 255
  of carnivores vs. vegetarians, 261
  cataracts and, 169
  reproductive health and, 178, 180
  undernourishment with, 14
Oxygen Radical Absorbance Capacity (ORAC). See ORAC scores
Oysters
  Oysters Sautéed in Asian Sauce, 311

P

Pain
  low-back, 280
  music reducing, 35
  from vitamin D deficiency, 41

Pancreatic cancer, preventing, 41, 233
Pantothenic acid. See Vitamin B5
Papain, 83, 85, 203
Papaya
  nutrients in, 83, 85, 203
  Papaya Ginger Smoothie, 318
  as superfood, 97
Parsley, nutrients in, 78
Parsnips, as superfood, 111
Peanuts, as superfood, 117
Pears, for weight loss, 328
Peas
  Broccoli and Pea Potage with Tarragon, 313
Pecans, as superfood, 118
Pectin, for weight loss, 256
Peppers
  red bell
    for immunity, 236
    for joint health, 206
    as superfood, 106
  Roasted Red Pepper and Crab Chowder, 319
Perspiration, calcium loss from, 226, 287
Phone calls, avoiding eating during, 266
Phosphorus
  bone health and, 217
  overview of, 51–52
Phytochemicals
  anthocyanins, 74–75, 132, 138, 151, 158
  carotenoids, 69–72, 129–30, 133, 151, 163
  fat-burning, 249
  flavanols, 75–77, 138, 154
  flavanones, 77, 77
  flavones, 78
  flavonoids, 73–74, 130, 133, 141
  flavonols, 80–81
  fruit enzymes, 83, 85
  functions of, 130
  glucosinolates, 82–83, 138, 138
  isoflavones, 79
  for joint health, 202
  overview of, 68–69
Phytoestrogens, isoflavones as, 79
Pineapple
  bromelain in, 83, 83, 203, 205
  for joint health, 205
  Pineapple Gazpacho, 308
  as superfood, 94
Pine nuts, as superfood, 118
Pinto beans, as superfood, 121
Pistachios, as superfood, 118
Plantains, as superfood, 96
Plant genetics, 4–5
Plants, minerals and pigments in, 129–30
Plums, as superfood, 101
PMS, vitamin D preventing, 42
Polyarthritis, preventing, 70
Polyunsaturated fats, 22, 245

Pomegranate, as superfood, 94
Portion control, 272, 275
Portion sizes, obesity from, 254
Portobello mushrooms. See Mushrooms, DOLE Portobello
Potassium
  for blood pressure control, 59, 153
  for bone health, 60, 61, 217, 223
  influencing gender of baby, 60, 177
  overview of, 59–60
  role of, in plants and animals, 129
Potatoes, as superfood, 109
Prebiotic fiber
  for bone health, 225
  for immunity, 236
Preeclampsia, 174, 177, 180
Pregnancy
  cravings during, 174
  diet during, 174, 183, 183
  fish eating during, 175
  morning sickness during, 175
  nutrients needed during
    antioxidants, 178
    betaine, 175
    calcium, 177
    choline, 39, 173, 175
    copper, 50, 177
    folate, 32, 175
    iodine, 178
    vitamin A, 25
    vitamin D, 177
    zinc, 178
  potassium and, 60, 177
  weight gain during, 174
Premature birth, preventing, 177
Prostate cancer, preventing, with
  fiber, 20
  green tea, 76–77
  lycopene, 70
  quercetin, 80, 81
  selenium, 61
  soy isoflavones, 79
  vegetables, 89
Prostatitis, quercetin preventing, 81
Protein(s)
  diets high in, 19, 264
  excess, effect on bone health, 217
  function of, 23
  good vs. bad sources of, 23, 23, 24
Prunes, as superfood, 95
Pumpkin, as superfood, 112

Q

Quercetin, health benefits of, 80–81, 132, 190, 232–33, 235
Quinoa
  Quinoa Salad, 316
  as superfood, 122

R

Radiology tests, obesity affecting, 252

Raspberries
    Raspberry Smoothie, 333
    as superfood, 98
RDAs, 90
Recipes. *See* Dole Diet, recipes for
Recommended dietary allowances (RDAs), 90
Red meat. *See* Meat, red
Reflux, from overeating, 259
Reproductive health. *See also* Pregnancy
    obesity and, 178, 180
    vegetables for, 89
Resistance training. *See* Strength training
Resistant starch. See also Prebiotic fiber
    in fruits and vegetables, 89, 236, 253, 318
Rheumatoid arthritis. *See also* Joint health; Osteoarthritis
    diet and, 201, 205, 210
    red meat and, 213
    selenium improving, 61, 210
    symptoms of, 201
    vitamin D preventing, 40
Riboflavin
    for eye health, 26, 167
    overview of, 26
Rice, brown, as superfood, 123
Rolls, Barbara J., 270–71, 303

S
Sablefish, as superfood, 115
Salads
    add-ins for, 167
    benefits of, 334
Salmon
    Atlantic, as superfood, 113
    Skillet-Blackened Salmon with Carrot Relish, 335
    Wild Salmon and Bean Stew, 341
Salt. *See* Salt restriction; Sodium
Salt restriction
    high blood pressure and, 62
    mortality and, 63
Sardines, as superfood, 114
Satiety
    from fish, 24, 91, 335
    posture and, 269
    slow eating for, 269
    volumetrics for, 270, 303
    from water content of food, 271
Saturated fats, 22, 145, 148, 213, 339
Scallops
    Bay Scallops with Green Beans, 339
Selenium
    in Brazil nuts, 61, 65, 210
    for CRP reduction, 155
    for eye health, 167
    for joint health, 210
    overview of, 60–62
Serotonin, depression and, 35
Serving size, vs. single serving, 91

Shrimp
    Sesame Ginger Frittata with Broccoli and Shrimp, 329
    as superfood, 115
Skin cancer
    preventing, with
        quercetin, 80
        zinc, 64
    selenium and, 61
Skin care, fruit enzymes for, 85
Skin health, nutrients for, 25, 38, 50, 64
Sleep, for immunity, 239
Sleep apnea, 151
Sleep loss, weight gain from, 269
Smokers
    beta-carotene supplements and, 72, 140
    vitamin C for, 36
Smoking, health risks from, 146, 147
Snoring, heart disease and, 151
Sodium. *See also* Salt restriction
    bone health and, 217
    high blood pressure and, 152, 152
    overview of, 62–63
Soup, for hunger control, 257, 271, 323
Soy foods
    for cancer prevention, 79
    for eye health, 169
Spaghetti squash, 130
Spinach
    for eye health, 166–67
    for immunity, 235
    Roasted Fennel Spinach Salad with Chicken, 336
    Springtime Spinach Salad, 334
    as superfood, 103
    Sweet Potato and Spinach Soup, 326
Sports gels, fruits vs., 289
Sports injuries, foods for recovering from, 288–89
Sports recovery, thiamin for, 26
Squash. *See also* Butternut squash
    spaghetti, 130
Stair climbing, improving fitness, 283
Stomach health, vitamin C for, 38
Strawberries, as superfood, 96
Strength training
    activities for, 159
    benefits of, 279–80, 281–82
        improved immunity, 235
        loss of abdominal fat, 257, 331
        osteoporosis prevention, 219, 220
    starting, 280–81, 282
    workout for, 292–95
Stress
    depleting vitamin B5, 29
    effect on immunity, 238
    exercise relieving, 147, 295
    heart disease from, 146, 158
Stretching exercises, 285, 286
Stroke
    deaths from, 146, 156

    preventing, 88, 150, 156, 158
    risk factors for, 147, 148, 152, 154, 155, 248, 252
Sugar
    effect on bone health, 217, 226
    increased consumption of, 14
Sulfur, for immunity, 236
Sunflower seeds, vitamin E in, 324
Sunlight
    beta-carotene and, 69
    cancer from underexposure to, 41
    for preventing high blood pressure, 40
    for vitamin D production, 17, 39, 177, 223, 304
Superfoods
    bean, 120–21
    fish, 113–15
    fruit, 93–102
    nut, 116–19
    vegetable, 103–13
    whole-grain, 122–23
Supplements
    antioxidant, 134, 140–41, 146, 187
    beta-carotene, 72, 140
    bromelain, 83
    calcium, 47, 141, 220
    choline, 173
    chromium, 48
    eye-health, 164
    heart-health, 145, 146
    joint-health, 203
    nutraceutical, 130, 132
    problems with, 15, 187, 333
    quercetin, 232
    vitamin E, 43, 141
Sweet potatoes
    as superfood, 105
    Sweet Potato and Spinach Soup, 326
Swiss chard, as superfood, 104

T
Tangerines, as superfood, 100
T cells
    aging and, 231–32
    low-fat diet and, 239
    stress and, 238
Tea
    health benefits from, 76–77, 138, 152, 239
    milk affecting antioxidants in, 140
    turmeric, 212
Thiamin, overview of, 25–26
Tomatoes
    for cardiovascular disease prevention, 70
    as superfood, 108
Toothpaste, danger from swallowing, 49
Trans fats, 22, 145, 148, 246, 332
Tuna, yellowfin, as superfood, 113
Turkey
    Almond Turkey Salad with Cranberry Vinaigrette, 325

Portobello Turkey Loaf, 322
Turkey, Avocado and Cheese Wrap, 331
Turmeric tea, 212

U
Undernourishment, with overweight, 14
Unsaturated fats, 22, 148, 151, 245, 339
Urinary tract infections, berries preventing, 75, 325
USDA Dietary Guidelines, 299, 299
Uterine cancer, obesity and, 249

V
Vegetable juice, for preventing Alzheimer's disease, 193
Vegetables. See also specific vegetables
antioxidants in, 133
baby, 182
cooking affecting nutrition of, 329
in Dole Diet, 315
health benefits from, 88–89, 159
anti-aging, 4, 7, 8, 88
for bones, 253, 253
for brain, 189–90
for heart, 145
for joints, 202–3
longevity, 7, 8
obesity prevention, 8, 159, 250
weight loss, 89, 128
inadequate consumption of, 14
increasing intake of, 140
low energy density of, 270–71
nutrients in peel of, 271
recommended servings of, 298, 299
replacing high-fat side dishes, 275
as superfoods, 103–13
washing, 141
Vegetarian diet. See also Vegetarians
health benefits from, 40, 155
Vegetarian protein
health benefits from, 89–90, 153
sources of, 23, 24, 90
Vegetarians. See also Vegetarian diet
intelligence of, 190
iron sources for, 54
weight control in, 261
Visceral fat, 257
Vitamin A
for eye health, 24, 163
for immunity, 25, 238
overview of, 24–25
Vitamin B1. See Thiamin
Vitamin B2. See Riboflavin
Vitamin B3. See Niacin
Vitamin B5
in mushrooms, 311
overview of, 29
Vitamin B6
homocysteine and, 30, 145, 146
overview of, 30–31
Vitamin B12

for bone health, 35, 223
homocysteine and, 35, 145, 223
overview of, 34–35
Vitamin C
for bone health, 36, 217, 224
for CRP reduction, 155
for eye health, 167
fat burning from, 36, 319
for heart health, 36, 205
for high blood pressure prevention, 153
for immunity, 236
for joint health, 36, 203, 205, 206
for LDL cholesterol reduction, 151
overview of, 35–38
for stroke prevention, 158
Vitamin D
for bone health, 40, 217, 223
overview of, 39–42
for pregnancy health, 177
from sunlight, 17, 39, 177, 223, 304
Vitamin D deficiency, 16–17, 41
Vitamin E
for brain health, 43, 193
for eye health, 167
for immunity, 43, 235
overview of, 42–43
sources of, 324
for stroke prevention, 158
Vitamin E supplements, 43, 141
Vitamin K
for bone health, 45, 224
for liver cancer prevention, 45, 224
overview of, 43–45
Volumetrics, for weight loss, 270, 271, 303

W
Walking
for brain health, 196
calorie burning from, 232
for immune function, 233
for preventing
colds, 232
osteoporosis, 220
workout for, 292
Walnuts
Apple and Walnut Salad, 338
as superfood, 119
Water
benefits of, 155, 255, 330
effect on energy density of food, 270
fluoridated, 49
satiety from, 271
Watermelon, as superfood, 100
Weight, charting of, 267
Weight-bearing exercise, increasing bone density, 219, 253, 257
Weight gain
from marriage, 269
during pregnancy, 174
from sleep loss, 269
Weight loss

affordability of, 265
calcium for, 47, 268–69
calorie burning needed for, 272
for diabetes prevention, 326
dietary changes for, 17, 258, 259, 261, 272, 308
Dole Diet for (see Dole Diet)
exercise for, 258, 261, 272, 287, 308
fruits and vegetables for, 89, 128, 328
handling setbacks in, 267
from high-flavor powders, 265
longevity increased by, 267
meal planning for, 269
motivation for, 245
pectin aiding, 256
setting goals for, 267
slow, benefits of, 272
volumetrics for, 270, 271, 303
Weight maintenance
best method of, 258, 275
weigh-ins for, 280
whole grains for, 316
Weight management
fiber for, 20
good fats for, 23
Weight training. See Strength training
Whole grains
antioxidants in, 133
as superfoods, 122–23
for weight maintenance, 316
Whole-wheat bread, as superfood, 123
Wild rice
Caribbean Beans and Wild Rice, 306
Wound healing
bromelain for, 85
exercise accelerating, 154
manganese for, 57
Wound infection, 253

Y
Yams, as superfood, 112
Yellowfin tuna, as superfood, 113
Yo-yo dieting, 267

Z
Zeaxanthin
for eye health, 72, 163, 167
sources of, 72, 164
Zeisel, Steven, 173
Zinc
for bone health, 217
copper absorption and, 50
for eye health, 169
for immunity, 238
overview of, 64–65
for pregnancy health, 178
Zinc lozenges, 65